This book is dedicated to my parents,
the late Emillie Anne and John T. Such,
and my husband, the late Edward E. Lockhart.
You always had faith in me and provided me with strength that
helped me realize anything is possible. "Pick yourself up, dust yourself
off, and keep on walking" enabled me to reach for the stars. Thank you.
I will forever hold you close to my heart.

Acknowledgments

Writing this book has been a long, challenging, but rewarding endeavor—a professional journey that would not have been possible without the constant understanding, patience, and encouragement of many individuals. First, I want to extend my deepest gratitude to my sister, Emillie (Mim) Such, for assuming many of my family responsibilities over the years so that I could finish this book. I will always appreciate your love, support, and understanding. Mim, you are allowed to talk about the book now. Second, I want to thank Ray McGill, whose love and presence in my life following difficult times provided me with the strength to move forward. You mean the world to me. Third, I want to extend a special "thank you" to my friends and colleagues, especially Lucy Werthman, Leni Resick, and Dr. Gladys Husted. You provided me with the encouragement to continue my work. Your enthusiasm always lifted my spirits and kept me moving forward. Fourth, I extend my thanks to Jane Bryce and my staff development colleagues at the University of Pittsburgh Medical Center, the former Eye and Ear Hospital, and Duquesne University School of Nursing. Together we learned to connect the worlds of education and clinical practice. Finally, I want thank Barb Sigler and Carmen Warner. Both of you gave me the chance to share my ideas with other nurses, and I appreciate your faith in me. A special thanks to the publishing staff at the Oncology Nursing Society for making this process a positive experience.

UNIT-BASED
STAFF DEVELOPMENT
for Clinical Nurses

Joan Such Lockhart, PhD, RN, CORLN, AOCN®, FAAN

Professor and Associate Dean
for Academic Affairs
Duquesne University School of Nursing
Pittsburgh, PA

Oncology Nursing Society
Pittsburgh, PA

ONS Publishing Division
Publisher: Leonard Mafrica, MBA, CAE
Director, Commercial Publishing: Barbara Sigler, RN, MNEd
Production Manager: Lisa M. George, BA
Technical Editor: Dorothy Mayernik, RN, MSN
Staff Editor: Lori Wilson, BA
Graphic Designer: Dany Sjoen

Unit-Based Staff Development for Clinical Nurses

Library of Congress Control Number: 2004104800

ISBN 1-890504-44-0

Publisher's Note

This book is published by the Oncology Nursing Society (ONS). ONS neither represents nor guarantees that the practices described herein will, if followed, ensure safe and effective patient care. The recommendations contained in this book reflect ONS's judgment regarding the state of general knowledge and practice in the field as of the date of publication. The recommendations may not be appropriate for use in all circumstances. Those who use this book should make their own determinations regarding specific safe and appropriate patient-care practices, taking into account the personnel, equipment, and practices available at the hospital or other facility at which they are located. The editors and publisher cannot be held responsible for any liability incurred as a consequence from the use or application of any of the contents of this book. Figures and tables are used as examples only. They are not meant to be all-inclusive, nor do they represent endorsement of any particular institution by ONS. Mention of specific products and opinions related to those products do not indicate or imply endorsement by ONS.

ONS publications are originally published in English. Permission has been granted by the ONS Board of Directors for foreign translation. (Individual tables and figures that are reprinted or adapted require additional permission from the original source.) However, because translations from English may not always be accurate or precise, ONS disclaims any responsibility for inaccuracies in words or meaning that may occur as a result of the translation. Readers relying on precise information should check the original English version.

Printed in the United States of America

Oncology Nursing Society
Integrity • Innovation • Stewardship • Advocacy • Excellence • Inclusiveness

CONTENTS

FOREWORD

The tremendous progress of technology and pharmacology in addressing a multitude of disease processes has greatly improved both the quality of life and the prognosis for individuals who suffer from various deviations from health. At the same time, the need for effective and caring nursing services for patients and their families has also increased remarkably. Each advance brings more complex and invasive implications for patients. Increasingly, these individuals and their families rely strongly on the ability of the nursing community to address their needs; protect them as they progress through various phases of illness; plan for their reentry to work, family roles, and social responsibilities; and advocate for their comfort and integrity throughout recovery processes. To accomplish the full dimension of these roles and meet the diversity of needs that patients present, nurses need to continually refine their skills, upgrade their knowledge, and enrich the basis of their practice.

This book provides a map to the personal and professional advancement of staff nurses and offers clinical leaders a framework to lead their staff to realizing their professional goals. Dr. Lockhart has provided a comprehensive guide for staff development clinicians to empower their staff in the achievement of their long-term professional goals. She has designed a text that incorporates a unit focus as well as an outward view of the nurse's broader role in the community and in the profession. In fact, the entire text is directed toward helping staff development personnel take the "proactive approach to the future," which is outlined in the final chapter.

It is a privilege for me to be among the first to congratulate Dr. Lockhart for her contribution to the profession and to the long-term development of nurses. It is evident that this text will serve as the guide and map to enrich professional nursing practice for many years to come.

Eileen H. Zungolo, EdD, RN, FAAN
Professor and Dean
Duquesne University School of Nursing
Pittsburgh, PA

PREFACE

Background: Clinical nurses in many healthcare organizations have assumed some educator roles previously performed by nurses in staff development departments. Nurses have often accomplished this in addition to their direct patient care responsibilities. This book is an attempt to blend the worlds of both clinical practice and education (i.e., staff development and academia) with the goal of strengthening the clinical and professional competencies of nurses who provide patient care. Promoting the continuing competency and lifelong learning of nurses is the primary focus of this book.

Target Audience: This book is a resource for nurses who have assumed the role of unit-based educator in their clinical settings, nurses whose career goals include becoming an educator in nursing staff development, or those who want to further develop their professional nursing role. This book provides clinical nurses with practical information about the key components of staff development (orientation, in-service education, and continuing education). It also serves as a guide for nurses who want to strengthen and expand their competencies related to their professional nursing role and progress in clinical advancement programs within their work settings.

This text is also a useful resource for senior undergraduate nursing students who are learning about the professional nursing role in transition or leadership courses. Graduate nursing students may also benefit from this book as they develop their role as nurse educator, nurse administrator, and various clinical practice roles.

Finally, nurse administrators and educators of healthcare organizations can rely on this book to as a resource to orient their clinical nurses to the educator role and to strengthen their competencies related to professional development.

Overview: This book consists of four units. The first three units focus on the staff development role of the unit-based educator, while the fourth chapter addresses various professional development activities. Although each chapter in this book stands alone, all of the chapters are related to one another.

Unit 1, Assuming the Role of a Unit-Based Clinical Educator, provides readers with a foundation for understanding the unit-based educator role. Chapter 1 provides readers with an overview of changes that have occurred in many healthcare organizations that resulted in the shifting of select staff development responsibilities to clinical nurses who provide direct patient care. Chapter 2 describes the roles and responsibilities of educators in nursing staff development departments. Chapter 3 focuses on the clinical nurse's role as a unit-based educator and includes strategies that nurses can use to prepare themselves for this new role.

Unit 2, Orienting Nursing Staff to the Clinical Unit, focuses on the orientation component of nursing staff development. Chapter 4 describes the process involved in developing a competency-based orientation program on a clinical unit, while Chapter 5 focuses on developing a unit-based clinical preceptorship program.

Unit 3, Developing Unit-Based Educational Programs, focuses on the second component of staff development, in-service education. Chapter 6 provides readers with a practical approach to assessing learning needs and developing an educational plan for several clinical units. Chapter 7 includes information to help staff learn how to develop, implement, and evaluate a unit-based in-service education offering.

Unit 4, Helping Staff Develop as Professionals, addresses various dimensions of the professional nursing role and focuses on activities often encouraged in clinical advancement programs. Chapter 8 discusses the importance of being active in professional nursing organizations. Chapter 9 covers publishing in healthcare journals and presents a practical 10-step process. Chapter 10 provides helpful strategies for developing presentations at professional meetings as well as for creating posters. Chapter 11 offers strategies for recording your professional achievements using a portfolio. Chapter 12 helps readers prepare a resume and cover letter that can be used when applying for school or a promotion. Chapter 13 provides readers with practical ways for encouraging staff to become involved in clinical research projects on a unit-based level. Chapter 14 reviews the steps of the third component of staff development, continuing education, and discusses what is involved in planning and implementing programs both within and outside the workplace. Last, Chapter 15 concludes the book by helping readers develop a professional career plan focused on the future.

UNIT 1

Assuming the Role of a Unit-Based Clinical Educator

CHAPTER 1

Gaining a Perspective on Trends in Nursing and Health Care

Nurses have witnessed the impact of social, political, and economic changes on the healthcare industry for nearly two decades. The implementation of legislative initiatives, such as diagnosis-related groups (DRGs) in the 1980s and managed care in the 1990s, resulted in financial constraints that have affected not only the structure and function of healthcare organizations but the healthcare professionals they employ (Hallam, 2001). Inpatient services shifted to less expensive treatments provided in outpatient, long-term care, and homecare settings (Hallam).

Recent evidence of a current and future nursing shortage (Robert Wood Johnson Foundation, 2002; U.S. Department of Health and Human Services, Health Resources and Services Administration, Bureau of Health Professions, 2000; U.S. General Accounting Office, 2001) has compounded the effect of these past initiatives. According to a recent workforce study, healthcare systems in the United States are expected to experience a 20% shortage in the number of nurses needed to provide patient care in 2020 (Buerhaus, Staiger, & Auerbach, 2000). A shortage of nurse aides also is expected (U.S. General Accounting Office). Reports of a similar shortage in the current and future supply of qualified nursing faculty also have implications for healthcare organizations that will need nurses to fill vacant positions (American Association of Colleges of Nursing, 2003).

There are several reasons why unit-based nurse educators need to recognize historical events that have shaped their healthcare organization and to anticipate future trends. This knowledge can help nurses understand the perspective and experiences of long-term employees of an institution and what they and new employees confront in the current workplace. This viewpoint can help clarify the nurse's role as a unit-based educator and determine the responsibilities in supporting these staff with change. This information can guide nurses as they assume a leadership position within their organization, helping them develop creative strategies to cope with current changes and be proactive with future initiatives.

This chapter will provide you with an overview of recent healthcare trends and strategies that healthcare organizations have developed to manage these challenges. It will describe the impact of these strategies on nursing staff development departments and the role of the unit-based educator.

Healthcare Organizations Respond to Change

Healthcare organizations have reacted to the changes mentioned in this chapter in a variety of ways. In fact, some agencies, such as small rural hospitals, were unable to maintain their financial viability and have not survived these decades of economic turmoil (Hallam, 2001). Many healthcare organizations have endured these changes by collaborating, partnering, and sharing either part or all of their services with other organizations.

Insightful healthcare organizations that have survived these restrictions have done so by reexamining the ways in which they internally functioned. These organizations constantly strive for ways to develop cost-effective and efficient means to maintain and/or attain quality patient care outcomes. Although numerous changes have occurred within healthcare organizations, five of them will be discussed in this chapter: financial streamlining; restructuring, downsizing, and rightsizing; work redesign and role changes; focus on cost-effective quality patient outcomes; and workforce redesign (see Figure 1-1).

Figure 1-1.
Changes in
Healthcare
Organizations

- Financial streamlining
- Restructuring, downsizing, and rightsizing
- Work redesign and role changes
- Focus on cost-effective quality patient outcomes
- Workforce redesign

Financial Streamlining

Healthcare reimbursement changes forced many healthcare administrators to review their existing financial policies and procedures. Managers who dealt with patient care services and clinical divisions, such as nursing, were asked to streamline their operating budgets, control unnecessary expenses, and seek untapped sources of revenue.

Major budgetary expenditures, such as salary and other personnel costs associated with healthcare workers, were targeted as costs that needed to be controlled. Departments were examined based on their operating costs and ability to generate additional revenue for the healthcare organization.

In addition to reducing direct labor costs, these reimbursement changes forced healthcare agencies to closely examine their expenses related to patient care services. As mentioned earlier in this chapter, many low-risk surgeries and treatments and invasive diagnostic procedures that were traditionally inpatient practices were modified using a more cost-effective outpatient approach (Hallam, 2001).

This shift in healthcare services resulted in a different inpatient profile. For example, individuals admitted to acute care agencies (hospitals) possessed higher acuity levels than in past years and, subsequently, required skilled and intensive nursing care. After a shortened length of stay in the hospital, some patients were discharged to other healthcare agencies that offered subacute, intermediate, or extended nursing care. Healthcare workers employed in these transitional units were expected to provide much of the nursing care previously performed in the acute care environment. In fact, some organizations added new clinical services, such as transition units, within their own systems to help patients to make this changeover from an acute care to a home setting. Other patients were discharged to their homes with or without homecare services.

Restructuring, Downsizing, and Rightsizing

Many chief operating officers (COOs) of healthcare organizations dealt with these financial constraints by focusing on the internal structure of their organizations and on the allocation of resources. For example, some COOs totally reorganized or redesigned their structures, whereas others chose to implement minor changes in their existing organizations. Decreases in hospital occupancy rates over the past decade (Hallam, 2001) influenced decisions like organizational downsizing or rightsizing, often resulting in the elimination of divisions and departments. Some positions, previously assumed by employees at these agencies, were reallocated or totally eliminated. In some instances, services such as laundry, dietary, and education were outsourced or contracted through external companies. Many healthcare organizations closed patient units and reduced their number of beds. Some departments that were nonrevenue generating or advisory in nature, like staff education, often faced negative consequences.

Healthcare organizations, confronted by the impact of managed care, focused their efforts on securing their share of the healthcare market. Many agencies diversified their services in an attempt to obtain more patients or clients (Shi & Singh, 2001). In an effort to compete with other healthcare organizations for customers, some hospitals diversified by expanding or shifting their services from inpatient admissions to include outpatient, subacute care, home health care, long-term care, ambulatory care, and community-based efforts.

Work Redesign and Role Changes

The restructuring and downsizing efforts that occurred in healthcare agencies also compelled healthcare administrators to examine how the work of the organization was being accomplished. As a result, many division or department managers were advised to take a closer look at how the work of their departments was being completed. Managers were encouraged to redesign the work in a manner that was cost saving, efficient, and effective. Frequently, all but essential financial and human resources were trimmed from budgets. Employees in these departments were encouraged to rethink their responsibilities and develop innovative ways to perform their jobs. They were asked to "work smarter, not harder" and "do more with less."

New paradigms or models that resulted from these work redesigns often changed the roles and responsibilities previously assumed by employees of these healthcare organizations. Although some workers could easily adjust to their new roles by making minor modifications in their daily activities, other workers faced major changes in their job responsibilities. Some employees needed to be cross-trained or retrained in order to gain the knowledge and skills required to function in their new positions.

Focus on Cost-Effective Quality Patient Outcomes

In concert with cost-effectiveness and efficiency, healthcare organizations focused their efforts on measuring and managing outcomes related to healthcare services, such as patient care (King, 2001). Healthcare workers employed by these agencies were challenged on a daily basis to provide quality patient care but with fewer resources. Managers were encouraged to make decisions using data-driven outcome measurements (King).

Existing system-wide quality control programs that focused on both the quality and the effectiveness of clinical services were enhanced within healthcare organizations (Shi & Singh, 2001). Managers were encouraged to not only improve the quality but also to reduce its associated costs. Outcomes management initiatives, referred to as total quality management (TQM), gained popularity (Shi & Singh). Because the primary focus of TQM is continuous improvement in all of the processes in which an organization is involved, managers and their employees were encouraged to improve their organizational performance on a daily basis.

For example, suppose the nursing staff on your unit wanted to improve its performance related to patient admissions. You would begin by breaking your existing admissions procedure down into its smallest components. While viewing the steps of this process, you decide which of the steps are essential, who should perform them, and how they can be implemented more efficiently and effectively. During this process, you discover that the staff repeated many steps without reasons, or perhaps you uncovered omissions in other departments that prevented your agency from reaching the best outcome. While working on this problem, you decide to investigate how other healthcare organizations that excel in the patient admission process perform. This process is referred to as "benchmarking" (Shi & Singh, 2001). Next, you use this information to refine the procedure of admitting patients at your workplace.

The significance of cost-effective quality patient care has led to the development and implementation of patient-centered and outcome-based tools, such as critical pathways and clinical practice guidelines (Shi & Singh, 2001). These items, developed with input by nurses, are useful not only to guide practice but also to reach clinical outcomes within prescribed time frames. Innovative patient care delivery models, such as case management, evolved and emphasized meeting patient outcomes within a specific time frame (Shi & Singh).

In their efforts to gain national recognition, some healthcare organizations have sought status in the Magnet Recognition Program, which was developed in 1994 by the American Nurses Credentialing Center (ANCC, 2002). This program, based on national standards of nursing practice and quality indicators, recognizes healthcare organizations that support professional nursing practice in their settings and offer excellent nursing care to their patients.

Workforce Redesign

Healthcare organizations have implemented a variety of initiatives in an attempt to cope with the current and future shortage of healthcare professionals, particularly their need for qualified RNs (U.S. General Accounting Office, 2001). Organizations have focused their efforts not only on recruiting new nurses but also on retaining existing nurses. Recruitment strategies have included initiatives such as creative hiring incentives, loan repayments for an employment commitment, internships, free licensure examination (NLCEX) review courses for new graduate nurses, RN refresher courses, and intensive orientations. Seasoned RNs already employed in these settings have an opportunity to advance themselves in direct patient care roles through innovative clinical advancement programs. Nurses required to develop knowledge and skills in a new specialty as the result of unit mergers are offered courses to help them with their cross-training efforts. Some employers, in an effort to strengthen their cadre of direct patient care workers, have developed partnerships with schools of nursing and other organizations to develop programs in which nursing assistants and licensed practical nurses can advance their careers.

Impact of Healthcare Trends on Clinical Nurses

The action taken by many healthcare agencies in response to these reimbursement changes influenced not only various departments within their organizations but also the nurses who staffed patient care units. Because almost 60% of the more than 2.2 million RNs employed in the United States work in hospital settings (U.S. Department of Health and Human Services, Health Resources and Services Administration, Bureau of Health Professions, 2000), these organizational changes have made a major impact on the nursing workforce. Downsizing resulted in the loss of jobs for some nurses, whereas other staff experienced challenges posed by being relocated to other units. In fact, more than 110,000 RNs in the United States reported that they changed their employer and/or position between 1995 and 1996 because of reorganization or cost-control efforts in the workplace (U.S. Department of Health and Human Services, 1997). Yet, other nurses continued to stay in their organizations and survived these downsizing and redesign efforts.

Although losing a job or even the threat of losing it can be an extremely stressful event for nurses, relocating to another clinical unit or position and developing new competencies for that role also can pose challenges. Many nurses have been asked to change their usual role and assume different, unfamiliar, or additional responsibilities. Healthcare trends have affected the role of the clinical nurse in a variety of ways, and four major role changes will be discussed in the section: emphasis on a holistic view of the organization; change in the work of the clinical nurse; altered patterns and mix of nursing staff; and increased professional expectations of the clinical nurse (see Figure 1-2).

> - Emphasis on a holistic view of the organization
> - Change in the work of the clinical nurse
> - Altered patterns and mix of nursing staff
> - Increased professional expectations of the clinical nurse

Figure 1-2. Impact of Healthcare Changes on the Clinical Nurse's Role

Emphasis on a Holistic View of the Organization

Many of the structural and functional changes made within healthcare agencies in response to external reimbursement issues suggest that workers employed in these settings need to acquire a holistic perspective of the organization in order to understand and foster its mission and goals. Because these changes impact each employee, it is important for staff members to not only understand the external environment but also to realize how it affects the organization's internal operations. For example, it is important for nurses to understand how various reimbursement policies in the external environment impact patient care services so they can find ways to adapt to these changes within their own organizations.

In addition to gaining a more global perspective of the organization, it was no longer acceptable or effective for nurses to work in isolation from other individuals, departments, or groups both inside and outside the work setting. An interdisciplinary perspective with the patient as the focus emerged. Nurses were expected to collaborate as part of an interdisciplinary team along with physical therapists, social workers, and speech therapists in developing an effective treatment plan for a patient. To facilitate this goal, some agencies implemented organization-wide and unit-based alliances or structures that encouraged participation in decision making within the organization or with partners in the community.

Although interdisciplinary teamwork among various healthcare personnel such as nurses, physicians, physical therapists, nutritionists, and social workers had previously existed within many healthcare agencies, effective collaboration among these individuals was now essential in this new managed care environment. It was also important for these healthcare workers to communicate with others within the organization who functioned in nondirect patient care roles. Therefore, nurses needed to extend their knowledge base beyond the bedside to include an awareness in areas such as computer technology, information systems, financial planning, and human resources.

Change in the Work of the Clinical Nurse

Many of the changes made by healthcare organizations had an impact at the patient unit level, subsequently affecting the work of nurses who staffed these areas. As mentioned earlier in this chapter, especially influenced were RNs who functioned as direct patient care providers or coordinators on clinical units.

The consolidation, relocation, and sometimes closing of patient care units forced some nurses to work on clinical units with patient populations that were sometimes unfamiliar to them. Because many patient care services shifted from traditional hospital-based environments to a managed care approach in ambulatory, homecare, and community-based settings, nurses also were needed to staff these areas. In fact, the largest growth in RN employment over the past two decades has occurred in community health, ambulatory care, and noninstitutional settings (U.S. Department of Health and Human Services, Health Resources and Services Administration, Bureau of Health Professions, 2000). Nurses not only had to adapt to new work environments and unfamiliar coworkers, but they also needed to gain the knowledge and skills necessary to effectively function in a new clinical specialty.

For example, some nurses who previously worked in acute care inpatient units and were relocated to outpatient areas needed to shift their perspective from tertiary care to health promotion and early detection activities. Other RNs, experienced in clinical specialties like otorhinolaryngology nursing, needed to quickly broaden their skills when their inpatient unit evolved into a same-day surgical unit with a general medical-surgical patient population.

While relocated nurses were dealing with these challenges, RNs who remained on their assigned units within acute care agencies also faced similar demands. Despite decreases in staff, these nurses were expected to provide direct care to patients who were often at a higher acuity level and whose length of stay was shortened.

Altered Patterns and Mix of Nursing Staff

While RNs were learning to care for patients under different conditions, they also encountered changes in both the patterns and mix of the healthcare workers with whom they provided care. Downsizing efforts in many healthcare agencies resulted in a decrease in total full-time–equivalent positions assigned to each clinical unit. In concert with the slogan "Do more with less," nurses were at risk for caring for a larger number of patients who were sicker and stayed a shorter period of time.

In addition to changing staffing patterns, restructuring and work redesigns also affected the total mix or type of healthcare workers who provided direct patient care services. A reduction in the number of RN positions often was accompanied by an increase in hiring of individuals to function as nurse aides (U.S. General Accounting Office, 2001), also referred to as assistive personnel (AP). These AP were hired as multiskilled workers who could assist with providing direct patient care.

These ancillary or auxiliary personnel, previously known as nursing assistants, nurse aides, or orderlies, were given a variety of titles, such as patient service technician (PST), patient care technician, or patient care partner. After downsizing efforts eliminated the positions of other allied healthcare workers, individuals functioning in jobs such as respiratory therapy technicians, dietary aides, unit secretaries, and patient escorts were frequently given the option to retrain and apply for some of these ancillary positions.

These PST positions were accompanied by a set of additional responsibilities that transformed these employees into unit-based multiskilled workers. This job change required PSTs to learn new tasks such as drawing blood samples, performing electrocardiograms, inserting urinary catheters, and other procedures previously assumed by other healthcare workers. Nurse educators and clinical nurses provided additional training to help PSTs become competent in these new tasks.

The creation of this new type of healthcare worker had direct implications for clinical nurses working on patient care units. RNs now needed to focus their efforts less on playing the role of provider of patient care and more on the role of manager of patient care. In addition to being expert clinicians, nurses needed to further develop their leadership, management, and teaching skills. Nurses were needed to direct, plan, organize, staff, and evaluate patient care activities, as well as provide many patient care services that could not be delivered by ancillary nursing personnel. Nurses also were required to supervise and assist with the training of PSTs.

Although some nurses are experienced in supervising the performance of ancillary personnel and providing training, others may need additional help in acquiring these skills. Differences in racial/ethnic backgrounds, educational preparation, and life experiences between RNs and AP may pose a challenge, so RNs need to understand the impact of such cultural differences. Nurse aides, orderlies, housekeepers, and janitors represent the most culturally diverse component of the hospital workforce and, in most cases, possess different backgrounds from RNs (Purnell & Paulanka, 1998). AP and RNs also can have different backgrounds compared to patients and families for whom they care. According to a national survey conducted in 2000, only 12.3% of the RNs licensed in the United States reported being from one or more racial/ethnic backgrounds (e.g., Hispanic; Black/African American; American Indian/Alaska Native; Asian; Native Hawaiian/Pacific Islander) (U.S. Department of Health and Human Services, Health Resources and Services Administration, Bureau of Health Professions, 2000). Cultural differences also pose an issue with the foreign-educated nurses who are being recruited to fill the vacant nursing positions in the United States (Purnell & Paulanka).

Nurses need to be effective in their clinical teaching and role-modeling behaviors to gain competence in working with a culturally diverse workforce (Purnell & Paulanka, 1998). Nurses need to develop expert communication skills in dealing with their coworkers, properly delegate clinical tasks, and supervise direct patient care activities. Potential workforce issues based on differences in cultural backgrounds between healthcare workers may exist in areas such as language and communication skills, healthcare practices, gender issues, and autonomy (Purnell & Paulanka).

Increased Professional Expectations of the Clinical Nurse

While nurses were experiencing changes at work that resulted from downsizing and restructuring, some organizations also increased their expectations of the professional behaviors of the nurses they employed. Healthcare agencies were competing against one another for patients and their anticipated revenue. Some organizations planned to positively influence their claim to the profits by marketing the talents of their nursing staff through programs such as the Magnet Recognition Program mentioned earlier in this chapter. Therefore, nurses in many institutions were encouraged to demonstrate behaviors and credentials that were not only valued by the organization but also highly regarded by the professional and lay communities.

These healthcare trends have had a tremendous impact on the way nurses practice in clinical settings. In addition to providing direct patient care, RNs are involved in a variety of other functions in the work setting. According to a recent National Sample Survey of Registered Nurses, most RNs (69%) reported they spent at least 50% of their work week in direct patient care activities, with the average time being approximately 63% of their work week (U.S. Department of Health and Human Services, Health Resources and Services Administration, Bureau of Health Professions, 2000). The remaining percentage of their time was dedicated to other activities, such as administration, supervision, consultation, teaching, and research.

Many healthcare agencies incorporated these professional expectations for clinical nurses into their organizational structure, with specific criteria integrated into documents such as position descriptions and performance appraisals. Clinical advancement or promotion within some organizations required nurses not only to demonstrate their clinical competency but also to demonstrate specific behavioral outcomes related to professional development.

Many of the skills identified by employers may be new and unfamiliar to nurses. Figure 1-3 illustrates some of the professional behaviors that may be expected of clinical nurses. Each of these topics will be discussed in greater detail in later chapters.

To help clinical nurses achieve these expected behaviors, nurse educators who worked in nursing staff development departments frequently offered learning activities that were needed to help staff acquire certain knowledge and skills. Professional development was viewed as an integral part of the staff educator's role (American Nurses Association [ANA], 2000) as they mentored clinical nurses.

Figure 1-3. Examples of Professional Behaviors Expected of Clinical Nurses

- Participate in orientation, in-service offerings, and continuing education programs.
- Serve as a preceptor to other nurses and nursing students on the clinical unit.
- Assist with the development and implementation of a competency program.
- Take part in community and professional nursing and healthcare organizations.
- Participate in nursing research.
- Write for publication.
- Present at professional nursing meetings and conferences (oral or poster).
- Attend continuing education programs related to a specialty area.
- Obtain and maintain nursing certification.
- Pursue an advanced degree in nursing (i.e., BSN, MSN, PhD).

Impact on Nurse Educators in Staff Development Departments

The restructuring efforts that occurred in healthcare agencies also affected departments that were responsible for providing nurses employed by these organizations with in-depth knowledge and skills needed to function competently in their jobs. In addition to providing both staff development and continuing education offerings, these departments were expected to assist nursing staff members in developing their expertise in professional development activities, such as publishing, understanding and applying nursing research, and designing presentations and posters for the local and professional community.

Staff development departments were affected by these changes in a variety of ways. These divisions, commonly referred to as Nursing Staff Development Departments (NSDDs), Nursing Education and Research Departments, or Nursing Professional Development Departments, were downsized, restructured, or, in some instances, eliminated. An overview of the major changes that affected both the structure and function of some staff development departments is depicted in Figure 1-4. These include restructuring and downsizing of departments, redesigning department priorities, and shifting and expanding roles. Each of these will be discussed further in the following section of this chapter.

> - Restructuring and downsizing of departments
> - Redesigning department priorities
> - Centralizing core functions
> - Decentralizing unit-based services
> - Shifting and expanding roles

Figure 1-4. Changes in Nursing Staff Development Departments

Restructuring and Downsizing of Departments

As mentioned earlier in this chapter, the restructuring efforts of healthcare organizations resulted in the downsizing of many NSDDs. Depending on the philosophy of their respective healthcare organization, managers of some NSDDs were asked by their supervisors to reduce the number of full-time–equivalent positions in their departments. They also were challenged to rethink the work of the department using the nursing staff that still remained. Managers of NSDDs in some healthcare organizations were asked to completely close their departments that previously existed as unique entities.

Redesigning Department Priorities

Downsizing efforts forced the managers of many NSDDs to redesign and shift the priorities of their departments based on the current needs and trends of their parent healthcare organization. Traditionally, the priorities of most NSDDs consisted of providing staff development services in the form of orientation, in-service offerings, and continuing education programs (ANA, 1992, 1994). In addition to these services, NSDDs also provided nurses with assistance in their overall professional development (ANA, 1992, 1994). These key components of NSDDs will be discussed in Chapter 2.

Despite various organizational changes, the need for staff development and continuing education of nurses continues to exist (ANA, 2000). For instance, while the shortage of new nurses reduced the demand for traditional orientation programs, RNs who were relocated to other patient units required educational support. These nurses needed to develop their knowledge and skills in order to function safely and competently on various specialized units.

Second, nursing staff who remained in their current positions needed assistance in maintaining and increasing their competencies related to clinical practice. Healthcare organizations have a responsibility to help staff to develop the skills required in a new work environment (American Hospital Association Strategic Policy Planning Committee, 2001). Therefore, a comprehensive staff development program that included competency testing, in-service educational activities, and continuing education programs was essential to help nurses to perform effectively and safely in their assigned positions. An increase in the number of ancillary nursing personnel to assist with patient care required RNs to refine their leadership and management skills, especially with regard to delegation and supervision. Educational requirements mandated by accreditation bodies such as the Joint Commission on Accreditation of Healthcare Organizations still existed and needed to be attained.

Third, nursing staff needed to function as effective members of their healthcare organizations as they extended their services into the community. Nurses needed to be skilled in providing community outreach and marketing their services.

Finally, many employers placed an increased value on the professional performance of nurses by including professional activities as criteria in merit evaluation and clinical advancement programs. Requirements for promotion often included formal academic activities, such as obtaining an advanced professional degree or certification, and informal initiatives, such as writing for publication, involvement in unit-based research, and professional and community presentations.

Centralizing Core Functions

The redesign of NSDDs often resulted in the centralization of several core functions assumed by staff development administrators and clinical educators who remained within the department after downsizing. These core functions involved decision making related to learning activities for nurses and the coordination of the responsibilities previously assumed by NSDDs. These nurses now concentrated more of their efforts on managing and facilitating staff education rather than providing it using a traditional approach. The role of the nursing staff development educator changed and included the roles of educator, facilitator, change agent, consultant, researcher, and leader (ANA, 2000). These multiple roles of the staff educator will be described in more detail in Chapters 2 and 3.

NSDDs made changes based on their needs and resources. For example, after redesign, some clinical educators focused on preparing many unit-based staff nurses to assume some of the roles and responsibilities of nursing staff development. They coordinated competency training on the units and served as resource persons. These educators often continued to coordinate the maintenance of records and reports for the department, served as contact persons for affiliating schools of nursing, and managed internship programs. Many nursing staff development educators also provided support by implementing programs to help nursing staff deal with the effects of organizational downsizing.

Decentralizing Unit-Based Services

Whereas some core functions were retained by clinical educators who remained in NSDDs, other services needed to be decentralized and assigned to other nurses, often clinical staff who worked on patient care units. Structures within the organization were created to facilitate communication between centralized personnel and unit representatives. Shared governance structures provided this opportunity through education councils. Clinical instructors in NSDDs were available to serve as advisors or resources to staff.

Some unit-based nurses helped in mentoring and cross-training other RNs who relocated to other clinical units. Because of their expertise, many unit-based nurses planned and implemented in-service programs and competency testing for their staff.

Shifting and Expanding Roles

The downsizing of NSDDs resulted in the shifting of some staff development responsibilities to other nurses within the organization. This approach to providing staff education is similar to that used by nurses in other countries where clinical nurses assume the responsibilities of the staff educator role by integrating them into their daily work (National Nursing Staff Development Organization, 2001). As the roles assumed by staff development educators changed, so did those of unit-based nurses who assumed many of the duties related to staff development and continuing education. These staff nurses had expanded their roles to include both patient care and staff education.

Need for Unit-Based Nurses to Prepare for New Roles and Functions

The constant nature of these changes also reinforces the importance for nurses to continuously focus on their professional development. Nurses must not only strive to maintain their current clinical competency but also to seek creative ways to maintain their marketability. They are expected to be proactive and acquire the competencies and attitudes currently valued by restructured healthcare organizations.

To survive as primary healthcare providers in this environment, it is vital that all nurses understand these changes, use flexible and innovative approaches to deal with them, and assume leadership roles in preparing creative strategies for the future. Rather than viewing these multiple healthcare changes as losses or threats, nurses must view these developments as opportunities for professional growth or as professional challenges and learn from them.

Changes that occurred within NSDDs and clinical units meant that select staff nurses needed to be prepared to assume the role of unit-based educator. Prior to this restructuring, many of these nurses functioned as assistant nurse managers, unit coordinators, or clinical staff nurses. As unit-based educators, these nurses not only needed to be competent in their clinical skills but also needed to understand and implement various staff development functions. In addition, unit-based educators needed to gain a perspective on their relationship with both staff development educators who still functioned in a centralized capacity and the NSDD itself, as it currently existed. Finally, unit-based educators needed to know how the personal and professional qualities and skills they already possessed could help them become successful as unit-based educators.

Although many of these staff nurses had the knowledge and skills needed to function as expert practitioners, few have been prepared with the knowledge and skills needed to function as unit-based educators. With a decrease in the number of staff development educators available to serve as mentors, clinical nurses often received little preparation for this educator role. Because of downsizing, staff also needed help with their professional development, specifically staff development and continuing education. These aspects of the staff development role will be discussed further in Chapters 2 and 3.

Summary

Almost two decades of healthcare changes have resulted in reorganization and downsizing of healthcare organizations. These changes also have resulted in multiple role adjustments for nurses employed in clinical practice settings, such as staff development and unit-based nurse educators. Changes in both organizations and nursing staff development departments have affected the roles and responsibilities of clinical staff nurses. Unit-based clinical nurse educators need to take a proactive approach and prepare themselves as they assume these responsibilities. They need to acquire the knowledge, skills, and attitudes to function effectively in a vital new role in the organization.

References

American Association of Colleges of Nursing. (2003, May). *Faculty shortages in baccalaureate and graduate nursing programs: Scope of the problem and strategies for expanding the supply.* Washington, DC: Author. Retrieved June 15, 2003, from http://www.aacn.nche.edu

American Hospital Association Strategic Policy Planning Committee. (2001, January 23). *Workforce supply for hospitals and health systems: Issues and recommendations.* Retrieved June 6, 2003, from http://www.y-axis.com/healthcare/Career/workforce-supply.shtml

American Nurses Association. (1992). *Roles and responsibilities for nursing continuing education and staff development across all settings.* Washington, DC: Author.

American Nurses Association. (1994). *Standards for nursing professional development: Continuing education and staff development.* Washington, DC: Author.

American Nurses Association. (2000). *Scope and standards of practice for nursing professional development.* Washington, DC: Author.

American Nurses Credentialing Center. (2002). *ANCC Magnet Recognition Program.* Retrieved June 15, 2003, from http://www.nursecredentialing.org/ANCC/magnet/About.htm

Buerhaus, P.I., Staiger, D.O., & Auerbach, D.I. (2000). Implications of an aging workforce. *JAMA, 283,* 2948–2954.

Hallam, K. (2001). Inpatient facilities and services. In L. Shi & D.A. Singh (Eds.), *Delivering health care in America* (2nd ed., pp. 270–311). Gaithersburg, MD: Aspen Publishers.

King, R. (2001). The future of health services delivery. In L. Shi & D.A. Singh (Eds.), *Delivering health care in America* (2nd ed., pp. 547–579). Gaithersburg, MD: Aspen Publishers.

National Nursing Staff Development Organization. (2001, July/August). President's message. Staff development: An international perspective. *TrendLines, 14*(4), 1–8.

Purnell, L.D., & Paulanka, B.J. (1998). *Transcultural health care: A culturally competent approach.* Philadelphia: F.A. Davis.

Robert Wood Johnson Foundation. (2002, April). *Health care's human crisis: The American nursing shortage.* Princeton, NJ: Author.

Shi, L., & Singh, D.A. (2001). *Delivering health care in America* (2nd ed.). Gaithersburg, MD: Aspen Publishers.

U.S. Department of Health and Human Services. (1997). *The registered nurse population: March 1996 findings from the national sample survey of registered nurses.* Rockville, MD: Author.

U.S. Department of Health and Human Services, Health Resources and Services Administration, Bureau of Health Professions. (2000, March). *The registered nurse populations: Findings from the national sample survey of registered nurses.* Retrieved December 17, 2003, from http://bhpr.hrsa.gov/healthworkforce/rnsurvey/default.htm

U.S. General Accounting Office. (2001, May 17). *Nursing workforce: Recruitment and retention of nurses and nurse aides is a growing concern.* Retrieved June 6, 2003, from http://www.gao.gov

CHAPTER 2

Understanding the Roles and Responsibilities of Nursing Staff Development

Chapter 1 described the impact of recent social, political, economic, and legislative changes on both the structure and function of healthcare organizations. The chapter also described how these movements affected the roles and responsibilities of clinical nurses who, in addition to providing direct patient care, were expected to assist with some of the educational activities previously assumed by staff development educators. In some organizations, this responsibility was delegated to nurse managers or clinical nurse specialists. Many clinical nurses who assumed this leadership role in education were designated as "unit-based educators."

As a unit-based educator, you will need to develop the knowledge, skills, and attitudes essential to this new role. First, you must gain a thorough understanding of what is involved in developing professional nurses and other healthcare workers, such as assistive personnel (AP). You also will need to be cognizant of the multiple roles previously assumed by nursing staff development educators and clarify the responsibilities that have been shifted to you at the unit level as a result of downsizing and restructuring.

Second, you will need to know who the learners are, what their particular learning style and needs are, and how to meet these needs. For example, helping graduate nurses learn clinical skills may differ from how you might assist experienced RNs or AP with learning new tasks. Regardless of the learner, you must know how and when to assess their learning needs and to design educational plans to meet these needs. You will need to evaluate if your educational activities made a difference in the learner's competencies and revise your teaching strategies accordingly.

Third, you must appreciate the reasons why it is essential to foster the professional development of clinical nurses and other healthcare workers. This requires you to be aware of nursing and healthcare trends, the goals and expectations of the organization in which you are employed, and the role of the staff educator.

Finally, you must realize when and how the learning activities can be accomplished, particularly within a unit-based perspective. This involves the use of active and creative teaching strategies, self-directed activities, flexible programming, and an understanding of the learners. These four areas will be discussed later in this chapter.

Identifying the Professional Development of Nurses

It is vital for clinical nurses employed in practice settings to constantly maintain or improve their competency as direct caregivers. In fact, graduation from nursing school marks only the beginning of a continuous, lifelong process of professional development expected of nurses (American Nurses Association [ANA], 2000). ANA, the professional nursing organization that establishes standards of practice and professional performance for nurses, supports this belief. ANA views the professional development of nurses as a "lifelong process of active participation by nurses in learning activities to assist in developing and maintaining their continuing competence, enhance their professional practice, and support achievement of career goals" (ANA, 2000, p. 1).

This process of nursing professional development is conceptualized as a framework consisting of three key educational components: staff development, continuing education, and academic education (ANA, 2000, p. 5). These three components and their relationships with each other are depicted in Figure 2-1. As pictured, these three components are related to each other and overlap.

Figure 2-1.
Framework for Nursing Professional Development

Note. From *Scope and Standards of Practice for Nursing Professional Development* (p. 5) by the American Nurses Association, 2000, Washington, DC: Author. Copyright 2000 by the American Nurses Association. Reprinted with permission.

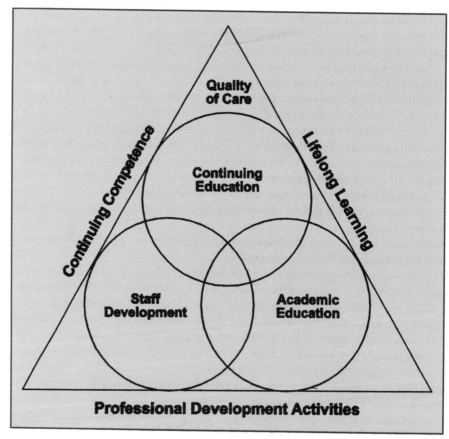

This chapter will focus primarily on the staff development component of nursing professional development. Although continuing education will be addressed, Chapter 14 will discuss the continuing education component in greater detail. Academic education will be included in Chapter 15 as it relates to career planning.

Nurses can become involved in this process of nursing professional development by participating in both formal and informal learning activities (ANA, 2000). Some examples of formal ways to pursue professional development include taking courses at a college or university or attending organized continuing education programs or workshops sponsored by professional groups or healthcare organizations. Other formal methods include participating in educational offerings sponsored by nursing staff development departments in the workplace or assisting with various research activities.

Nurses can pursue a variety of informal strategies to ensure their professional development, such as reading professional books and journal articles or participating in self-directed learning activities (DiMauro, 2000). Other informal methods such as being involved in clinical research, consulting, and participating in professional nursing organizations also can help nurses develop themselves professionally (DiMauro).

With the variety of activities available to foster the professional development of nurses, it is important to understand who is responsible for promoting this professional development. Although the primary responsibility for lifelong learning is that of the individual nurse, healthcare organizations that employ these nurses have a responsibility to assist them with this goal within the workplace (ANA, 2000). Other sources of support include professional nursing organizations, regulatory groups, and schools of nursing (ANA, 2000).

To better understand the process of nursing professional development that will be described in this chapter, start by envisioning the big picture of the nursing profession. Think how you, in the role of a professional nurse, have a responsibility to contribute to the nursing profession and develop it during your career. Remember that the primary outcome of professional development in nurses is quality patient care. Next, think about yourself hired in a particular position within a healthcare organization. You have a job description that outlines the behaviors that you are expected to perform.

Although these two situations appear as separate entities, the second case is actually part of the big picture of your contribution to the nursing profession. The duties you perform at work on a daily basis have the potential to make a difference for the patients for whom you provide care, other nurses at your workplace, and the nursing profession in general.

Both perspectives, you as a member of the nursing profession and you as a nurse employed within a particular healthcare organization, involve assuming certain roles and responsibilities. Career landmarks, such as graduating from a nursing program and then successfully passing your nursing licensure examination, indicate that you possess a minimal degree of competency as an RN. In order to maintain and improve your performance and level of competency, you must continue to participate in learning activities.

As each component of the professional development process is presented in this chapter, try to remember some of the educational experiences you have had since graduation. First, recall your experience when you were initially hired, or reflect upon your observations in the clinical setting when you functioned as a student nurse. Try to remember what kind of educational offerings were available to you and the nursing staff who worked on the patient units. Recalling these kinds of experiences will help you to not only make sense of the professional development process but also to gain a holistic perspective of the organization that was described in Chapter 1.

Defining Nursing Staff Development

As mentioned earlier in this chapter, staff development is one of three components that comprise the framework for nursing professional development (ANA, 2000). According to the National Nursing Staff Development Organization (NNSDO), staff development is the "systematic process of assessment, planning, development, and evaluation that enhances the performance or professional development of healthcare providers and their continuing competence" (NNSDO, 1999, p.1).

Staff development activities, often provided by employers, are designed to assist nurses with their performance related to their job or position in the workplace; the focus is on competency assessment and development (ANA, 2000). Although some staff development learning activities have the potential to benefit nurses regardless of where they are employed, these offerings are primarily aimed at helping nurses with their performance in the workplace. However, one of the anticipated outcomes of providing staff development is an increase in the professional development and competency levels of nurses (ANA, 2000). These outcomes, in turn, directly influence the quality of care nurses provide for patients.

Staff development includes three main activities: orientation, in-service education, and continuing education (ANA, 2000) (see Figure 2-2). An overview of each of these components of staff development will be discussed next in this chapter. Chapters 4 and 5 will elaborate on orientation, Chapters 6 and 7 will focus on in-service education, and Chapter 14 will discuss continuing education.

Figure 2-2.
Key Components of Nursing Staff Development

- Orientation
- In-service education
- Continuing education

Note. Based on information from American Nurses Association, 2000.

Orientation

The orientation component of staff development is the process of introducing nursing staff to information they need to carry out their assigned roles and responsibilities in the workplace (ANA, 2000). This is the part of the nursing professional development that usually is implemented by the employer in the work environment (ANA, 2000). Orientation programs include information such as the organization's "philosophy, goals, policies, role expectations, and other factors necessary to function in a specific work setting" (ANA, 2000, p. 6).

Nurses participate in an orientation program when they are first hired. They may receive another orientation during their employment at the agency when their assigned role, responsibilities, or practice setting changes (ANA, 2000). Chapter 1 described the experiences of RNs who were reassigned to other patient care units following organizational downsizing and structuring. This change created a need for these nurses to be cross-trained or retrained to perform competently in their new positions and environment. Therefore, these nurses participated in a second orientation program, often conducted on the clinical unit, to help them learn how to provide safe, quality nursing care for patients in this new setting.

Orientation also is needed when nurses assume a new position within the organization that is very different from their previous one. For example, a nurse who shifts roles from that of a clinical staff nurse on an inpatient unit to the coordinator of an ambulatory care clinic would benefit from participating in an orientation program.

Orientation helps nurses become socialized into the organization (ANA, 2000), assisting them to understand how they can become a valued member of their organization. Second, orientation helps new employees understand the culture or environment of the healthcare organization (ANA, 2000) because it highlights the performance criteria that are valued by their employers and the organization. Nurses can use this information to focus their career planning efforts toward developing these skills. Third, orientation focuses on assessing, validating, and developing competencies in nurses (ANA, 2000).

During the orientation process, nurses are tested on their knowledge and skills that are essential to performance in their role. Competency testing to assess and validate a nurse's performance level often is initiated during orientation and repeated at predetermined, regular intervals during his or her employment. Competency testing will be discussed in greater detail in Chapter 4.

Orientation programs vary in length, content, and methods. Some organizations sponsor house-wide orientation sessions that are open to all new employees, followed by a special program dedicated to nurses. After attending these general orientation sessions, nurses usually participate in unit-based learning activities aimed at helping them to understand their expected behaviors related to direct patient care on the clinical unit. Orientation that occurs in the unit-based setting often is guided by an experienced nurse who serves as a preceptor or mentor to the new nurse, referred to as an orientee. The roles and responsibilities of preceptors will be described in more detail in Chapter 5.

In-Service Education

The second component of nursing staff development is in-service education. In-service education consists of "learning experiences provided in the work setting for the purpose of assisting staff members in performing their assigned functions in that particular agency or institution" (ANA, 2000, p. 24). Similar to orientation, in-service offerings usually are sponsored by employers to help their nurses perform according to their position description and to help these nurses "acquire, maintain, or increase their competence" in that environment (ANA, 2000, p. 6). In-service education is warranted not only for nurses who hold current positions but also for nurses who experienced a change in their roles and responsibilities within that organization.

Whereas orientation programs can take a few days to several weeks, in-service programs usually are brief sessions, often lasting 15–30 minutes but no longer than one hour. Topics for in-service sessions often include those mandated by the institution or required by external accreditation and regulatory agencies. Regardless of the source, these educational programs should be based on a thorough assessment that reflects the input and learning needs of the staff.

In-service offerings can be presented in a variety of ways, depending on the preference of the organization. For instance, some agencies schedule in-service sessions in a centralized location so that all interested staff can attend. Other workplaces integrate in-service offerings into the daily schedule on a unit-based level. It is important to consider active teaching strategies that permit nurses to learn in a self-paced, independent fashion, such as posters, computer-based exercises and simulations, Internet-based programs, programmed instruction modules, videotapes, and audiotapes.

For example, suppose you work as a home health nurse. You may participate in in-service sessions that reflect topics related to the clients for whom you provide care, or maybe an in-service session is scheduled to review the major points of a new insurance documentation form or to familiarize you to a new type of peripheral IV catheter that many of your clients have in place.

In-service education will be discussed further in Chapters 6 and 7. Chapter 6 will help you develop an educational plan for in-service offerings on your clinical unit that is based on a systematic needs assessment. Chapter 7 focuses on how to actually develop and present a unit-based in-service offering.

Continuing Education

The third component of staff development, continuing education, was addressed earlier in this chapter as being a separate entity from that of staff development, with a portion of continuing education overlapping the staff development domain (ANA, 2000). This overlap implies that there is a continuing education component in staff development activities, such as with orientation and in-service education. Likewise, there is a portion of continuing education in academic education (ANA, 2000). Although this portion of continuing education that lies within the domain of staff development is part of the process of nursing professional development, it contributes to the competency of nurses employed by the healthcare organization. Chapter 14 will focus on continuing education both within and outside the workplace.

Clarifying the Roles Assumed by Staff Development Educators

As mentioned in Chapter 1, the role of the staff development educator has undergone reevaluation at many healthcare organizations across the United States. In concert with role changes, many staff development educators experienced title changes following their organization's restructuring efforts. These changes included titles such as staff development instructor, clinical educator, staff development specialist, or professional development specialist. Regardless of the title given to the staff development educator role, it is important for you, as a unit-based educator, to understand the expectations of the various educator roles within your own organization.

ANA uses the term "nursing professional development educator" in its current publications (ANA, 2000), replacing the title of "continuing education/staff development educator" that was previously used (ANA, 1992, 1994). ANA defines the nursing professional development educator as a "registered nurse whose practice is in nursing education and who facilitates lifelong learning in a variety of healthcare, educational, and academic settings" (ANA, 2000, p. 25). Although the responsibility for providing staff development programs for workers employed by healthcare organizations was traditionally assumed by nurses hired as staff development educators, a variety of creative partnerships have resulted in unique staff educator roles.

Nursing professional development educators function within six primary roles that often overlap with each other: educator, facilitator, change agent, consultant, researcher, and leader (ANA, 2000) (see Figure 2-3). These six roles, derived from standards of practice of professional development, demand different skill sets of nurses who function as staff educators (ANA, 2000).

To be effective within each of these six roles, staff development educators need to develop the knowledge, skills, and attitudes required by this specialty. ANA currently recommends nursing professional development educators be educated at the graduate level in nursing (ANA, 2000). If the nurse has a graduate degree in another related field, then the undergraduate degree must be in nursing (ANA, 2000).

- Educator
- Facilitator
- Change agent
- Consultant
- Researcher
- Leader

Figure 2-3.
Major Roles Assumed by Nursing Professional Development Educators

Note. Based on information from American Nurses Association, 2000.

Formal learning opportunities, such as graduate programs in nursing education, are available through degree-granting institutions, such as schools of nursing. Expertise in nursing staff development can be nurtured through informal avenues, such as continuing education programs offered by professional nursing organizations, experiential learning activities guided by a mentor in the workplace, and independent study offerings such as texts, journals, and media sources.

Staff development educators need to gain this expertise and add it to their existing competencies as clinical nurses. Both of these backgrounds are needed for staff development educators to be successful in their roles. It is important to remember, however, that being a skilled clinician does not automatically make a nurse a competent staff development educator (Bonnel & Starling, 2003).

Educator

An obvious role assumed by nurses in staff development is that of educator, especially related to the components of orientation, in-service education, and continuing education (ANA, 2000). This role includes overseeing the entire educational process, from conducting a needs assessment to planning, implementing, and evaluating offerings. It is expected that staff educators understand curriculum design, active teaching-learning strategies, testing and measurement issues, educational research, and technology in order to function effectively in this role (ANA, 2000).

As educators, nurses who provide staff development education need to create an atmosphere that is conducive to staff learning and to incorporate adult learning principles in their offerings (ANA, 2000). More information about the use of adult learning principles in staff development and continuing education will be provided in Chapter 3.

Nurses in nursing staff development departments (NSDDs) can fulfill their role as educators in various ways. They can serve as direct providers of learning activities. For example, they can develop and present a program themselves on topics such as how to detect abnormal breath sounds in clients with chronic obstructive lung disease. They can implement this role with nurses in a variety of environments, such as in a classroom or unit conference room, at the patient's bedside, in the client's home, or in an office setting in an ambulatory care clinic. Educators also need to use self-directed strategies in their teaching, such as computer-based instruction, that will provide learners with flexibility and independence.

Second, they can contact other professionals who are experts on a chosen topic to fulfill this role of educator. For instance, an NSDD instructor may ask a nurse in the IV therapy department to present an in-service offering on changing central venous catheter dressings on patients. In this situation, in addition to providing staff with an educational offering, the presenter also learns more about the role of the educator.

Staff development instructors often demonstrate the role of educator through informal methods. During their daily interactions with staff, patients, and families on the unit, educators frequently role model positive professional behaviors that other nurses can imitate and use in their work.

Third, clinical instructors in staff development can help other nurses within the organization learn to teach other staff, patients, and families. For example, staff development educators can help staff nurses to present unit-based in-service offerings or participate in orientation and continuing education programs. Nurses can learn to develop a unit-based education plan based on a thorough needs assessment, implement the plan, and evaluate the plan's effectiveness on patient outcomes.

Facilitator

Staff development educators serve in the role of facilitator within their organization (ANA, 2000), especially in the context of the teaching-learning process. For example, educators guide staff to play an active role in identifying and meeting their learning needs based on organizational and professional goals. Educators also are expected to promote team building among learners within the organization.

Change Agent

Staff development educators are expected to assume the role of change agent in a healthcare organization (ANA, 2000). They can accomplish this by identifying change within the organization, helping to implement changes, and supporting clinical staff as they attempt to adjust to these changes. This role is essential in light of the trends that have occurred in health care over recent years. For example, staff development educators can be instrumental in helping nurses learn new clinical skills as the result of a unit merger or manage a multiple-patient assignment as a result of the nursing shortage.

In addition to implementing change within the organization, staff development educators also are expected to serve as change agents through their professional development activities (ANA, 2000). This can occur within the local community or regional, national, and international levels.

Consultant

The fourth role that staff development educators assume is that of consultant to individuals both within the organization and in the local and professional community (ANA, 2000). They informally assist nursing staff within the workplace with activities that help them develop as professionals. These activities can be integrated into their daily interactions with individual staff or shared with groups of nurses in scheduled educational offerings. Some endeavors include helping nurses learn how to publish in professional journals, developing oral or poster presentations for a conference, or applying research findings on the clinical unit. Staff development educators often are instrumental in developing staff as unit-based educators, preceptors, and mentors for other nurses. Also, staff development educators are expected to be accessible resources to nurses who wish to advance both within their healthcare organization and in their professional nursing careers.

Staff development educators can serve as consultants, on a more formal basis, by providing professional or expert advice on topics such as those that have been previously mentioned (ANA, 2000). Although the formal role of consultant can be enacted within the workplace, it often is shared with community and professional organizations. For example, the nurse with expertise in staff development might serve as a consultant to another healthcare agency that needs help in developing a clinical competency program for nurses; or perhaps the agency wants assistance in designing a unit-based clinical research program, like the one you developed at your workplace.

Chapter 8 will focus more on the nurse's role in community and professional activities. In that chapter, the role of consultant is addressed for all nurses, including those assuming staff development roles.

Researcher

Staff development educators function within the role of researcher (ANA, 2000). This role of researcher in staff development can be viewed within a broad perspective and applies to the development of the educator as well as the clinical staff nurses. Staff educators are expected to conduct research related to their role in education, apply these findings to their teaching-learning, and evaluate the outcomes of their teaching on learners. Brazil, Jewell, Lyle, Zuraw, and Stanton (1998) provided an example of assessing the impact of staff development on nursing practice following a geriatric nursing education program. Increases in learners' knowledge of gerontology problems and their ability to assess patients, plan, and chart nursing interventions were significant results of the educational program.

Staff development educators also need to assist clinical nurses as they participate in the research process, apply findings to patient care, and share the results of unit-based research efforts through methods such as standards, policies, publications, and presentations. These aspects of the researcher role will be discussed further in Chapter 13.

Educators in NSDDs can foster research participation within healthcare organizations by providing staff with needs-based educational offerings related to research. This can consist of unit-based sessions called journal clubs in which staff meet and discuss the findings of research articles based on a chosen clinical topic. Educators also can help staff incorporate relevant research findings into practice standards on the clinical unit.

The instructor can coordinate liaisons between staff and research faculty in affiliating schools of nursing so that nurses can acquire hands-on research expertise. This connection can provide staff nurses with an opportunity to actively participate in research under the guidance of an experienced research mentor.

Staff development educators can encourage staff participation in research by guiding them as they attempt to analyze a problem or incident. The educators within their own departments as well as on the clinical units can model this process.

Next, staff development instructors and clinical nurses can use relevant research findings in their daily practice (ANA, 2000). For example, educators can integrate findings from published research and quality assurance investigations into educational offerings, standards of care, policies, and procedures.

Finally, staff development instructors must support dissemination of research findings. Research findings can be communicated using creative strategies, such as unit-based journal clubs in which clinical nurses focus on select research articles. Other methods include networking at professional nursing meetings, developing and reading research-based publications, and sharing research projects with the nursing community through oral presentations and posters. Chapter 13 will describe strategies that can be used by both staff development educators and clinical nurses to facilitate a unit-based research program.

Leader

In addition to being educators, nurses in NSDDs frequently assume the role of leader within both the organization and the NSDD (ANA, 2000). Educators support the mission and goals of the organization by offering suitable educational programs. They also assume a leadership role in their own professional development, including active participation both within the organization and in professional nursing and community groups. Within this role of leader, educators coordinate the educational experiences and learning activities of nursing staff. For instance, they organize continuing education programs for the agency and professional community and orchestrate an education plan for specialty patient units. Staff development instructors also design the schedule and content of orientation programs.

Instructors in NSDDs also participate in various administrative functions that are associated with either directing a department or being a member of a staff development department (ANA, 2000). These include activities such as organizing and preparing documentation related to staff development offerings, evaluating staff within the department, and developing and managing departmental resources (human and fiscal). Staff educators play an important role in seeking outside funding sources, such as education and research grants, to support programs offered by the department. Instructors assume a leadership role in coordinating the clinical placement of nursing students with faculty from affiliating schools of nursing and managing student internship programs for the healthcare organization.

Questioning the Development of Nursing Staff

Why should healthcare organizations be concerned with the professional development of the nursing staff they employ? Why should they sponsor various staff development and continuing education offerings? Although several sources, such as professional nursing organizations and accreditation agencies, support the need for staff development to occur, it is important to remember that the ultimate goal of professional development is to provide quality care and positive health outcomes for patients.

Standards of Nursing Practice and Professional Performance

ANA serves as the national professional organization for nurses and represents and guides them on a variety of professional nursing and healthcare issues (ANA, 2000). One of ANA's primary functions is to develop standards for professional nursing practice, such as its *Standards of Clinical Nursing Practice* (ANA, 1998). This document outlines eight Standards of Professional Performance that describe a "competent level of behavior" expected by professional nurses in the clinical setting (ANA, 1998, p. 4).

Similarly, ANA developed standards of practice and professional performance for nursing professional development educators in its *Scope and Standards of Practice for Nursing Professional Development* (ANA, 2000). These guidelines outline the specific expectations of educators.

Healthcare organizations that base their nursing staff education programs on these professional standards and criteria maximize their potential success in providing educational offerings that are tailored to meeting the specific learning needs of staff within their agencies. This approach also supports their endeavor to positively influence patient outcomes.

Accreditation of Healthcare Organizations

Similar to schools of nursing, healthcare organizations request to be reviewed by a nonprofit accrediting organization. Using pre-established standards and criteria, the Joint Commission on Accreditation of Healthcare Organizations (JCAHO) evaluates the quality of services and level of performance in specific areas that are being provided by healthcare organizations (JCAHO, 2003). These standards are "maximum achievable performance expectations for activities that affect patient care" (JCAHO). With particular respect to continuing education, JCAHO mandates provision of education and training designed to maintain and improve the knowledge and skills of all personnel.

Rather than focusing on the processes used in education, JCAHO standards emphasize the impact of educational offerings on patient outcomes (JCAHO, 2003). Interdisciplinary collaboration, rather than traditional departmental perspectives, is encouraged. This poses several implications for the education of all healthcare workers employed within an institution.

Because the final outcomes of the JCAHO evaluation are made readily available to consumers through its Web site, healthcare organizations that attain a quality rating benefit from their compliance when JCAHO standards are made public. A positive JCAHO evaluation sends a message to the public that the institution strives for excellence in patient care and that consumers are valued.

Goals of the Healthcare Organization

As discussed in Chapter 1, many organizations are trying to survive in the current healthcare market and are constantly competing against other agencies for patients. Faced with this challenge, healthcare organizations develop goals for themselves and their constituents that include providing quality patient care services and attaining positive patient outcomes. Professional development in the form of staff development and continuing education exists as one method for nurses to meet this challenge and to reach this goal of quality care. Education also has the potential to serve as a recruitment and retention strategy for organizations and often is used as a marketing feature.

Consumer Rights to Quality Care

Consumers have a right to receive quality care when they enter a healthcare institution. They deserve to be cared for by nurses and other healthcare professionals who are knowledgeable in their practice, exhibit competent clinical skills, and demonstrate professional behaviors and a caring concern. Therefore, providing nurses with opportunities for professional development is an essential step in accomplishing this outcome.

Targeting Learners

Nursing staff development educators frequently are involved in orientations, in-service offerings, and continuing education programs designed not only for nursing staff but also for other individuals who do not provide patient care services. It is important for staff educators to know who their learners are. For instance, educators employed in some healthcare organizations are responsible for developing programs that are open to hospital-wide employees, patients, and individuals and groups in the community (ANA, 2000). This aspect of the staff development educator role has important implications for how educators assess, plan, implement, and evaluate educational offerings. Because learners often include healthcare workers, such as clinical nurses, AP, affiliating faculty and students, and patients, the needs of these groups will be discussed.

Unit-Based Clinical Staff

This chapter has focused on the various components of professional development, such as staff development and continuing education, that staff development educators provide for clinical nurses. Similar offerings may be furnished to AP or other multiskilled workers so they can develop the knowledge, skills, and attitudes they need to provide quality patient care. The educator's responsibility also may extend to, and include, training and developing unit secretaries, receptionists, volunteers, and foreign-educated nurses.

Affiliating Nursing Students and Faculty

As mentioned earlier, nursing staff development educators often are responsible for coordinating unit placements for nursing students who come to the agency for their clinical experience. Students may be accompanied to the site with their clinical instructor or require placement with a staff nurse who serves as a preceptor. Just as with newly hired employees, these individuals must be oriented to the organization and clinical unit, informed of its clinical policies and procedures, and updated on its documentation guidelines. Some healthcare organizations also validate the clinical knowledge and skills of faculty through competency testing. Staff development instructors also need to understand the course objectives outlined for each group of students so that proper clinical placement will enable students to meet these goals. All of these measures help visitors to the healthcare organization maintain quality patient care.

Consumers of Health Care

Individuals, families, and community groups who enter the healthcare system have a right to receive quality health care. Healthcare workers who possess competency in their clinical skills offer consumers an opportunity to obtain quality care and, hopefully, improved outcomes.

Assessing When Staff Development Is Needed

Paper #3

In most healthcare organizations, nurses provide patient care 24 hours a day. However, staff development educators frequently are directly available to nursing staff fewer than 8–12 hours per day.

Although orientation, in-service offerings, and continuing education programs are intended to provide nurses with the knowledge and skills they need to deliver competent nursing care, it is not uncommon for nurses to occasionally encounter patient care situations that are unfamiliar to them. These circumstances offer nurses little or no advanced notice and deny them the option to delay interventions and wait for guidance from an instructor.

Paper 2 - Scenario ō HO nurse as a bedside learning opportunity

Because these clinical scenarios occur, it is important for nurses who function as staff development educators to anticipate these critical situations and take a proactive approach in dealing with them. How can one instructor accommodate meeting the multiple and constant learning needs of staff? The options that follow, such as time, priorities, coverage, and mentoring, can offer some practical suggestions.

Determine Peak Times for Staff Development

Start by tracking the peak times in which the direct services of staff development educators may be needed on clinical units. Although educators traditionally have worked during the daylight hours, recent organizational changes at the unit level suggest that this practice may need to be reexamined. This is especially true because changes frequently have affected both patient care needs and the availability of resources. With limited resources available to them, staff educators need to match what assets they have with times of peak demands for staff learning that occur on the clinical units.

For example, suppose you are the staff development educator responsible for meeting the learning needs of staff on a surgical unit. Most postoperative patients traditionally returned from the postanesthesia room (PAR) before 3 pm. Because your unit recently merged with another surgical unit, there has been an increase in the number of surgical cases on two of the five days per week. To deal with this increase in patients, surgeons have scheduled operating room cases that begin later in the day. This resulted in patients returning from the PAR to the clinical unit as late as 8 pm.

Given these changes, it may be warranted to reevaluate your accessibility to staff during the evening hours on those two days. This is especially appropriate if you recently acquired new nursing staff that needs cross-training or retraining. Once these nurses are comfortable with their new environment, you may choose to re-evaluate your schedule. Therefore, it is important to be flexible and make informed decisions that respond to the learning needs of the staff, or consider making more independent learning modules, such as computer simulations, available to nursing staff in need of a quick review.

Paper #3 Ind. learning module only why not to use salin.

Set Priorities

Another important approach to meeting staff needs with limited resources is to prioritize learning needs and to remain open and flexible. Categorizing needs based on their urgency or criticality will be discussed further in regard to planning in-service offerings in Chapters 6 and 7.

Network for 24-Hour Coverage

Because there is often only one nurse who functions as a staff development educator for one or more units, try developing a network of experts that can help meet some of the staff's learning needs 24 hours a day. Start by developing a group of staff development experts on the unit. Identify nurses who demonstrate positive behaviors, such as expert clinical skills, as well as excellent interpersonal and critical-thinking skills. These nurses also should be willing to mentor other staff and act as professional role models. Ways to develop a unit-based education network will be provided in Chapter 4.

In addition to facilitating staff access to human resources, it also is helpful to establish staff's availability to print and media resources on the clinical unit. For example, develop a system through which staff can access reference texts, videos, Internet resources, computer programs, and other printed resources as the need arises.

Paper 3 to dis. info.

What to D in paper 2 — No on-line resources for Staff + family.

Mentoring Clinical Staff

It is important for staff development educators to mentor clinical staff who are appropriate candidates for the role of unit-based clinical educator. Being an expert practitioner does not mean a nurse can automatically function as an educator. Nurses need to develop their role of educator over time. This includes having them learn about what is involved in staff development, as discussed throughout this chapter, and how to function within this role. This latter aspect will be discussed in Chapter 3.

Summary

This chapter described the professional development of nurses and focused on one of its primary components, staff development. The roles and responsibilities of staff development educators as educators, facilitators, change agents, consultants, researchers, and leaders also were explained within the context of healthcare settings. Suggestions were made for nurses who assume the role of unit-based educator in the clinical setting.

References

American Nurses Association. (1992). *Roles and responsibilities for nursing continuing education and staff development across all settings.* Washington, DC: Author.

American Nurses Association. (1994). *Standards for nursing professional development: Continuing education and staff development.* Washington, DC: Author.

American Nurses Association. (1998). *Standards of clinical nursing practice* (2nd ed.). Washington, DC: Author.

American Nurses Association. (2000). *Scope and standards of practice for nursing professional development.* Washington, DC: Author.

Bonnel, W., & Starling, C. (2003). Nurse educator shortage: New program approach. *Kansas Nurse, 78*(3), 1–2.

Brazil, K., Jewell, A., Lyle, C., Zuraw, L., & Stanton, S. (1998). Assessing the impact of staff development on nursing practice. *Journal for Nurses in Staff Development, 14,* 198–204.

DiMauro, N.M. (2000). Continuous professional development. *Journal of Continuing Education in Nursing, 31*(2), 59–62.

Joint Commission on Accreditation of Healthcare Organizations. (2003). *Facts about Joint Commission accreditation.* Retrieved June 18, 2003, from www.jcaho.org/accredited+organizations/publicing+your+accreditation/facts+about

National Nursing Staff Development Organization. (1999). *Strategic plan 2000.* Pensacola, FL: Author.

CHAPTER 3

Managing Your Responsibilities as a Unit-Based Educator: Getting Prepared for the Role

As the recently designated educator for your clinical unit, take a minute to reflect on the information you have learned so far from Chapters 1 and 2. First, you gained insight into current healthcare trends, how these trends have impacted your organization, and how these changes have affected the traditional roles and responsibilities of both clinical staff nurses and nursing staff development educators. Second, you developed an understanding of what is meant by the term "nursing professional development" and understood its importance for nurses and nursing staff development educators.

In Chapter 2 you also learned how helpful and important a well-planned orientation program is for staff nurses, who find themselves assigned to a new role and additional responsibilities on the clinical unit. Chapter 3 will assist you in designing a personal orientation to help you be successful in your new role as unit-based educator. More information on developing an orientation program for newly employed nursing staff, faculty, and nursing students will be discussed in Chapter 4.

Taking on new or added responsibilities may feel overwhelming at first, so you will want to prepare for this in advance. Before you implement your role as a unit-based staff educator, you will need to gather key information about your role and responsibilities, then analyze, organize, and plan your work. Include in your plan a way to evaluate your effectiveness in your new role.

Each of these steps will require you to review essential print materials and documents and meet with key people both within and outside your organization. These actions will help you obtain and clarify information regarding your responsibilities. Perform a self-assessment that will help you inventory the knowledge, skills, and attitudes that you will need to develop in order to be successful in your new role.

Gather Key Information About Your Role and Responsibilities

Before you begin functioning as a unit-based educator, gather information about your new position from an organizational perspective. Learn about your workplace starting with a view of the total organization. Then, get more specific and learn about your division or department, for example the nursing department, followed by the Nursing Staff Development Department (NSDD) and the clinical unit(s) to which you are assigned as an educator. As you survey your organization using this process, collect data that can help you understand and clarify your new responsibilities.

Information that you obtain from this organizational assessment will help you understand the beliefs, values, and planned direction of the organization for one to possibly three years in the future. Keep this information in mind as you develop your educational goals at a unit-based level. Because resources such as money, personnel, and administrative support are frequently allocated to departments based on organizational goals, it is to your advantage to relate your specific goals of unit-based staff education to those of the clinical unit, division or department, and organization.

Understand the Structure and Function of Your Organization

Learn as much as you can about your healthcare organization from a general perspective. This can be accomplished in a variety of ways. First, understand your organization's history, especially how your workplace was before recent changes in restructuring occurred. This will give you insight into how to help staff to deal with the changes that have occurred over past years. Investigate the organization's vision, mission, philosophy, strategic goals, and objectives. These features can provide you with information about the direction of the organization and what is valued. Become familiar with policies, procedures, and rules that relate to your role as a unit-based educator. These will be discussed in more detail related to the NSDD in the section that follows. Learn the names of key individuals within your organization, especially those with whom you may interface in your new role.

Before you explore your role on the clinical unit(s) to which you are assigned, focus on the division or department in which your new role resides. Next, repeat the process described previously. For example, if your unit-based educator position is associated with a centralized NSDD or a Nursing Education and Research Department under the direction of the Clinical Services Division or Nursing Department, investigate both of these departments. As you learn about them, try to understand the overall impact that recent structuring changes have had on their system, such as the way departments are divided and staffed, and daily operations. Learn the names of key individuals who are responsible for implementing the department's goals and understand their responsibilities. Meet with them to clarify how you, as a unit-based educator, fit into these departments and can participate in meeting departmental goals and objectives.

Because you play a significant role in helping the NSDD attain its educational goals targeted to healthcare staff, it is important for you to understand specific aspects of this department. This information can provide you with the context on which to base your role so that your work is congruent with that of the department. Start this process by learning about the following four components that comprise the NSDD's plan: (a) the department's vision and mission statements, (b) philosophy, (c) goals and objectives, and (d) policies and procedures. Focus on other features of the NSDD that will help you in your role, such as its educational design, documentation and record-keeping system, and available resources.

Vision and Mission Statements

Start learning about the plan by reviewing the vision and mission statements of the NSDD. The vision statement, if available, describes what the department ultimately expects to become in the future. An example of a vision statement for a NSDD is illustrated in Figure 3-1. Use this vision statement as you attempt to blend your aspirations as a unit-based educator on the clinical unit(s) with those of the department and organization. This strategy will help you move in the same direction as your guiding department and meet your professional development goals.

> To be a recognized provider of quality and cost-effective educational programs and services for healthcare employees in our healthcare organization and for professionals and laypersons in the regional community

Figure 3-1.
Sample Vision Statement for a Nursing Staff Development Department

The mission statement of the NSDD may sometimes include the vision but actually focuses on the reason why the department exists; it addresses the department's specific aims or function (Marquis & Huston, 1998). The mission statement is very important because it sets the tone for the NSDD's philosophy, goals, objectives, policies, and procedures. An example of a mission statement for a NSDD is provided in Figure 3-2.

Use the mission statement in a similar manner as its vision. These statements will tell you how the department

> The mission of this department is to provide quality, cost-effective educational offerings and professional development activities that are based on latest knowledge, foster quality patient care, and support the goals of the nursing profession and this healthcare organization.

Figure 3-2.
Sample Mission Statement for a Nursing Staff Development Department

perceives itself and what services it offers. This information can help you clarify the boundaries of your role as a unit-based educator and guide you in preparing for it. For example, after reading these statements, ask yourself the following questions: Is the main intention of the department to provide education that assists with the professional development of nursing staff? Does its purpose include other services, such as assisting with nursing research or community outreach? Is education defined with emphasis on orientation, in-service education, or continuing education?

Philosophy

Closely examine the philosophy of the NSDD. The philosophy should reflect the department's vision and mission statements (Marquis & Huston, 1998). The philosophy also should tell you what the department's beliefs are regarding key concepts, such as the learner, the nurse educator, the teaching-learning process and environment, and professional development (American Nurses Association [ANA], 1994). It is important for you to be aware of the philosophy because it reflects what the NSDD values and guides nurse educators employed by the department as they perform their daily work. It is essential that you, as a unit-based educator, not only understand the department's philosophy but also agree to work within its scope.

Determine how the department's philosophy compares with your personal philosophy. If you feel uncomfortable with these beliefs or perform your job in opposition to the department's philosophy, you run the risk of experiencing emotional strain and conflict within yourself, between you and other educators, and within the NSDD itself.

The philosophy should clarify who the learner is and the degree to which the learner is involved in the teaching-learning process. Knowing the scope of your learners is especially important if your organization has multiple centers or several affiliations within the community. Some places consider the learner to include all employees within the institution, whereas others limit learners to nursing staff or all healthcare workers, such as nurses, assistive personnel (AP), unit secretaries, physical and occupational therapists, and social workers. Some agencies also include patients, families, and the lay community among their learners. This topic is addressed further in Chapters 6 and 7.

Discover what role learners are expected to play in the teaching-learning process, especially related to their professional development. For example, discover if learners are expected to assume total responsibility for meeting their learning needs or if the NSDD determines this. Find out if nursing staff play an active role in educating their peers or if all education offerings will be performed by nurse educators like yourself.

Within this philosophy, understand how NSDD educators perceive and enact the roles of the "learner" and "educator" at your workplace. For instance, although some departmental philosophies may depict the nurse educator as a facilitator of learning, actual practice may reflect the role of educator as the expert or sole bearer of knowledge. Investigate if differences in learning based on cultural and ethnic diversities are accounted for in educational activities.

Become familiar with the standards used by the NSDD to guide practice and professional performance. Standards of practice are statements developed by experts in the nursing profession upon which the quality of services, such as education or nursing care, is evaluated (ANA, 2000). Standards of professional performance describe a "competent level of behavior in the professional role" (ANA, 2000, p. 26). The observed performance and work by educators in the NSDD are judged according to these standards. Chapter 2 addressed national standards used by staff development departments, such as the ANA's *Scope and Standards of Practice for Nursing Professional Development* (2000) and *Standards of Clinical Nursing Practice* (1998).

In addition to standards, you need to familiarize yourself with the latest expectations of the accreditation agencies that evaluate your organization on education and staff performance, such as the Joint Commission on Accreditation of Healthcare Organizations (JCAHO, 2003). Your nurse manager, nurse educator, or agency librarian can help you locate relevant portions of the JCAHO guidelines.

Goals and Objectives—The Strategic Plan

Familiarize yourself with the strategic plan developed by the NSDD. This plan guides the activities or work of the department over a specified period of time and determines how resources will be distributed, how responsibilities will be delegated, and what time period will be used (Marquis & Huston, 1998). Focus on the specific priorities identified by the department, especially the long- and short-term goals based on these needs. Although long-term goals traditionally guided a department's activities over a long period of time, rapid changes in healthcare organizations have changed this time range to include a more moderate span (5–10 years) (Marquis & Huston). Ask your unit manager about the time span for long-term goals adopted by your healthcare organization. In most organizations, a "year" refers to the fiscal year that coincides with the organization's budget period, usually beginning June 30 and going to July 1 the following year. The NSDD identifies several goals to be accomplished over a one-year period and often prioritizes them. Limited departmental resources often are allocated based on these priorities.

Next, carefully review the short-term goals developed for the current year. Each goal should be accompanied by observable measurements (outcomes) that indicate successful attainment of the goal, actions needed to help the department meet the goal, and assigned responsibility for these actions. Goal setting will be discussed further in Chapters 6 and 7.

The strategic plan of the NSDD is very similar to a care plan for patients. Both need to be flexible and accommodate changes as they arise. Goals are developed based on needs identified from a variety of sources, including those you have observed and those expressed by the patient and family. These goals are patient-centered, realistic, measurable, and attainable. Specific interventions are identified to help the patient meet these goals. Specific observable outcomes or measures indicate successful attainment of each goal.

Because goals outlined in the strategic plan guide both the efforts and resources of the NSDD, it is logical for your unit-based goals to be congruent with and reflect those of the department. It also is important that your work matches the department's plan for educational activities because your role is an extension of the NSDD.

Policies and Procedures

Review the NSDD's policies and procedures. These statements should be consistent with the vision, mission, and philosophy of the nursing department because they direct the work of the NSDD. They also should reflect priorities expressed by national professional standards, such as ANA, and external accreditation agencies, such as JCAHO. Similar to its philosophy, policies and procedures should guide you in your unit-based role and communication with other educators. Policies and procedures also enable members of the organization to work together to meet departmental goals.

After reviewing these policies and procedures, note which ones directly apply to you in your role as a unit-based educator. As you develop your role, decide if new policies and procedures need to be developed to guide your activities on the clinical unit. Suggested policies and procedures will be discussed later as they relate to specific staff development components, such as orientation (Chapter 4), preceptorships (Chapter 5), and continuing education (Chapter 14).

Educational Design

Learn more about the educational design used by educators in the NSDD (ANA, 1994). The design is the department's plan for providing instruction and includes several key features that are indicated in Figure 3-3. It is important to note how learners at your workplace participate in each phase of the educational design (ANA, 1994). As a unit-based educator, you need to gain an understanding of the components of the design and how it should be reflected in your role. Each of these elements will be briefly described in the section that follows.

Description of Targeted Learners: First, investigate to whom the NSDD in your organization is responsible for providing instruction. Chapter 2 discussed groups of nursing personnel employed by their organizations for which NSDDs are often responsible: RNs, licensed practical and licensed vocational nurses (LPNs and LVNs), AP, nursing assistants (NAs), and unit secretaries. Other nursing personnel who interface with the NSDD include faculty and nursing students from affiliating schools of nursing. These schools prepare students at various entry levels into the nursing profession, such as diploma, associate, and baccalaureate degrees.

Figure 3-3.
Key Features of an
Educational Design
for a Nursing Staff
Development
Department

Note. Based on information from American Nurses Association, 1994.

- Assessment of learning needs
- Description of targeted learners
- Objectives
- Outline of content
- Teaching strategies
- Evaluation strategies
- Available resources and physical facilities for learning

If your NSDD also includes non-nursing personnel among its targeted learners, find out which individuals comprise this group. For example, your NSDD may provide educational services for patients who use your healthcare organization, their families, and individuals living in the community. Perhaps educators in your NSDD teach all agency employees cardiopulmonary resuscitation or offer classes in conflict management. Find out if this is also part of your role as a unit-based educator.

Once you know which people the educators in the NSDD identify as their "learners," find out who comprises your own set of "learners." Next, learn more about their roles and responsibilities within your organization if you are not already familiar with them. For example, if you are responsible for the staff development needs of AP and LPNs/LVNs, be sure you understand their job expectations on the unit. You can learn about their current role by reviewing their job descriptions. The nurse manager of the unit can provide you with information about any anticipated changes in their roles in the future. If you are not familiar with staff on your assigned clinical unit(s), spend some time with them on the unit to get to know them as professionals. This also will give you an opportunity to clarify your role as unit-based educator.

Assessment of Learning Needs: Now that you know who the NSDD views as its learners, discover more about the process the department uses to determine the staff's learning needs. Conducting a needs assessment helps nurse educators determine actual competencies of learners related to specific areas. Results are compared with competencies that the organization wants their employees to possess in order to provide safe, quality patient care. Educators obtain these desired behaviors using multiple sources as mentioned in Chapter 2, such as position descriptions, professional nursing standards, healthcare trends, and criteria determined by regulatory and accreditation agencies. The outcomes obtained through conducting a needs assessment are used to help educators in your organization plan and implement educational activities for the target learners. It is important that you uncover how the learning needs of staff working on your clinical unit are assessed and how you can access this information. If a needs assessment has not been conducted on your unit, then you will need to do this to develop your plan for unit-based educational activities. Chapters 6 and 7 will help you learn how to conduct a needs assessment.

To understand how needs assessment helps employees and the ways that they are used by educators within healthcare organizations, think about this process within each of the components of nursing staff development: orientation, in-service education, and continuing education (ANA, 2000). Chapter 2 emphasized the professional development of nurses as being a process that is not only composed of various components but also one that is continuous and lifelong (ANA, 2000). However, to help nursing staff with this process, NSDD educators often divide the needs assessment process related to professional development down into smaller, more manageable segments. Because the learning needs and competencies of nursing staff need to be continually developed and maintained (ANA, 2000), healthcare organizations regularly assess these skills. This is one reason why NSDDs often collect, organize, and record each worker's learning needs, educational ac-

tivities, and competencies according to the components of nursing staff development mentioned earlier. The results, although often categorized, still need to be
viewed as an integrated whole within each employee's continuous process of professional development within your organization.

For example, Chapter 2 described how orientation helps prepare new employees to fulfill their assigned roles and responsibilities in the workplace (ANA, 2000).
Because orientation focuses on a person's specific role within the agency, a position (job) description can serve as a foundation for determining successful performance or desired competencies. When a group of new nurses is hired, their skills
are evaluated based on expectations identified in their position descriptions. Assessment of the actual skills of new staff helps determine what competencies need
to be developed during orientation. Helping individual staff develop these desired
competencies will enable them to function effectively in their role. Actual competencies of employees are determined when they are hired using a variety of methods, such as self-assessments, written tests, and observation of skills. Any differences observed between demonstrated behaviors versus desired behaviors should
be considered as learning needs (ANA, 2000).

Similarly, Chapter 2 described the purpose of in-service educational activities
to "assist nurses as they perform their assigned functions in that particular agency
or institution" (ANA, 2000, p. 24). Suppose a physician tells your nurse manager
and you that a new chemotherapy drug will be part of a clinical protocol used for
patients admitted to your clinical unit. Existing staff members on your unit already are skilled in administering chemotherapy drugs but are unfamiliar with
this drug and its nursing implications. Use this identified learning need to help
existing staff develop competencies in administering this drug, assess and manage
potential side effects, and provide appropriate patient education. A unit-based in-
service program would be an appropriate strategy to accomplish this goal. When
any new nurses are hired for your unit, include a review of this drug as part of the
planned educational program.

Details about how to assess the learning needs of nursing staff related to each
of the components of nursing staff development will be discussed later throughout this book. Chapter 4 will explain ways to assess the learning needs of new staff
during orientation, whereas Chapters 6 and 14 will focus on determining learning
needs for existing experienced unit staff through in-service education offerings
and continuing education, respectively.

While reviewing this information, be sure to discover the process used by your
own organization to assess learning needs, how it prioritizes needs based on limited resources, and ways learners have input into this process. Also, observe what
kinds of methods are used to collect this information, such as written surveys or
unit-based focus groups, and when the learning needs assessment is conducted.
Discover how this needs assessment is used to develop educational activities aimed
at correcting any deficiencies. Finally, investigate your role in this process and
how it impacts your work on your clinical unit(s).

Components of Educational Offerings: Based on data received from the needs
assessment, educators develop various educational offerings aimed at strengthening the skills of targeted learners. Be sure to review the main components of this
process used by educators in the NSDD as they plan each educational activity.
These items include objectives, content, teaching strategies, and evaluation methods (ANA, 2000). Determine if principles of adult learning and education are
considered when these educational activities are designed (ANA, 2000). Find out

what your role is in this operation. More details about this process, such as developing a teaching plan, are discussed in Chapter 7. The following example is provided to clarify this process.

Suppose that changing a laryngectomy tube is an expected clinical skill for nurses who work on your unit. Because only a few nurses can successfully perform this skill, you identify this as a learning need for select staff nurses. Before you begin to help these nurses develop this competency, you create a plan to teach this skill. You begin this process by identifying a few objectives that describe key behaviors you expect nurses to demonstrate after receiving your instruction. Next, you outline content that will help these nurses meet these objectives and choose teaching strategies you will use to convey this information. For example, you plan to demonstrate the procedure of changing a tube and then have the nurses repeat this demonstration as you observe their technique, or instead of demonstrating the procedure, you may have them view a videotape of this procedure. After the program, you evaluate each nurse's ability to meet the objectives and provide him or her with feedback to guide their performance. You also obtain their response about the program and your teaching skills.

Ask educators in the NSDD what mechanisms they use to communicate their educational offerings to nursing staff, especially how they identify and inform those nurses who urgently need to develop these competencies. Determine if the notification process is conducted in a way that gives nurse managers sufficient time to provide coverage for patient care activities as these nurses attend programs. Find out if staff members are expected to seek out these learning experiences themselves once they obtain permission from their nurse manager, or if you as the unit-based educator are responsible for coordinating this procedure in collaboration with the staff and unit manager.

Resources Available for Educational Activities

Educators, including those in the NSDD and yourself on the clinical unit, need access to various resources and facilities for implementing educational activities to meet goals and objectives (ANA, 2000). Managers of NSDDs and clinical units develop a financial plan each fiscal year that will enable their department to meet their goals and objectives. However, they may ask for your input on their plan from a unit-based perspective. Because resources often are limited in most healthcare organizations, you will need to be creative in developing cost-effective educational activities that successfully develop staff competencies.

To provide appropriate advice to managers regarding the resources you will need to be successful in your role as unit-based educator, you will need to understand several things. These include learning what the term "resources" means, anticipating resources you will need to carry out your responsibilities, and knowing what existing resources are already available to you.

To learn more about resources, think of them according to three categories: human, fiscal, and material. Human resources consist of people and the services they provide. Fiscal resources are monies that can be allocated for expenditures, such as conference fees, refreshments at receptions, and printing costs for brochures or handouts. Material resources include office supplies, computer hardware and software, and teaching models. Table 3-1 illustrates various resources you may need as a unit-based educator. This table also indicates how each resource can potentially contribute to your unit's educational goals. Because requesting all of these resources may be unrealistic in today's healthcare setting, you will need to prioritize them based

Resource	Examples	Purpose Related to Unit-Based Educational Goals
		Table 3-1. Examples of Resources Needed for Unit-Based Educational Activities
Human	Secretarial support	Assist in preparing documents, keeping records, duplicating materials, and scheduling rooms.
	Audiovisual technician	Deliver audiovisual equipment and assist with operating equipment.
	Graphics	Help prepare slides and posters for teaching and presentations.
	Expert presenters	Assist with presenting educational content.
	Expert scholars (research and publication)	Provide consultation with unit-based research and publication efforts of staff.
Fiscal	Monies	Registration fees for conferences both internal and external to organization Purchase of unit-based reference books and teaching models and materials Support rewards and incentives for preceptors Fund unit-based celebrations and meetings. Assist with cost of mailings to external agencies.
Material	Supplies	Access to teaching models and supplies, audiovisual materials, office supplies, staff and patient education materials
	Equipment	Access to audiovisual equipment, computer hardware and software, and duplication machines
	Facilities/space	Access to teaching space (classroom, skills laboratory), storage of teaching materials, and office space for unit-based educator

on your goals. This task may be easier to accomplish after you have conducted a self-assessment regarding the skills you need in your new role, completed a needs assessment for your clinical unit, and prioritized your goals.

Keep in mind that resources may be available from sources both within and outside your organization. For example, in your role as unit-based educator, you may have access to resources from various places: within your organization (e.g., library, public relations), within the NSDD (e.g., teaching models, secretarial support), or on your clinical unit (e.g., conference rooms, duplication services). You also may have access to resources outside your organization, such as faculty expertise or classrooms at affiliating schools of nursing and other related agencies. Because resources can be found in a variety of places, it is necessary for you to meet with individuals in these departments to discuss their availability.

Documentation, Record Keeping, and Reports

Familiarize yourself with the documentation system adopted by nurse educators in the NSDD and the overall record-keeping system used to track educational activities. Professional nursing organizations, such as ANA (2000), and accreditation agencies, such as JCAHO (2003), suggest having systems in place that also reflect organizational goals. Learn which reports educators need to generate as well as those they use that are issued by other departments. As you obtain this information, think about the implications for you in the role of unit-based educator.

To better understand the documentation and record-keeping system used by nurse educators in your healthcare agency, try contrasting the system with tools you use in patient care. For example, compare a patient's chart with the professional record of a staff nurse on your unit. Just as the patient record provides you with information about the health status of the patient, the professional record of a staff nurse informs you about his or her professional development or "educational health" in your agency.

The patient chart, whether constructed of paper or computer files, contains various forms that are organized in a standard sequence and kept on the clinical unit. Each form in the chart is used for a designated purpose. Patient data are documented in an objective manner based on agency policies and professional standards. Information found in the patient's chart helps the nurse plan nursing care and evaluate its effectiveness based on patient outcomes. Because the content of the patient chart is considered confidential, only certain healthcare workers are permitted to access it.

Data from the patient's record may be used to generate various reports referred to by others within the healthcare agency, such as staff who study agency infection rates or deal with insurance or government agencies. Others use these reports to make informed decisions that have the potential to influence a variety of individuals, such as patients, unit staff, and educators. These reports also can impact the unit, department, and healthcare organization.

The staff nurse's professional record is similar to that of a patient chart in that it contains notations about the nurse's competencies related to his or her role on the unit and the effectiveness of educational activities he or she attended in an effort to strengthen these abilities. Educators or preceptors write objective notations about the nurse's progress at time intervals determined by departmental policies and procedures. Data contained in staff records are considered confidential and need to be accessed by those with permission (ANA, 2000).

The same as with patient records, various reports are generated based on data obtained from the professional records of staff nurses. These reports are used to make decisions that can influence various individuals and departments as well as organizational goals (ANA, 2000). Although some reports focus on individual staff, others may reflect data based on groups of healthcare workers or staff on particular clinical units.

For example, a staff nurse may need access to a list of recent continuing education programs attended and contact hours earned in order to apply for recertification in a clinical specialty, to develop a resume, or to create a portfolio for promotion. To complete a periodic performance evaluation for a staff nurse, a nurse manager might need information about each nurse's clinical competency testing, performance as a unit-based preceptor, and performance as a presenter in unit-based in-service and continuing education programs. A healthcare organization may develop reports for accreditation purposes to monitor staff's learning needs.

NSDDs often use different approaches to develop a record-keeping system, so be sure to find out what method is used at your organization. Some organizations maintain their records using hard copies and self-designed computer databases, whereas others have purchased commercially produced learning management systems. In addition to keeping data by each staff member organized, the department also may develop records that reflect the work (programs) of educators in the NSDD. For example, the NSDD may document the number of orientations, in-service education offerings, and continuing education programs in a fiscal year, along with the number and type of healthcare workers who attend each educational activity. This type of information is helpful in developing reports for the administrator in the nursing division or for developing a fiscal plan for the department.

Regardless of what type of documentation, record-keeping system, or reports the NSDD generates, you will want to learn more about each process and the key participants responsible. Ask where records are stored, how they can be retrieved, and who has permission to access them. For example, in some organizations, staff records are maintained in the appropriate unit manager's office, whereas other agencies keep all records in the NSDD. As mentioned earlier, some departments maintain data about the professional development of staff in a computerized database for easy storage and retrieval.

Now that you understand the documentation and record-keeping system from the perspective of the nurse educator in your NSDD, think about your participation in this process from a unit-based level. Find out which aspects of the staff development process you will be responsible for documenting and your role in the overall record-keeping system of the NSDD. Inquire about what reports you need to generate, for whom, and how often. Additional guidance regarding documentation and record keeping will be discussed in Chapter 4 on orientation, Chapter 7 on unit-based in-service education, and Chapter 15 on continuing education programs.

Clarify Your Role as a Unit-Based Educator in the Clinical Setting

Once you have an understanding of the organization, nursing department, and NSDD, then you can focus on the clinical unit to which you are assigned as a unit-based educator. If you are responsible for more than one clinical unit, be sure to examine each of them, especially if they are not familiar to you. Clarify your role as a unit-based educator with your immediate supervisor and review the performance standards and expectations listed in your position (job) description. Depending on your organization, your supervisor might be the nurse manager of your unit or the manager or educator in the NSDD.

Start by discovering what organizational changes have affected the unit over recent years and what the strategic goals are for the unit. Obtain this information from the nurse manager of the clinical unit and the NSDD educator, if appropriate. Spend some time on the unit observing the nursing care and talking with the staff if you have not done this as a staff nurse. Find answers to questions that were posed earlier in this chapter.

Find out how the unit is structured and how it functions. Ask how staff members on the clinical unit implement the vision, mission, philosophy, and goals of the organization and nursing department. Focus on any unit-specific policies and procedures. Learn more information about workers who comprise the unit's staff, including their names, positions, and strengths they add to the unit. Try to determine which staff members might be considered the unit's "stars," because they will undoubtedly help you meet the unit's education goals.

Try to understand the unit manager's and staff's philosophy of professional staff development, much like what was described earlier in this chapter. Compare their philosophies with those of the NSDD and your own. Determine the staff's past and current learning needs. Investigate available unit-based resources that will maximize your role as unit-based educator. For example, do the unit's staff nurses perceive the importance of lifelong professional development, or do they feel they already have attained the competencies they will need to care for patients? How do staff members view their role in the teaching-learning process? Is their role one of personal responsibility and active participation, or do they view their role in education as a passive one directed by the staff development educator? These are just samples of questions you should attempt to investigate to help you plan your approach.

Next, clarify your role and responsibilities as unit-based staff educator. Start by finding your position on the department's organizational chart, and notice the authority and communication lines between you and others. Determine the person to whom you are responsible and accountable. Locate individuals who hold positions similar to yours and those people for whom you are responsible in terms of helping them meet their learning needs. Set some time aside to meet with these individuals and to ask questions.

While comparing the data contained in your job description, validate to whom you directly report, such as the nurse manager or staff development educator. Check if you report to more than one manager, especially if you are the educator for more than one unit or if you also perform direct patient care activities. If you report to more than one person, be sure you know what aspect of your job is reported to whom.

Closely examine your job description and the specific performance standards and expectations listed for both unit-based educator and other roles you assume. Be sure to seek clarification from your supervisor about each expectation and discuss realistic ways to manage multiple roles. Note if your staff development responsibilities include all aspects of professional development for staff or if they are confined to single components of staff development, such as orientation or in-service education offerings. Discuss additional department or organization committees to which you may be assigned because of your new role. Be sure to clarify any vague statements with your supervisor, especially if you have multiple roles that are composed of a combination of advisory and line authority. Finally, understand how you are evaluated and the procedure and expectations that you should follow.

Conduct a Self-Assessment for Your Role as Unit-Based Educator

Once you have investigated the organization, nursing department, NSDD, and clinical unit(s), spend some time reflecting on your own beliefs about education. Uncover what you value as important in the teaching-learning process and how you envision your role as unit-based educator. Compare your philosophy of professional development with that of the NSDD and your clinical unit, which ultimately guides the direction of education activities at your workplace.

Next, conduct a self-assessment of your qualities so that you can compare them with those needed in your new role as unit-based educator. Start by making a list of your personal and professional strengths, such as knowledge you have on special topics, your expertise in performing skills, and attitudes or beliefs. Figure 3-4 lists some examples of desired qualities of unit-based educators.

Remember to include caregiver abilities, such as your coordination, interpersonal, and critical-thinking skills, that are highly valued as a unit-based educator.

Keep your personal qualities in mind also, such as your flexibility, creativity, and optimism. For example, you might be a good listener or able to lead groups. Perhaps you excel at handling medical equipment needed to care for patients on your unit. It might be that you are good at providing homecare instructions to patients and families. All of these skills should be included in your list of strengths.

Second, use your new position description as a guide to create a second list that contains knowledge, skills, and attitudes that you perceive are needed to be successful as a unit-based educator. Arrange this list in order of importance, starting with the most important quality and ending the list with the least important. Obtain this information from others in your organization (e.g., nurse managers, educators in the NSDD, other unit-based educators within your organization). Ask your co-workers to give you feedback about skills in which you excel. Seek help from nursing publications on this topic, your colleagues who work at other agencies, and faculty from affiliating schools of nursing. Note how the abilities that you need to function as a unit-based educator parallel with skills required in your clinical staff nurse role.

Knowledge
• Teaching-learning process
• Adult learning principles and learning styles
• Clinical skills
• Implementing change
• Understanding of professional activities (e.g., research, publication)
Skills
• Self-directed and dependable
• Negotiation
• Conflict management
• Problem-solving
• Developing an agenda and running a meeting
• Communication and interpersonal skills
• Organization and managing time effectively
• Leadership management
Attitudes
• Seeks learning experiences
• Treats all staff fairly and with respect
• Creates a positive work environment
• Possesses an optimistic perspective

Figure 3-4.
Examples of Desired Qualities of Unit-Based Educators

Determine Unit-Based Staff Development Needs

To carry out your role as unit-based educator, it is essential that you have information regarding the staff development needs of nursing staff on your unit, related to both educational and professional development. These identified needs will guide you as you develop educational goals for the unit staff and a plan to meet these learning needs. You also will need to evaluate the effectiveness of your unit-based education plan.

Educational Needs

Learn how your organization determines the learning needs of nursing staff who work on your unit. This duty may be the responsibility of the educator in your centralized NSDD, your unit's nurse manager, or yours as a unit-based educator.

Learning needs of staff are determined using a variety of sources and approaches and will be described in later chapters that discuss orientation (Chapter 4), inservice education (Chapters 6 and 7), and continuing education (Chapter 14). However, it is helpful to compile an ongoing master list of learning needs. As learning needs become evident on a daily basis, add them to the list, upgrading their urgency as needed. In addition to conducting formal needs assessment surveys, be sure to use feedback that you obtain from meeting with key individuals in your agency, such as the educator in the NSDD, your nurse manager, and other unit-based educators. Spend some time meeting with unit staff to understand their perspective of their learning needs.

Professional Development Needs

In addition to your role as educator, you may be asked to assist staff development educators in activities that reflect their multiple roles mentioned earlier in Chapter 2: educator, facilitator, change agent, consultant, researcher, and leader (ANA, 2000). This information may be available from the NSDD educator or nurse manager and should reflect the direction of the organization and, therefore, your professional development plan.

For example, your nursing department may need you to help staff members develop formal presentations or prepare manuscripts for publication, or you may be advised to encourage staff participation in clinical research projects or in continuing education programs for the local community. If your nursing department has a clinical advancement program, you may need to assist clinical nurses in developing their resumes and portfolios. All of these responsibilities are reviewed later in this text. If you have never performed some of these activities yourself, then it is important to include them as part of your own professional development.

Analyze, Organize, and Plan Your Work

Once you have gathered information about your own learning needs and those of the staff on your clinical unit(s), spend some time analyzing and organizing it. Start by focusing on your needs first and then the staff development needs for the unit.

Develop a Plan for Self-Development

After you have collected data about yourself and your role, compare both lists of qualities. Determine the qualities that are desired, the ones you already demonstrate, and those you do not yet have. Label those you already possess as being excellent (3), adequate (2), or not adequate (1). Although you probably have excellent clinical skills, it is likely that your new unit-based educator skills are not as fully developed at this point in your career.

Use this information to develop a professional career plan that will help you meet your goal of strengthening the qualities you listed as being adequate (2) or inadequate (1). Because it is unrealistic to imagine that you can develop all these competencies immediately, use the priority order in which they are arranged to help you determine which skills to develop first. Investigate various resources both within and outside your healthcare organization that can help you attain these goals. Possible sources that can help you develop in the role of unit-based educator include mentors, professional nursing organizations, formal and informal educational offerings, and other colleagues. Career planning will be discussed in more detail in Chapter 15.

Mentors

Identify one or more individuals who can serve as mentors for you. These mentors can help you improve your skills as unit-based educator. You may choose individuals at your workplace whom you admire and already have a comfortable relationship with, such as an educator in the NSDD, your unit manager, or a more experienced unit-based educator. Your mentor may work outside of your agency. For example, you might choose to ask your favorite nurse faculty from the school of nursing you attended or a colleague who works at another organization.

Professional Nursing Organizations

Try joining a professional nursing organization whose mission is related to your learning needs. Clinically oriented nursing organizations, such as the American Association of Critical Care Nurses or the Association of Operating Room Nurses, offer educational programs that focus on topics related to clinical nursing practice, and they frequently sponsor educational activities that target the needs of staff educators. Other organizations, such as Sigma Theta Tau International, offer professional development programs for nurses in diverse roles (e.g., clinical practice, education, research, administration). Some nursing organizations, such as the National Nursing Staff Development Organization, are entirely dedicated to meeting the needs of nurses who function as staff educators in healthcare settings.

In addition to their programs, take advantage of the many networking opportunities these organizations provide, especially through conferences or special interest groups. Explore the organization's products, like their books, journals, newsletters, and electronic and Internet resources. Many national organizations have local chapters that enable nurses to actively participate at an affordable cost. Investigate other nursing journals that focus on your role as a unit-based educator, such as *Journal for Nurses in Staff Development* or the *Journal of Continuing Education in Nursing*.

Formal and Informal Educational Offerings

In addition to educational offerings sponsored by professional nursing organizations, consider attending continuing education programs presented by others, such as your workplace or affiliating schools of nursing. Consider enrolling in formal courses for academic credit that focus on the educator role, or ask nursing faculty from affiliating schools of nursing to present a series of in-service education offerings for a group of unit-based educators at your agency in return for serving as preceptors for their students. Be sure to utilize less formal educational activities, such as books, journals, videos, and computer-assisted instruction.

Colleagues

Along with these various resources, remember that your colleagues who hold similar positions to yours also can provide support. Think about developing a unit-based educator support group in your organization or communication pathways through e-mail.

Develop a Plan for Unit-Based Staff Development

After you develop a plan to strengthen your competencies as a unit-based educator, prepare a plan to meet the staff development needs of the unit's clinical staff. Start this process by analyzing and organizing the data you obtained about the staff's learning needs from various sources. Then develop several goals or objectives (outcomes) you hope to accomplish within the year.

Although you want a holistic perspective of each staff member's competencies related to patient care needs on the clinical unit, this may be an overwhelming task. To make your work more manageable, try organizing your work into smaller and more realistic components. Select a method that facilitates your unit-based record-keeping and reporting systems and matches your work with any centralized education efforts. Your method also should be cost effective.

One approach you can choose is to categorize the unit's education plan into the three components of staff development, which are mentioned in Chapter 2: orientation, in-service education, and continuing education (ANA, 2000). Begin by sorting individual learning needs (competencies), included in your master list, into like categories based on similar topics. Because you have limited resources, organize these needs in order of their priority. Develop goals and objectives (outcomes) you hope to accomplish that will enable staff to meet this need. Sort each category along with its goals into the educational approach (e.g., orientation, in-service education, continuing education) that might best meet these goals. Specific descriptions about ways to meet learning needs will be covered in Chapter 4 (orientation), Chapters 6 and 7 (in-service education), and Chapter 14 (continuing education). Because the learning needs of staff are constant and changing, try to visualize your efforts as an educational plan in progress.

Suppose all staff nurses on your unit will need to perform venipunctures on patients to obtain blood specimens during the unit's evening shift. This need was brought to your attention by the unit's nurse manager, who communicated a recent departmental decision and policy change. Because of organizational restructuring, the staff members who routinely provided this service from a centralized location were transferred to an ambulatory patient setting. The responsibility for drawing blood samples must be assumed by nurses on your clinical unit three months from now.

Following the approach just described, you decide that a unit-based in-service education program is the best way for staff to learn to master this skill. None of the existing staff know how to perform venipunctures but do have prior knowledge concerning its complications. This brief in-service session will be sufficient time for you to review the procedure, discuss key issues, and provide a demonstration on a model arm. There also will be time for you to guide staff as they provide a return demonstration. This unit-based session will be easier for staff to attend while they are providing patient care. To help staff master their venipuncture skills, you later team each nurse with a phlebotomist for a brief but intensive practicum. Because it is unrealistic to expect all staff to attend these sessions at one time, you initially target nurses who need to master this skill first, such as nurses who work the evening shift. After demonstrating competence in venipunctures, these nurses can become the "experts" who will be responsible for teaching remaining staff. This cost-effective approach will not only meet the learning needs of the staff but also will help staff develop their unit-based presentation and preceptor skills.

Develop a Communication System

As a unit-based educator, it is important that you communicate with various individuals both inside and outside the organization. This will not only help you meet your goals but also will provide all staff with a sense of commitment to the educational activities of the unit. Because of this, be sure to consider key individuals with whom you will need to communicate on a regular basis and available strategies to accomplish this.

Start by making a list of these individuals and the communication methods available in your organization. Try meeting with these individuals to determine the most effective approach. For example, you may want to have monthly meetings with your nurse manager or staff educator to update them on the progress of the unit-based activities. Perhaps you can rely on e-mail to share changes in between meetings. If all staff have access to e-mail, then consider regular updates about the unit's educational activities. Also consider traditional methods, such as face-to-face meetings, posters, signs, written memos, communication books, and newsletters. You will need to decide what the most effective approach will be based on your organization.

In addition to these communication systems, be sure to let staff know the best way to contact you if you are not on the clinical unit (e.g., voice message, pager, e-mail). Keep them abreast of your schedule and who will handle your responsibilities when you are away.

Capitalize on the Strengths of the Unit Staff

As mentioned in Chapter 2, meeting the education needs of staff on the clinical unit is a 24-hour responsibility. Because of this, it is important that you develop creative strategies that will not only deal with this time frame but also will contribute to the professional development of staff. For example, think of including staff in helping to meet the educational goals of the unit by developing an education committee on your unit. This committee can consist of staff who are interested or staff you select who will assist you with the planning and implementation of educational activities on the unit. The development of a preceptorship program, as discussed in Chapter 5, is another example. In developing these approaches, be sure to match the strengths and interests of the staff with the tasks, if possible. This is another reason why it is important for you to be familiar with unit staff, including their strengths, needs for improvement, motivation, and professional goals.

Evaluate Your Effectiveness in Meeting Goals

Similar to a patient's plan of care, develop a plan to evaluate how effective your interventions were in meeting both your personal goals and the unit's staff development goals. Evaluate your progress at the end of the (fiscal) year prior to developing a new plan for the following year. However, tracking your progress on an ongoing basis (i.e., monthly) will enable you to revise your plan if it is not on target.

Evaluation of Personal Goals as a Unit-Based Educator

Earlier in this chapter you inventoried your personal and professional qualities and compared them with those needed to be effective in the role of unit-based educator. Using your prioritized list as a guide, you developed realistic career goals to accomplish during the year along with strategies.

Spend some time each month reviewing your personal plan and deciding if you are heading in the right direction. Take this opportunity to revise your plan if it is unrealistic or if unexpected opportunities to develop other skills arise. You may decide that skills other than the ones you had previously identified should be a priority to develop. Conduct a final evaluation at the end of the year before you develop next year's plan.

In addition to your self-evaluation, obtain feedback from others about your performance. The nurse educator in the NSDD, your unit manager, and other experienced unit-based educators may be most helpful. Incorporate feedback you receive during your formal performance evaluation, and make changes as needed.

Evaluation of Unit-Based Staff Development Goals

In addition to your personal goals, evaluate those goals created for the staff development needs of unit personnel. Track your progress monthly, and make needed revisions. Conduct a summary evaluation annually before you design a plan for the following year.

For example, suppose one of your goals was to develop a preceptor preparation program for your unit. Evaluate your progress on this project each month based on the specific measurements you outlined from the start. If you find that you are off course one month, revise your approach, as needed, to get back on track.

In addition to collecting objective data about unit-based educational activities, obtain input from others on the unit, such as the staff and nurse manager. The staff can provide you with their perspective about meeting their learning needs. The unit manager gives you feedback based on unit reports, such as patient satisfaction surveys, patient outcomes, performance indicators, competencies, and incident reports. Chapters presented later in this book will focus on evaluating specific goals and learning objectives of orientation, in-service education, and continuing education.

Summary

In getting prepared for the role of unit-based educator, you need to gather information about your organization and department, the nursing education department, and the clinical unit(s) to which you are assigned. You also need to conduct a self-assessment based on your performance expectations, and develop a realistic plan for professional development. After you assess your unit-based staff development needs, prioritize these needs and develop a plan based on analysis of these data. Implement this plan by motivating staff and dealing effectively with conflict. Finally, develop a systematic feedback of both your performance as an educator and how well the educational offering met its goal of improving competency of the learners.

References

American Nurses Association. (1994). *Standards for nursing professional development: Continuing education and staff development*. Washington, DC: Author.

American Nurses Association. (1998). *Standards of clinical nursing practice*. Washington, DC: Author.

American Nurses Association. (2000). *Scope and standards of practice for nursing professional development*. Washington, DC: Author.

Joint Commission on Accreditation of Healthcare Organization. (2003). *Facts about Joint Commission Accreditation*. Retrieved June 18, 2003, from www.jcaho.org/ accredited+organizations/publicizing+your+accreditation/facts+about

Marquis, B.L., & Huston, C.J. (1998). *Management decision making for nurses: 124 case studies* (3rd ed.). Philadelphia: Lippincott Williams & Wilkins.

UNIT 2

Orienting Nursing Staff to the Clinical Unit

CHAPTER 4

Developing a Competency-Based Orientation Program for Nursing Staff on a Clinical Unit

The staff development domain within the American Nurses Association (ANA) Framework for Nursing Professional Development (ANA, 2000) was described earlier within Chapter 2. That chapter described nursing staff development as a separate domain of nursing professional development yet one that is related, in some aspects, to the other two domains of the framework: continuing education (CE) and academic education (ANA, 2000). Figure 2-1 in Chapter 2 illustrates the relationship among these three domains.

The staff development domain includes three primary educational activities: orientation, in-service education activities, and CE programs (ANA, 2000). Each of these activities focuses on assessing, validating, and developing the competencies of nurses employed by healthcare organizations (ANA, 2000). Orientation will be the focus of this chapter, whereas in-service educational activities and CE programs will be discussed in Chapters 7 and 14, respectively.

As a unit-based educator, it is important for you to understand the orientation component of nursing staff development and your specific role and responsibilities related to orientation activities within your healthcare organization. Understanding this information will help you coordinate your unit-based orientation efforts with your agency's centralized staff development activities. This also will help you determine what to include in your unit-based orientation program and how to plan, organize, implement, and evaluate it.

Unit-based educators also need to understand continuing competence through all staff development activities and the important role it plays in promoting safe, quality health care for patients. This focus of continuing competence in staff development will be discussed in the next section of this chapter followed by a discussion of competency within the context of orientation.

Continuing Competence and Nursing Staff Development

Continuing competence and lifelong learning are the primary aims of professional development activities for nurses (ANA, 2000). The ultimate goal of professional nursing development is to ensure that consumers receive safe, quality health care provided by competent nurses (ANA, 2000).

Eichelberger and Hewlett (1999) described this need to ensure nurses' competencies as a quandary for the nursing profession, especially in light of the current healthcare situation. These authors advocate core competency statements for nurses

51

based on the *five rights:* "assuring the *right* nurse with the *right* preparation for the *right* patient in the *right* setting at the *right* cost" (p. 204).

Clarifying the Meanings of *Competence, Competency,* and *Continuing Competence*

Unit-based educators involved in staff development activities such as orientation, in-service education, and CE need to understand the meaning of continuing competence to promote it in nurses employed by their healthcare organizations. Staff development educators also need to be familiar with the various standards and outcome criteria that focus on competencies in professional nurses.

The terms *competence* and *competency* refer to the "determination of an individual's capabilities to perform up to defined expectations" (Joint Commission on Accreditation of Healthcare Organizations [JCAHO], 2003, p. 347). *Continuing competence,* as defined by ANA, is the "ongoing professional nursing competence according to level of expertise, responsibility, and domains of practice as evidenced by behavior based on beliefs, attitudes, and knowledge matched to and in the context of a set of expected outcomes as defined by nursing scope of practice, policy, code of ethics, standards, guidelines, and benchmarks that ensure safe performance of professional activities" (ANA, 2000, p. 23).

Continuing competence is important so that nurses are able to provide safe, quality nursing care to their patients, who have a right to expect this level of care in healthcare organizations (ANA, 2000). In fact, continuing competence is not only a key feature of nursing professionalism but also is a way that the nursing profession is held accountable to society (ANA, 2000).

Assuming Responsibility for Continuing Competence of Nurses

Although nurses assume primary responsibility for ensuring their own continuing competence, others also participate in this obligation (ANA, 2000). Those partners who help nurses with their competencies include professional nursing organizations, their employers, regulatory agencies, credentialing bodies (ANA, 2000), and nurse educators (Exstrom, 2001).

Nurses

Professional nurses are expected to be self-directed learners (ANA, 2000). They are expected to recognize their own learning needs and demonstrate this initiative by actively participating in appropriate educational experiences that will help them maintain their continuing competence (ANA, 2000; Exstrom, 2001). Nurses have a professional responsibility to keep abreast of the nurse practice act in the state where they are licensed to practice as a RN. Nurses can demonstrate their continuing competency using a variety of options, which will be discussed later in this chapter.

Professional Nursing Associations and Organizations

Professional nursing associations and organizations also assume responsibility for the continuing competence of RNs. ANA has developed standards of practice and professional performance for the nursing profession (ANA, 2000), such as its *Standards of Clinical Nursing Practice* (ANA, 1998). Standards of nursing practice describe a "level of care or performance common to the profession of nursing by which the quality of nursing practice can be judged or reassured" (ANA, 2000, p. 26). Standards of professional performance describe a "competent level of behavior in the professional role, including activities related to quality of care, performance appraisal, education, collegiality, ethics, collaboration, research, and resource utilization" (ANA, 2000, p. 26).

For example, a professional practice standard in ANA's document states that nurses should "acquire and maintain current knowledge and competency in nursing practice as a professional practice" (ANA, 1998, p. 12). Clinical nurses are expected to adhere to this standard and demonstrate it by seeking and participating in appropriate educational offerings to maintain their current competencies.

ANA also assumes responsibility for the continuing competence of nurses through its involvement in the legislative and health policy arenas, CE and nursing certification efforts, and research in this area (ANA, 2000).

Many specialty nursing organizations, such as the Oncology Nursing Society (ONS), also have developed standards of practice for its members (ANA & ONS, 1996; ONS, 2003). The ONS standards, like those of ANA, emphasize the individual nurse's responsibility in continuing competence. In addition, ONS sponsors CE activities and provides various materials and learning opportunities to help oncology nurses maintain or develop the knowledge, skills, and values that are essential in cancer care. The Oncology Nursing Certification Corporation, the certifying corporation of ONS, provides opportunities for oncology nurses to demonstrate their competency in oncology nursing through the certification process.

Employers of Nurses

Healthcare organizations, such as hospitals, are responsible for establishing a work environment that makes it possible for their patients to receive safe, quality care from competent nurses (ANA, 2000; Exstrom, 2001). Hospitals use various strategies to accomplish this goal, such as providing for sufficient staffing on clinical units, sponsoring staff development programs for nurses to maintain their competencies, and assessing and validating nurses' competencies (ANA, 2000).

Hospitals are responsible for determining the competency of the nurses they hire prior to employment, upon hire during orientation, and on a regular, ongoing basis (JCAHO, 2003). This information will be discussed in detail later in this chapter.

Accreditation Agencies

Accrediting agencies, such as JCAHO, also take responsibility for ensuring the continuing competency of nurses employed by healthcare organizations (ANA, 2000). The mission of JCAHO is to "continually improve the safety and quality of care provided to the public" (JCAHO, 2003, p. ii). JCAHO supports improved performance by establishing accreditation standards that address competence (JCAHO). Therefore, hospitals voluntarily seeking accreditation from JCAHO need to comply with these standards.

JCAHO addresses the issue of competency through several standards, especially in the "Management of Human Resources" section of its hospital accreditation manual (JCAHO, 2003). Competency is addressed in other sections of the JCAHO manual as well. Figure 4-1 identifies several key standards that relate to competencies. Each of these standards is accompanied by an intent that

Figure 4-1.
Joint Commission
on Accreditation
of Healthcare
Organizations:
Human Resource
Standards That Re-
fer to Competency
of Employees

Note. From 2003 Hos-
pital Accreditation
Standards: Accredita-
tion Policies, Stan-
dards, Intent State-
ments (p. 244) by the
Joint Commission on
Accreditation of
Healthcare Organiza-
tions, 2003, Oakbrook
Terrace, IL: Author.
Copyright 2003 by
Joint Comission Re-
sources. Reprinted
with permission.

HR.3: The leaders ensure that the competence of all staff members is assessed, maintained, demonstrated, and improved continually.

HR.4: An orientation process provides initial job training and information and assesses the staff's ability to fulfill specified responsibilities.

HR.4.2: Ongoing in-service and other education and training maintain and improve staff competence and support an interdisciplinary approach to patient care.

HR.4.3: The hospital regularly collects aggregate data on competence patterns and trends to identify and respond to the staff's learning needs.

explains the rationale and significance of the standard and ways that hospitals can demonstrate the standard (JCAHO).

Regulatory Agencies

Regulatory agencies, such as state boards of nursing, take responsibility for nurses' continuing competency through their licensing process (ANA, 2000; Exstrom, 2001). The state board of nursing issues licenses to graduate nurses (GNs) who successfully pass the licensure examination (NCLEX-RN). The board also grants relicensure to experienced nurses who meet their state's requirements. State boards of nursing "interpret, administer, and enforce nursing practice acts and rules and regulations" (ANA, 2000, p. 32). Nurses can meet requirements for continuing competency through active participation in CE programs (Exstrom) or multiple validation options in some states (McGuire & Weisenbeck, 2001).

The Occupational Safety and Health Administration (OSHA) also supports this need for competency by establishing guidelines for healthcare organizations (OSHA, 2003). These guidelines protect nurses from injuring themselves while providing patient care, with the expectation that they will function safely and without injury in the work setting.

Nurse Educators

Nurse educators in schools of nursing also contribute to the competency of nurses through offering nursing students an up-to-date curriculum, evaluating student performance throughout the program, and serving as role models for students (Exstrom, 2001). Nurse educators also contribute to the continuing competence of practicing nurses by sponsoring CE programs.

Orientation Component of Staff Development

ANA defines orientation as the "process of introducing nursing staff to the philosophy, goals, policies, procedures, role expectations, and other factors needed to function in a specific work setting" (ANA, 2000, p. 25). The orientation process provides newly employed nurses with information and experiences to function effectively in their assigned roles within an organization (ANA, 2000).

New GNs often comprise a large portion of nurses who participate in nursing orientation activities, but experienced nurses may attend an orientation program if they change jobs, change their roles or responsibilities within the same organization, or are reassigned to a new clinical unit or department. Staff development educators also may be responsible for developing orientation programs for other individuals who work at their organization or for members of the professional community (ANA, 2000). The specific learning needs of each of these groups of orientees will be discussed later in this chapter.

Purposes of Orientation

Orientations focus on three main purposes: competency, socialization, and role transition (ANA, 2000). The primary emphasis during orientation is on assessing, validating, and developing specific competencies in nurses that are needed for them to effectively function in the roles for which they were hired. Second, orientation socializes new employees to the work environment and helps orientees understand what is expected of them. Third, orientation programs help nurses, especially GNs, ease their transition from being a student nurse to assuming the role of a professional nurse in a healthcare setting.

Orientations also play an important role in helping healthcare organizations in not only recruiting new nurses to the organization but also in retaining the nurses they currently employ. For example, newly hired nurses who experience educational support, guidance, and a positive work environment may be more likely to stay at that organization than nurses who have a negative experience upon hire. The availability of a well-developed orientation program guided by experienced preceptors may encourage a nurse to seek employment at that organization.

Competency-Based Orientation Programs

Many healthcare organizations use a competency-based approach when orienting new nurse employees (Abruzzese, 1996). This type of orientation emphasizes the outcomes expected of the orientee as a result of the orientation program rather than focusing on the knowledge that the orientee possesses about performing the job (Alspach, 1996). The outcome of a competency-based orientation (CBO) program is the ability of the orientee to carry out the specific responsibilities defined in his or her job description (Abruzzese).

In a CBO, the healthcare organization determines a set of competencies (knowledge, skills, or values) that all orientees must adequately demonstrate before they are determined to be qualified to provide safe, quality care to patients within that organization without the supervision of a preceptor (Alspach, 1996). Demonstration of these competencies indicates that the orientee has successfully completed orientation.

A variety of competency programs have been reported in the nursing literature. Whereas some programs have focused on strengthening the nursing care received by age-specific groups of patients, such as adults and children (Beauman, 2001), others have dealt with specialty units, such as emergency departments (Gurney, 2002; Proehl, 2002), critical care units (Leonard & Plotnikoff, 2000), and medical/oncology units (Johnson, Opfer, VanCura, & Williams, 2000). Some organizations have developed competencies in specific areas that support the goals of the healthcare organization, such as chemotherapy administration (Kanaskie & Arnold, 1999), IV therapy in home care (Rudzik, 1999), genetics (Jenkins, 2002), culturally congruent (Leonard & Plotnikoff) and age-specific nursing care (Marrone, 1999), and computer skills (Miller & Arquiza, 1999).

Orientees may progress through a CBO at different rates (Amerson, 2002). Once orientees attain specific competencies, they advance to the next phase of the orientation program that poses a new list of competencies for them to demonstrate. Orientees are expected to attend various educational activities of the orientation program that address the competencies that they are unable to demonstrate adequately.

Performance-Based Development System

The performance-based development system (PBDS), a more developed CBO, focuses on management and clinical competencies and criterion-based performance standards (Abruzzese, 1996). A PBDS based on a model developed by del Bueno (1997) describes competency as having three overlapping dimensions applied within the context of a given situation: critical thinking skills, interpersonal skills, and technical skills (del Bueno, Weeks, & Brown-Stewart, 1987). In this system, both new and experienced nurses demonstrate their competencies in assessment centers during the orientation period before they provide patient care on the clinical units (Abruzzese). These centers actively engage learners through the use of videotaped scenarios, simulations, self-learning packets, and other active learning exercises. Although this system may be costly for its initial upstart, it offers the benefit of a decreased orientation time for nurses (Abruzzese).

Orientation Pathways for Newly Hired Nurses

Several authors have applied the concept of critical pathways used in patient care to the orientation process experienced by the newly hired nurse (Bumgarner & Biggerstaff, 2000; Francis & Batsie, 1998; Johnston & Ferraro, 2001). These orientation pathways offer advantages to nurse orientees, preceptors, and the healthcare organization.

For example, orientation pathways provide a framework that promotes individualized orientation based on the nurse's past clinical experience, while focusing on specific job expectations related to patient care (Johnston & Ferraro, 2001). They also help educators identify competencies that need to be strengthened, along with target dates (Johnston & Ferraro). Orientation pathways also serve as a guide or road map for preceptors and orientees as they provide direct patient care, promoting critical thinking skills and application of the nursing process (Bumgarner & Biggerstaff, 2000). Pathways also have been reported to positively impact job satisfaction and retention (Bumgarner & Biggerstaff).

Advantages of Competency-Based Orientations

CBOs offer several advantages to the orientee, preceptor, and healthcare organization. First, by focusing on the learning needs and abilities of individual learners, CBOs allow experienced RNs to demonstrate their fundamental nursing competencies within a short period of time. GNs, with less nursing experience, have an opportunity to validate those competencies with which they are most familiar and then develop new competencies at their own pace. Orientees can identify their own strengths and weaknesses based on their performance related to the evaluation criteria needed to meet the competency. Although most CBOs do not have specific time limitations, some experts suggest using target dates to help the orientee complete the orientation program within a reasonable time period after being hired (Abruzzese, 1996).

Second, CBOs provide preceptors with clearly defined expectations of orientees during their clinical experience on the unit (Abruzzese, 1996). This feature of CBOs minimizes the chance that preceptors and other staff may provide inconsistent information to the orientees.

Third, because CBOs reduce the amount of time that experienced orientees may spend in orientation, they often can offer a cost savings to healthcare organizations (Abruzzese, 1996). The competency statements and critical behaviors recorded as part of the orientees' competency validation process provide organizations with a performance document—evidence that orientees demonstrated safe, quality care at that time (Abruzzese). This recording system complies with JCAHO standards mentioned earlier in this chapter.

Disadvantages of Competency-Based Orientations

CBOs also pose some disadvantages. For example, preceptors should be familiar with the main concepts of CBOs and consistently hold orientees to the same performance outcomes (Alspach, 1996). Second, although each clinical unit within a healthcare organization may identify unique competencies based on its needs, all clinical units within that organization should use a similar format and approach to verify nurses' competencies. Finally, the majority of competencies should focus on essential high-risk procedures, despite their volume. This last feature of competencies will be explained further in the section that follows.

Developing Competencies for a Competency-Based Orientation Program

Nurses begin their professional development with their basic nursing education program in a school of nursing and continue developing themselves throughout their nursing careers by participating in educational activities within the domains of staff development, CE, and academic preparation. Although GNs are expected to have demonstrated select competencies prior to being employed by a healthcare organization, these competencies may need to be validated or further developed upon hire. Although passing the NCLEX-RN is one way that GNs can demonstrate their current nursing knowledge, it does not ensure competency (Cooper, 2002). Employers also require experienced nurses to validate their competencies during the orientation period in order to verify that they can function safely in their role at that organization.

Before implementing a CBO program, you will need to identify key competencies that you expect all nurses to successfully demonstrate by the end of the orientation program. You will need to develop a process to evaluate or validate these competencies in nurses and provide them with various learning options so they can develop or strengthen them. Each of these elements will be discussed in the following section of this chapter.

Identify Relevant Competencies

The first step in developing a CBO program is to identify the competencies that you expect all nurse orientees to demonstrate by the end of the orientation program (Alspach, 1996). You can identify these competencies through a variety of sources. Then, you will need to organize these competencies in order of their importance within the context of ensuring safe, quality patient care at your healthcare organization.

Sources for Competencies

Ideas for competencies can come from a variety of sources, such as nursing staff, the healthcare organization, and external agencies. You can use a variety of methods to retrieve this information, including interviews, focus groups, and surveys.

Nursing Staff

Nurses, including nurse managers, staff educators, and unit staff, are excellent resources for identifying competencies that should be included in an orientation program (Exstrom, 2001). Because nurse managers evaluate the performance of nursing staff and manage patient care issues on the unit, they are in a prime position to identify competencies that are vital to safe, quality patient care. Results of patient satisfaction surveys, quality assurance reports, policies and procedures, and incident reports often provide ideas for competencies.

Nurses in leadership roles can be instrumental in identifying competencies needed by staff nurses who are assuming leadership roles. For example, Connelly (1998) identified specific competencies needed to assume the charge nurse role and cited barriers and facilitators to this role. Data were collected through interviews with 42 staff nurses who often served as charge nurses on their clinical units. Findings revealed 52 competencies that were categorized into four groups: clinical/technical, critical thinking, organizational, and human relations skills. Findings have implications for educators who orient staff nurses to the charge nurse role and who promote continuing competence through ongoing in-service and CE programs.

Staff development educators, including unit-based educators, play an important role in determining baseline competencies that orientees must demonstrate before the conclusion of the orientation. These competencies often reflect expectations outlined in the orientee's job description but can include competencies identified through past orientations. For example, LaDuke (2001) described an alternative strategy used to determine competencies based on the Nursing Interventions Classification. Educators are responsible for providing orientees with various learning opportunities to help them develop their competencies and successfully complete the orientation program.

As a unit-based educator, encourage nursing staff on your clinical unit to identify the specific competencies that orientees need to demonstrate before the conclusion of the unit-based orientation. Cooper (2002) described an approach in which all nursing staff had input in identifying the competencies required for their unit's orientation program. A group of staff nurses from diverse levels brainstormed possible competencies that they believed new nurses should possess at the completion of orientation. Next, they ranked these competencies according to their importance and sought input from other unit staff before developing the details of these competencies and determining ways to evaluate them. Obtaining input from all staff is important because nurses who work during the night hours may experience different learning needs than nurses who staff the unit during the day (Glass & Todd-Atkinson, 1999).

Accreditation and Regulatory Agencies

As mentioned earlier in this chapter, JCAHO shares in the responsibility for assuring the public of safe, quality nursing care through its published accreditation standards (JCAHO, 2003). Although JCAHO allows hospitals to develop their own systems to assess, validate, and appraise the competencies of nursing staff, orientees are expected to demonstrate competence in "job-related aspects of patient safety" (JCAHO, p. 248). These aspects can include topics such as fire safety, life safety, safety and security, hazardous materials and waste, infection control, restraints, medication errors, patient falls, and pain management.

Because nursing care should be adapted to a patient's age, nurses need to onstrate age-specific competencies (JCAHO, 2003). For example, a nurse sh consider the age of a cardiac arrest victim (i.e., infant, child, or adult) when viding cardiopulmonary resuscitation (CPR).

Hospitals have the flexibility to determine the age ranges and labels for age-specific group they recognize (Cooper, 2002). For example, a pediatric hospital may choose to use the following age-specific categories and designate age ranges for them: neonate, infant, toddler, preschool, school age, adolescent, and adult.

OSHA focuses on the prevention of injury and death in the workplace (OSHA, 2003). OSHA's protective standards can be a valuable source of expected competencies for nurses. These topics may overlap with those of JCAHO and include job safety and health, protective equipment, blood-borne pathogens, emergency evacuation, ergonomics, and hazardous chemicals.

A variety of other licensing and certifying agencies also can serve as sources of ideas for competencies. As a unit-based educator, speak with leaders at your healthcare organization to determine what these ideas may be.

Prioritizing and Organizing Competencies

After identifying a list of competencies that nurse orientees need to demonstrate before completing the orientation program, prioritize this list of competencies in order of importance for your setting. Consider the risk, volume, and problem areas among the criteria when ranking your competencies (Cooper, 2002).

Most healthcare organizations include 8–16 job expectations of nurses that comprise either high-risk/high-volume or high-risk/low-volume competencies that are congruent with the organization's standards, policies, and procedures (Krozek & Scoggins, 2000). Organizations usually do not include competencies in each area of the nurse's job requirements. Each of these types of competencies will be discussed in the section that follows.

High-Risk, High-Volume Competencies

High-risk competencies are those (knowledge, skills, and attitudes) that can cause serious damage to patients or nurses if performed incorrectly. If the nurse performs this high-risk competency every day (high-volume), then the competency should be included among the baseline competencies demonstrated during orientation rather than in an annual competency review (Cooper, 2002). Some organizations refer to these competencies as "essential" competencies.

For example, nurses who work on a surgical head and neck unit perform tracheostomy care every day. If they do not perform it correctly, then the patient may experience difficulty breathing, a condition that may greatly worsen over time. Nurses who are hired to work on this unit should demonstrate this skill as part of their unit-based orientation program. Because these nurses perform tracheostomy care daily, this competency may not be included in their annual competency review.

High-Risk, Low-Volume Competencies

High-risk, low-volume competencies are those (knowledge, skills, and attitudes) that could pose harm to the patient if a nurse performed them incorrectly, but they are not performed often on the unit (Cooper, 2002). High-risk, low-volume competencies may be reviewed during an annual competency event to ensure that nurses will be able to perform these skills well, if and when the situation arises.

For example, some patients admitted to the surgical head and neck unit require chest tubes after surgery. This event does not occur often, but, when it occurs, nurses who work on that unit need to know how to safely care for these patients. If the nurse does not perform this care appropriately, the patients could suffer serious consequences, including death. You may decide to include this competency during orientation, but, at minimum, it should be included in an annual review.

Problem-Prone Areas

Some ideas for competencies arise from sources internal to the healthcare organization, such as incident or quality assurance reports (Cooper, 2002). For example, a clinical unit may have had several medication errors related to incorrect dosage calculations or a high incidence of wound infections in postoperative patients. These incidents may require investigation regarding factors that contributed to their causes and may warrant further education of staff through in-service education or CE programs.

Writing Competency Statements and Evaluation Criteria

After organizing your list of competencies, you will need to write them using the proper format. Each competency consists of a competency statement with a set of evaluation criteria, also referred to by some authors as critical behaviors (Abruzzese, 1996; Cooper, 2002) or performance criteria (Alspach, 1996).

Competency Statements

A competency statement describes the specific areas of competence included in an orientation program (Alspach, 1996) and defines the outcomes that the orientees need to demonstrate (Abruzzese, 1996; Cooper, 2002). For example, a competency statement targeted to nurse orientees assigned to a surgical head and neck unit may read, "Provides nursing care to patients following head and neck surgery."

Evaluation Criteria

The second part of a competency statement consists of a set of evaluation criteria, critical behaviors (Abruzzese, 1996; Cooper, 2002), or performance criteria (Alspach, 1996). These criteria describe the behaviors or actions the orientee needs to "demonstrate as evidence of competency in a particular area" (Alspach, p. 89). In an orientation program, preceptors observe these behaviors and determine if the orientee's performance is acceptable related to the competency (Alspach). For example, evaluation criteria for the competency statement mentioned earlier may include the following: "Develops a plan of care that includes assessing potential complications of surgery: airway obstruction, bleeding from the surgical incision, wound infection, fistula formation, and fluid and electrolyte problems."

Essential Elements

Evaluation criteria (performance criteria) should include several elements in order to be deemed acceptable (Alspach, 1996). For example, each criterion must be learner-centered and describe a single behavior in measurable and observable terms (Alspach). Critical behaviors begin with an action verb, such as the ones listed in Table 7-1 in Chapter 7. Second, each criterion should be described clearly enough so that the orientee and preceptor will understand the specific behavior that is being evaluated (Alspach). Third, criteria need to include any conditions that may be placed on the orientee's performance, such as demonstrating the expected behavior after attending an educational session on nursing care.

Fourth, criteria should include a performance standard that provides the preceptor with a baseline against which the orientee's behavior can be deemed acceptable (Alspach, 1996). A standard may include requiring the orientee to perform the expected behavior within the first 15 minutes of the patient's arrival to the clinical unit after surgery. Finally, only the key aspects of the behavior should be included in performance criteria (Alspach). Additional words that do not contribute to the criteria create confusion.

Comparison With Educational Objectives

Evaluation criteria, critical behaviors, or performance criteria are somewhat similar to patient-centered objectives or educational objectives that nurses develop for unit-based in-service education and CE programs. This latter type of objective will be discussed in Chapters 7 and 14, respectively.

Some educators advocate that competencies should reflect the three domains of learning described by Bloom, Englehart, and Furst (1956) that are used in developing educational objectives: cognitive, psychomotor, and affective (Exstrom, 2001). These domains were applied to the development of competencies more than 15 years ago (del Bueno et al., 1987). Other educators claim that competencies should not be based on these separate domains but rather should be integrated (Alspach, 1996). More information about these three domains of learning will be discussed later in Chapter 7.

Evaluation criteria (critical behaviors) differ from objectives in several ways (Alspach, 1996) and should not be replaced with objectives. For example, critical behaviors focus on the orientee's behavior rather than the orientee's knowledge of the behavior, much like objectives do (Abruzzese, 1996; Alspach). Second, critical behaviors are evaluated in clinical settings by preceptors who often use a performance checklist as an assessment tool. Conversely, objectives often are assessed in a classroom setting by educators using a written examination (Alspach). Third, critical behaviors relate directly to the performance expectations contained in the orientee's job description, unlike objectives, which may or may not refer to a specific role (Alspach).

Assessing Competencies

After developing your competencies, determine a way to assess these behaviors in orientees. Because the purpose of competency assessment is to determine if orientees can perform their assigned jobs (Alspach, 1996), you will need to develop assessment tools that will help you evaluate this.

Assessment Tools

As mentioned earlier in this chapter, competencies generally focus on what the orientee does rather than on what the orientee knows (Alspach, 1996). Therefore, competencies should focus on the behaviors (actions) demonstrated by the orientees rather than on the knowledge that the orientee possesses. This latter form of competencies should be kept to a minimum in a CBO (Alspach).

Written Examinations: Although written examinations may be used in a classroom setting to assess competencies that are cognitive (knowledge-based) in nature (Exstrom, 2001), some educators do not choose tests as a preferred assessment tool in a CBO (Alspach, 1996). Alspach also advised that if written examinations are needed to assess particular competencies, they should not comprise a major portion of the orientee's assessment.

Oermann, Truesdell, and Ziolkowski (2000) described the benefits of using context-dependent test items to evaluate critical thinking in nurses. These authors suggested their use in competency testing, for orientation, and by preceptors for guiding learners in a formative way.

Checklists: Because most competencies focus on specific behaviors that the orientee must demonstrate, performance checklists are the preferred assessment tools to evaluate the achievement of competencies (Alspach, 1996). These checklists may be referred to by different names, depending on the healthcare organization. Preceptors use checklists to assess the orientees' behaviors as they provide direct patient care on the clinical unit or as they demonstrate behaviors in a setting or situation that simulates the clinical unit (Alspach).

Jones, Cason, and Mancini (2002) supported the value of using simulated conditions compared with actual patient care situations to assess competencies in a recent study. Evaluation of 35 sets of observations related to both knowledge and skill performance in 368 nurses demonstrated that these two approaches were equally valid strategies to assess nurses' competence.

For example, a preceptor can observe an orientee performing a dressing change on a real patient or assess the orientee's performance of this skill on a mannequin in a nursing skills laboratory. Orientees also could demonstrate their CPR skills on a mannequin rather than in the clinical unit using a real patient.

The clinical setting is the preferred setting for assessing competencies because it best reflects the orientee's ability to function appropriately in the clinical setting (Alspach, 1996). Clinical simulations will be discussed further in Chapter 7.

Performance checklists may vary among organizations but usually are prepared using a table or grid format (Alspach, 1996). Each competency statement and associated set of evaluation criteria (critical behaviors or performance criteria) is listed with areas for the preceptor to document the orientee's attainment of each performance criteria and to identify the method used to assess the competency (e.g., documentation, observation, written examination). The preceptor's assessment needs to indicate whether the behavior was observed, but it should not reflect a rating or a grade (Alspach). The preceptor, as the evaluator, is required to provide his or her signature and date for each criterion that was observed. The signature indicates that the preceptor observed the orientee demonstrating the behavior appropriately on that date but does not guarantee the orientee's continuing competency.

Documenting Competency Assessments

Various reasons for assessing the competence of nursing staff were mentioned earlier in this chapter. The possible learners whose competencies need to be documented during orientation will be discussed later in this chapter.

Although the nurse manager is ultimately responsible for ensuring that the "competence of all nursing staff is assessed, maintained, demonstrated, and improved continually" (JCAHO, 2003, p. 247), other individuals, such as unit-based educators and preceptors who are experienced assessing competencies, may assist the manager in this overwhelming task. Hospitals need to determine the competency of their employees prior to and during their employment (Alspach, 1996; JCAHO).

Credentials and Qualifications

The nurse's credentials and qualifications usually are verified by the human resource department at the nurse's pre-employment interview or prior to orientation. These credentials and qualifications include evidence of the nurse's education and training, RN license, certifications, and references reflecting past experience (Alspach, 1996; JCAHO, 2003). These credentials and qualifications are based on the prerequisites identified in the nurse's job description.

Competency

Baseline During Orientation

Depending on the healthcare organization, new nurse employees usually attend various orientation sessions, such as organization-wide, departmental, specialty, and unit-based programs. During this orientation period, the organization assesses the nurses' competencies based on specific job duties. Some organizations ask orientees to complete a checklist indicating their familiarity with select skills. Because this checklist represents the perceptions of the orientee, these skills need to be validated before assuming competency.

In the event that an orientee does not successfully attain a competency, the preceptor should discuss the situation with the orientee, together identify specific learning needs, develop an action plan to remedy these deficiencies, and continue to support and guide the orientee. The orientee may need to review the competency though a learning activity or may need the preceptor's support to reduce anxiety experienced while demonstrating the competency. If the orientee does not successfully attain the expected competencies after repeated support, the orientee may face dismissal.

Annual Reviews

In addition to demonstrating competencies during the initial orientation period, the orientee may be required by the healthcare organization to demonstrate select competencies, such as during an annual review, on a regular basis (JCAHO, 2003). These reviews frequently are scheduled during the time of the employee's annual performance appraisal and are associated with it. If the nurse does not perform satisfactorily during this annual review, then an action plan may be developed to assist the nurse in strengthening any deficiencies. Although these annual competencies are based on the nurse's job description, they may change each year based on unit priorities, such as the introduction of new equipment or new findings from incident and quality assurance reports.

After orientation, staff educators help nurses continue to acquire, maintain, and increase their competencies through staff development activities, such as in-service education and CE programs (ANA, 2000). Both in-service education and CE programs will be discussed later in Chapters 7 and 14, respectively. Nurses also can accomplish this through CE programs outside the realm of their employer and through academic education, such as attending formal programs sponsored by schools of nursing. Nurses also can obtain certification in their clinical area through a professional organization that "validates a nurse's qualifications, knowledge, and practice" in a specific area of nursing (ANA, 2000, p. 23).

Aggregate Data on Competence Patterns and Trends

JCAHO requires hospitals to "regularly collect aggregate data on competence patterns and trends to identify and respond to staff's learning needs" (JCAHO, 2003, p. 244). This information may be collected by the nurse manager with the help of unit-based educators using a variety of sources, such as performance evaluations, performance improvement reports, staff surveys, needs assessments, and outcomes of staff development programs. These data should be analyzed, noting patterns and trends. Problem areas may be remedied by various staff development activities. These reports need to be communicated to the hospital's governing body at least yearly (JCAHO).

Record-Keeping System

Competency documents, regardless of their type, should be considered confidential and treated accordingly in the clinical setting. Competency documents need to be stored in a place that enables these records to be accessible by those who need them, such as the preceptor, unit-based educator, and nurse manager, and easily retrievable. Information about the orientee's qualifications may be kept in a confidential employee file in the human resource department, and the nurse manager on the clinical unit may maintain competency assessments. This allows the manager to access these records for performance evaluations.

Developing Creative Activities for Orientees to Demonstrate and Develop Competencies

Unit-based educators should develop a variety of learning activities that orientees and other nursing staff can use to demonstrate and develop their behaviors included in competencies (Abruzzese, 1996). These activities should be creative and cost-effective and encourage self-directed learning. Examples of learning activities include videotapes, review of print materials, self-learning packets, games, puzzles, posters, computer-assisted instruction, skill demonstrations, and bedside clinical teaching rounds (Guin, Counsell, & Briggs, 2002). Chapter 7 will review these in more detail.

For example, Clutter (2001) described the creation of an innovative competency day skills fair targeted at nurses in emergency trauma departments. This fair not only served as a strategy to validate and strengthen these nurses' continuing competencies but also provided a fun atmosphere for learning. These events were based on rotating themes, such as a MASH unit and a tropical island adventure, and offered games and prizes to participants as they demonstrated their competencies.

Jones, Jasperson, and Gusa (2000) used a game approach by developing the Cranial Nerve Wheel of Competencies to validate the cranial nerve knowledge competencies of neuroscience intensive care nurses. Nurses were given the option of attending a class on cranial nerves and reviewing written materials prior to being tested. Participants favored this innovative testing over a written examination yet found it appropriately challenging.

Fostering Adult Learning During Orientation

Adults, similar to orientees hired by your healthcare organization, view and comprehend the learning experience in different ways than children and adolescents (Knowles, 1990). These differences require unit-based educators to not only develop educational activities that will appeal to adult learners but also to develop teaching skills that will encourage successful learning.

Information about adult learning will help you assess the orientees' learning needs, clarify both your role and the role of the learners, and develop creative strategies to help learners attain their orientation and professional goals. This information also will help you encourage orientees to be self-directed learners, supporting their professional responsibility for continuing competence and lifelong learning.

Unit-based educators also have the responsibility for ensuring that nursing staff on the unit, particularly preceptors who work in partnership with orientees, understand how adults learn and how they can develop their skills as clinical teachers. The skills that preceptors develop can be used in a variety of staff development activities that involve adult learners, such as orientation, in-service education, and CE programs.

Hohler (2003) described a preceptor program in perioperative nursing that incorporated key principles of adult learning. This program provided an atmosphere that enabled new nurses to develop their competencies within an environment of trust and respect.

Andragogy and Adult Learning Principles

Andragogy is a term used by educators to describe the "art and science of helping adults learn" (Knowles, 1980, p. 43). Andragogy is based on a philosophy and set of learning assumptions that can help guide unit-based educators, preceptors, and others who are involved in teaching adult learners in the work setting. Educators need to apply these principles when planning and implementing orientation programs, as well as other staff development activities, such as in-service education and CE programs. Adult learning principles support the staff development educator's role of being a facilitator of learning rather than serving as an expert on a topic and providing information to learners. Each of these assumptions will be described in the following section of this chapter, with suggestions offered for unit-based educators and preceptors.

Need to Know

Adults need to know why they are expected to learn something before they will do it (Knowles, 1990). They also need to realize the benefits of learning and the negative consequences that may result from not learning.

Unit-based educators need to clarify the purposes of an orientation program to newly employed nurses and how they can benefit from participating in this program. Conversely, orientees need to understand the negative consequences of not participating in orientation. For example, explain how the orientation program is designed to help them develop key competencies to provide safe, quality care to patients as expected in their job descriptions. Discuss how orientation will help them become socialized to the work environment and give them a sense of belonging. Provide orientees with frequent and continuous feedback on their progress in meeting these goals through written and verbal evaluation and counseling (Hohler, 2003).

Self-Concept and Self-Directedness

Adults have a general need to be self-directed in their learning (Knowles, 1990). They know what they want to learn and when they need to learn it. Unit-based educators need to work collaboratively with orientees when assessing learning needs and developing a plan that includes experiences that build upon each individual's career goals. Provide orientees with a variety of learning options from which to choose. Encourage their responsibility for, and active participation in, the learning experience. Allow them to make choices, when available, and provide them with information about various options (Hohler, 2003). Avoid telling orientees what to do or imposing your own beliefs on them. This principle of adult learning is congruent with ANA's emphasis on self-directed lifelong learning and continuing competence in nurses (ANA, 2000).

Experience

Adults are a product of their life's experiences (Knowles, 1990). The experiences among adult learners are diverse and can influence their learning in either positive or negative ways. Adults recall their life experiences when learning; therefore, past experiences are a good resource for learning (Knowles, 1990).

Unit-based educators need to encourage orientees to share their experiences with others during the orientation program. Express your appreciation and respect for the various experiences shared by the learners. Educators need to consider these life experiences when assessing the orientee's learning needs for orientation and build on these experiences through experiential learning activities (Hohler, 2003), such as clinical practice or reality-based simulations. Encourage peer learning and group discussions of clinical issues.

Educators should help orientees perform a self-evaluation of their learning needs in light of their past experiences. These may include helping them realize possible biases that they may have developed over time and the consideration of new ideas and alternative ways of thinking (Knowles, 1990).

Readiness to Learn

Adults are ready to learn when a need exists for them to know this information, such as in assuming a new role in life (Knowles, 1990). Adults also may be ready to learn if they realize they lack knowledge in a specific area or if they need to perform something more effectively (Knowles, 1990).

Unit-based educators should time learning experiences for orientees with their readiness to learn (Knowles, 1990). Conducting a self-assessment at the beginning of orientation will help orientees realize any gaps in what they are expected to demonstrate. Review the job expectations with them to help them realize what competencies they need to learn for this role. Promote the orientees' readiness to learn by having them spend some time working alongside experienced nurses who are good role models. Develop a trusting relationship with orientees by providing them with learning information and experiences when they need it (Hohler, 2003). Allow orientees the opportunity to apply and demonstrate their skills as soon as they learn them.

Orientation to Learning

Adults' orientation to learning is task-centered, problem-centered, or life-centered rather than subject-centered (Knowles, 1990). Adults are motivated to learn something if they perceive that it will help them perform the task or deal with problems they may confront.

Unit-based educators need to provide orientees with experiential learning activities that they can readily apply and use to solve problems in clinical practice. This approach to learning is congruent with CBOs that focus on the learners' performance. Use realistic scenarios when assessing and developing competencies, and allow orientees to advance at their own pace as they progress toward meeting goals.

Motivation to Learn

Adults are motivated to learn something largely by internal factors, such as their desire for self-esteem, recognition, job satisfaction, improved quality of life, and increased self-confidence (Knowles, 1990). However, sometimes adults are motivated by external factors, such as obtaining a better job, getting promoted, or gaining a higher salary.

Unit-based educators can use these internal sources to motivate orientees to learn during orientation and other staff development activities. Educators also should demonstrate respect toward orientees and their expertise and knowledge and recognize their accomplishments. Educators need to create an atmosphere on the clinical unit that is conducive to learning and fosters mutual trust and respect (Hohler, 2003). Hohler also suggested encouraging staff to extend their hospitality to orientees through simple gestures that will give them a feeling of belonging to the unit, such as inviting them to join the staff for lunch and breaks.

Understanding the Unique Needs of Learners in Orientation Programs

As mentioned in Chapter 1, recent changes in healthcare organizations have affected the nature of the work performed by nurses and other healthcare workers. These changes, in turn, have influenced what nurses need to learn to deliver competent nursing care to patients and to assume leadership roles among a team of diverse healthcare workers. Staff development educators need to create innovative approaches that will help nursing staff meet their learning needs.

Chapter 1 explained the impact of organizational restructuring efforts on centralized staff development departments. Some staff development departments were totally eliminated, whereas other departments drastically reduced their centralized manpower of staff development educators. Nurses who provided direct patient care on clinical units often were asked to assume the role of staff development educator on the clinical unit and to carry out many of the education-related responsibilities previously performed by centralized staff development educators.

Unit-based educators frequently assume responsibility for orienting nursing staff. As a unit-based educator, you may be involved with particular aspects of the orientation process or be totally responsible for the orientation of new nursing staff to your clinical unit.

Nurses who assume the unit-based educator role may be responsible for meeting the learning needs of various healthcare professionals. You need to understand the background and learning needs of the workers you will encounter during the unit-based orientation process. Figure 4-2 lists the types of healthcare workers you may encounter during orientation. The learning needs of each group and suggestions for the unit-based educator are provided in the following section. Regardless of the orientee's background, your focus should be on helping him or her provide safe, quality care to patients.

Figure 4-2.
Possible
Employees
Encountered
in a Nursing
Orientation

- Newly hired nurses (graduate and experienced nurses)
- Nurses from other units (cross-trained or retrained)
- Nurses assuming a new role on a familiar unit (charge nurse or unit-based educator)
- Foreign-educated nurses
- Nursing faculty
- Nursing students
- Student externs
- Licensed practical and licensed vocational nurses
- Assistive personnel and nursing assistants
- Healthcare workers from disciplines other than nursing
- Volunteers on clinical units
- Forensic personnel on clinical units

Professional Nurses

Most healthcare organizations currently hire both inexperienced GNs and more experienced RNs. These nurses possess varied work histories, clinical competencies, educational preparation, and specialty interests. Regardless of their background, newly hired nurses need information to help them understand the healthcare organization and enable them to contribute to its goals (ANA, 2000). These new employees need to learn how to function safely and effectively in their assigned roles on the clinical unit (ANA, 2000). These roles may vary and can include such roles as direct patient care provider, educator, researcher, or manager.

Nurses with diverse backgrounds have unique learning needs that often pose challenges for the unit-based educator. Although these nurses have a set of common learning needs based on the fact that they are new employees within the same healthcare organization, each nurse has unique learning needs that should be addressed during the orientation program.

Newly Hired Graduate Nurses

Inexperienced nurses, such as GNs, have learning needs that differ from those of more experienced RNs. As mentioned earlier in this chapter, GNs need your guidance in making the transition from being a student nurse to assuming the professional nurse role. This process of role transition takes time and support from preceptors and other colleagues on the clinical unit. Being a professional nurse may be the first time GNs have provided patient care without the supervision of their nursing instructor or preceptor.

This experience may elicit mixed feelings among the new GNs. Although new graduates may find excitement in finally meeting their goal of being a professional nurse, they also may be anxious, afraid of failing, and overwhelmed by the reality of the work environment. Oermann and Garvin (2002) examined the stress experienced by 46 GNs during their initial employment as professional nurses. Analysis of data obtained from these nurses who completed a Clinical Stress Questionnaire revealed that these nurses experienced 20 different emotions during that time. In addition to these stressors, newly hired GNs who are unsuccessful in passing their NCLEX-RN during the orientation period also may experience emotional issues (Poorman, Mastorovich, & Webb, 2002). Unit-based educators and preceptors can play a significant role in helping GNs deal with these emotions and in mentoring these new orientees during orientation.

Godinez, Schweiger, Gruver, and Ryan (1999) also studied the role transition of 27 GNs during their first three weeks of orientation. Content analysis of weekly feedback sheets from these GNs and their preceptors was used to develop a model that represented the role transition process. This model contained five themes:

Real Nurse Work; Guidance; Transitional Processes; Institutional Context; and Interpersonal Dynamics. Role transition was understood to be a dynamic and interactive process that occurred between the preceptor and the GN. The preceptor's clinical mentoring influenced the GN's ability to progress during this transition. Interpersonal dynamics among the GN, preceptor, and other staff nurses on the clinical unit influenced the role transition process.

New graduates also may differ from more experienced nurses regarding their mastery of clinical skills. For example, some nurse managers in healthcare agencies may claim that GNs need assistance with improving their skills, such as organizing care for multiple patient assignments, setting priorities, and delegating tasks to other members of the healthcare team. Some GNs may need help perfecting their fundamental nursing skills and in gaining self-confidence in performing procedures (e.g., inserting an indwelling urinary catheter, providing discharge instructions, administering injections). GNs also may need help in mastering specialty skills, such as suctioning a tracheostomy tube or interpreting a patient's heart rhythm on an electrocardiogram (EKG) tracing.

Some GNs may have worked as nursing assistants (NAs) or externs while enrolled in their nursing program, mastered their fundamental nursing skills, and understand unit routines. Extern programs usually are offered during the summer months when students may not be enrolled in classes, whereas others may be scheduled year-round (Johnson, 2001). Students are paired with preceptors in the clinical units and have an opportunity to perform hands-on nursing skills. This experience not only helps students develop their nursing skills and self-confidence but also helps them realize the importance of lifelong learning and the value of mentoring others.

Newly Hired Experienced Nurses

Experienced nurses, on the other hand, also present challenges to unit-based educators. These RNs may require your help as they assume the role of a professional nurse in an unfamiliar healthcare setting. Depending on the quality of their prior professional experiences, these seasoned nurses are most likely proficient in basic nursing skills, unlike GNs, and may progress more rapidly through the orientation process. Instead, experienced nurses may need help on learning how to adjust to their new work environment and developing new competencies required on a specialty unit.

Employed, Experienced Nurses Assuming New Roles and Responsibilities

Chapter 1 described how healthcare structuring resulted in the reassignment of some experienced nurses and other healthcare workers to unfamiliar patient care units. Some nurses were reassigned to units similar to their previous clinical specialty, whereas others faced providing nursing care to patients on clinical units within an entirely different specialty.

Some experienced RNs need to be cross-trained to new but related patient care units (Miller, Flynn, & Umadac, 1998). In order to function safely and effectively on these units, nurses may need to develop additional clinical competencies specific to the units. A group of part-time nurses, often referred to as prn staff or casual pool staff, usually are assigned to various units throughout the healthcare organization based on staffing needs. Some organizations contract with private agencies that provide nurses to supplement an organization's staffing pool on a prn basis. These contracted (agency) nurses also need to be oriented to their roles and responsibilities on their assigned unit in order to function effectively.

Nurses who are retrained or cross-trained need time to adjust to their new role, work setting, and coworkers and to gain the knowledge and clinical skills that are vital on the specialty unit. For example, suppose a nurse experienced in caring for patients with ear, nose, and throat (ENT) conditions is asked to cross-train and function on a head and neck surgical unit within the same organization. Although the nurse may be proficient in caring for ENT patients, the nurse is unfamiliar with the core knowledge and competencies related to this new specialty. To function effectively in the same position but in a different setting, this nurse needs an orientation program to the head and neck unit that focuses on these competencies.

In another example, an experienced intensive care unit (ICU) nurse is reassigned to a medical-surgical unit. Although this nurse may be proficient in organizing and performing multiple tasks for one or two critically ill patients, this nurse may need assistance and time to adapt to providing nursing care to five or more patients who have a lower level of acuity than patients in the ICU.

Although nurses who are asked to provide nursing care to patients on a new unit need to be oriented to their unfamiliar setting, nurses who are familiar to the organization but change their roles and responsibilities also require an orientation to function effectively in that role (ANA, 2000). For example, think about a clinical staff nurse who accepts a nurse manager position within an organization. Even if this nurse is familiar with the organization or the clinical unit, the nurse may need to learn about the organization and unit from the perspective of this new position. Because the work of a staff nurse is quite different when compared to that of a nurse manager, so is the focus of the learning need. A nurse with several years of clinical experience may need assistance in mastering the management skills required of a nurse manager, whereas a staff nurse must focus on perfecting direct patient care skills.

Unit-based educators need to understand the emotions that experienced RNs who are cross-trained or retrained may feel. These nurses may experience fear of losing their jobs, regaining a new identity, or meeting new coworkers. You can be instrumental in helping these nurses become socialized to their new work environment and feeling valued within the organization.

Foreign-Educated Nurses

As mentioned in Chapter 1, the nursing shortage in the United States has forced some healthcare organizations to hire foreign-educated nurses and other healthcare workers (Purnell & Paulanka, 1998). This hiring practice poses some unique workforce problems for nurse managers and staff development educators in areas such as language and interpersonal communication, differences in gender roles, educational preparation as a nurse, and perspectives in heathcare practices (Purnell & Paulanka). Unit-based educators need to consider these potential barriers during the employee's orientation and help foreign-educated nurses to understand not only the healthcare organization in which they are employed but also American culture, its healthcare system, and its expectations of nurses (Amerson, 2002). Educators also need to help nursing staff strengthen their cultural competence within this diverse work environment.

Licensed Practical/Vocational Nurses, Assistive Personnel, and Nursing Assistants

Recent changes in healthcare reimbursement led many healthcare administrators to reexamine both the number and mix of healthcare workers who provide patient care. Some organizations changed their staffing patterns by increasing their pool of licensed practical and licensed vocational nurses (LPNs and LVNs), assistive personnel (AP), and NAs to assist with patient care. The multiple tasks often included among the responsibilities of AP are drawing blood, inserting urinary catheters, and performing EKGs. These procedures are often more than what is expected of NAs.

Unit-based educators need to understand potential issues they may face in working with NAs during the orientation program and provide them with proper assistance and guidance. Although individuals who are hired for NA positions are expected to have a high school diploma or an equivalent, they may possess various levels of literacy (Benjamin, 1997). These literacy issues, especially in reading and math skills, may hinder their performance in the NA role. Therefore, it is important that you explore the availability of appropriate resources in your organization that can support these individuals so they can develop these skills.

As a unit-based educator, you may be expected to develop a unit-based orientation program for LPNs, AP, or NAs who are newly hired or need to be cross-trained to your clinical unit. Consider several key points in planning your program.

First, understand the role expectations and responsibilities of LPNs, AP, and NAs by reviewing their job descriptions and any related policies and procedures in your organization. It is important to remember that although AP and NAs may be able to perform the various tasks assigned to them, they may not understand the reasoning behind why and when these tasks need to be performed (Benjamin, 1997). Nurses can minimize this problem by providing clear and simple explanations of medical terms and patient situations.

Second, realize the strength of the life experiences that these healthcare workers bring with them to their job when planning their orientation. Build upon these experiences in their orientation classes and clinical experiences.

Third, create a work environment in which LPNs, AP, and NAs feel valued for the services they perform for patients on the clinical unit and have a sense of the important role they play on the healthcare team. Create an environment in which they feel comfortable to discuss their learning needs with you and the staff, including ways to meet these learning needs.

Finally, develop an orientation program that is tailored to an appropriate educational level for specific learners so that they will be successful in developing the competencies they need to function effectively in their roles. Provide them with explanations of medical terms or the rationale behind why particular clinical decisions are made by nurses when a patient's condition changes. These healthcare workers need to function effectively as team members on the clinical unit.

Interdisciplinary Healthcare Workers

In addition to orienting staff nurses, LPNs, and AP, unit-based educators often have an opportunity to work with healthcare workers from disciplines other than nursing. These individuals include professionals such as physicians, physical therapists, social workers, respiratory therapists, and nutritionists. You may be responsible for orienting these individuals after they are hired or if they are reassigned to your clinical unit.

As with healthcare workers mentioned earlier in this chapter, it is important to develop a mutual understanding of the contributions that each discipline makes to patient outcomes. This experience is a unique opportunity to develop a collaborative relationship and understand each other's role in patient care from an interdisciplinary perspective. This approach also can help identify immediate learning needs that can be addressed during orientation or later through in-service education (see Chapter 7). Increases in patient acuity combined with shortened lengths of stay make this partnership essential in order to have a coordinated, effective, and efficient healthcare team.

Faculty and Students From Affiliating Schools of Nursing

In addition to orienting GNs and RNs employed by your organization, staff development educators also may be responsible for the continuing competency of other healthcare workers both within the agency and in the community (ANA, 2000). For example, many healthcare organizations have legal affiliations (contracts) with schools of nursing that allow their faculty and nursing students to use their settings for their clinical experiences. Some agencies, in fact, serve as clinical sites for several schools of nursing simultaneously, with each school assigned to a particular clinical unit on designated days and times.

Nursing Students in Academic Courses

Nursing students are assigned to clinical units based on the focus and clinical objectives of the courses in which they are enrolled. Each course usually has a clinical focus, such as acute care of adults or care of children, as well as specific course and clinical objectives that the student must attain by the completion of the course.

For example, students enrolled in an adult medical-surgical course might be assigned to a patient care unit that admits patients with these conditions. Students receive classroom instruction provided by faculty on the nursing care of these patients. They often receive clinical skills training in a clinical skills laboratory at the school of nursing. Students are supervised by faculty members who evaluate each student based on the clinical objectives. Each course has a required number of clinical hours that students need to complete, determined by academic credits. Clinical courses and credit hours often vary among schools of nursing.

Nursing Students in Extern Programs

Some nursing students participate in specially designed programs sponsored by healthcare agencies called extern programs (Johnson, 2001), described earlier in this chapter. These programs, usually offered to students during the summer months before their senior year of school, provide students with an opportunity to team with experienced staff nurses while perfecting their clinical skills. Students who function in these learning roles also are paid a stipend or salary.

Extern programs offer several advantages to both the student and healthcare organization sponsoring the program. First, the experiential nature of this learning experience helps nursing students develop their clinical competencies and socializes them to the work environment, easing their transition to the professional nursing role. They have an opportunity to work closely with experienced staff nurses who serve as preceptors and observe their professional behaviors, knowledge, and values. This experience can increase students' self-esteem and professional autonomy and strengthen their organizational management skills.

Healthcare organizations also reap benefits from this arrangement. The extern program is viewed as a recruitment strategy. Students who return to the organization as employees following graduation already are somewhat familiar with the organization and may require less orientation time. Weigh the costs of this program against the benefit of easing the shortage of specialty nurses.

Faculty

Unit-based educators in staff development often are involved in orienting faculty from various schools of nursing to their healthcare organization. Administrators of schools of nursing determine which course faculty members teach based on their educational preparation and clinical expertise. Faculty members who teach the clinical component of a nursing course may be employed either on a full-time (FT) or part-time (PT) basis. FT faculty, such as clinical staff in healthcare organizations, assume multiple roles, including teaching in the classroom setting, publishing, conducting research, presenting at conferences, and serving on various school, university, and professional committees. FT faculty members often participate in more than one clinical course during an academic year. PT faculty members usually are hired on a per semester basis to supervise students in the clinical setting. In addition, both FT and PT faculty often work per diem in a clinical setting in order to maintain their clinical competencies.

Although faculty members on the clinical unit often supervise nursing students, students enrolled in senior-level courses are frequently paired with experienced nurses in a special learning partnership called a preceptorship. In this arrangement, a staff nurse (preceptor) directly supervises the clinical learning of a student nurse, called a preceptee. Preceptor arrangements also are used with newly hired nurses during orientation. More information about preceptor programs will be discussed in Chapter 5.

Although faculty and students from schools of nursing are not employees when working within the context of an academic course, they still need to be oriented to the organization and the clinical unit to which they are assigned. Because their time at a clinical setting often lasts less than a semester, orientation programs targeted to these groups need to be provided in a concise, creative, and timely manner. In some organizations, faculties attend the orientation and are responsible for sharing this information with students.

Healthcare agencies usually identify a contact person who acts as a liaison between faculty at schools of nursing and the healthcare organization. This person, who may or may not be the unit-based educator, is responsible for communicating with faculty and arranging the clinical placements for students. The liaison, in conjunction with the unit-based educator and nurse manager, may schedule unit-based orientations and select qualified preceptors for these nursing students. Unit-based educators may or may not be asked to provide formal and informal feedback concerning the performance of graduates from a particular school of nursing as part of the school's program evaluation process.

As a unit-based educator working with faculty and students from various schools of nursing, you need to be familiar with each school of nursing's scheduled dates and times on the clinical units, faculty and students assigned to the units, clinical course objectives, and students' level of performance.

Confusion can result on the clinical unit when staff members assume that nursing students from various schools possess similar skills, clinical interests, and learning needs. Ask faculty to share course profiles and clinical expectations with nursing staff on the unit. Meet with faculty prior to the scheduled clinical rotation to clarify role expectations and to discuss learning needs of students. Ask faculty to post students' weekly clinical objectives on the assignment board on the unit so that staff can help them meet their learning needs. Meet with faculty before the start of the clinical experience and communicate regularly. Help faculty and students feel welcome on the clinical unit, and offer your services as a resource for them.

Volunteers

Other individuals, such as volunteers, also require orientation to function effectively in their role within the healthcare organization (JCAHO, 2003). Volunteers need to demonstrate competence in patient care skills that they are expected to perform, including safety and infection control procedures (JCAHO).

Forensic Personnel

Forensic personnel without clinical backgrounds (e.g., guards, correctional officers) also need to be oriented to their responsibilities in patient care settings (JCAHO, 2003). For example, these individuals need to understand appropriate ways to interact with patients, respond to unexpected clinical events, and follow appropriate communication lines with hospital staff. Forensic officers also need to understand the differences between "administrative and clinical seclusion and restraint" (JCAHO, p. 248).

Unit-based educators need to develop creative strategies that can help forensic personnel develop the knowledge and skills they need to function effectively in the healthcare setting. One healthcare organization developed a brochure to orient forensic personnel ("First Hand," 2002).

Gathering Information About Orientation Programs at Your Organization

Now that you, as a unit-based educator, have an idea about the possible learners with whom you may interface in your orientation program, gather additional information about the orientation program offered at both organizational and departmental levels before developing your unit-based orientation program. Clarify the process that new employees experience once they are hired and before they arrive on your unit. Contact appropriate representatives in your organization and arrange to attend these programs, or meet with them to discuss the purpose and specific content of these orientation programs.

Learning about the organization's orientation programs can benefit both you and the new nursing employees. Although this task may seem time-consuming, it can help you to clarify your unit-based orientation and coordinate your unit-based program with the organization-wide and nursing department orientations. Knowing the competencies that new employees have already attained before they arrive on your clinical unit will help you in focusing on unit-specific competencies.

Second, careful review of the entire orientation process will enable you to reduce duplication among these orientations, saving the organization both time and money. For example, new employees can complete the orientation in less time and assume their responsibilities in providing patient care.

Third, being familiar with other orientations also can assist you in identifying learning needs of nursing staff that can be addressed through other staff development activities, such as in-service education and CE programs. Conversely, you may realize the need for some topics, currently delivered through in-service education and CE programs, to be moved to the orientation phase. This advantage is especially helpful given the limited resources (nursing staff and time) available to you on the clinical unit.

Fourth, gaining an organizational perspective of the orientation programs can make you aware of resources that may be available to you at the unit-based level. These resources may include items such as guest speakers, audiovisual equipment, supplies, and assessment and evaluation documents.

Finally, reviewing the orientation process at your organization can help you develop professionally as a unit-based educator. For example, it gives you an opportunity to observe the teaching skills of various experts within your organization so that you can model these behaviors. It also provides you with the opportunity to network with other educators and offer your expertise in these orientation programs.

Organization-Wide Orientation Programs

The orientation process that new nursing employees experience may vary among healthcare organizations. Most organizations require all new employees to attend an organization-wide (institution-wide or hospital-wide) orientation program. All employees who are hired to work in various roles, positions, and departments within the organization attend this program.

The primary purpose of the organization-wide orientation program is to introduce all new employees to the organization's mission, philosophy, goals, and objectives. This orientation also includes a review of key policies, procedures, and rules and regulations that affect all employees, not just those who provide direct patient care services. Various topics that are mandated by the healthcare organization's accreditation and regulatory agencies are included in this orientation program (O'Shea & Smith, 2002). These topics usually include a review of the organization's fire, safety, infection control, and emergency procedures. Figure 4-3 lists examples of content areas that are commonly reviewed during an organization-wide orientation program.

The organization-wide orientation is usually the time when employers verify

- Welcome and introduction to organization-level personnel
- Mission, values, and vision statements of the organization
- Philosophy of the organization
- Goals and objectives
- Policies and procedures
- Rules and regulations
- Strategic plan of the organization
- Payroll compensation and benefits
- Tour of physical layout of organization
- Communication systems (e-mail, telephone, fax, newsletter, paging system)
- Fire and safety procedures (drug-free workplace, smoking policy, hazardous substances)
- Emergency disaster plan, emergency numbers, and procedures
- Employee accident and illness procedures
- Universal precautions
- Health promotion services
- System-wide expected behaviors (customer relations, communication skills, quality services)
- Diversity in the workplace

Figure 4-3. Content That May Be Included in an Organization-Wide Orientation Program

the credentials and job requirements of new employees. For nurses, this may include providing their display portion of their current RN license and other documents needed to complete their employee file, such as evidence of current immunizations and drug testing. This also may be the time when new employees obtain their photo identification badges and complete paperwork related to parking, payroll, and benefits.

The length of this organization-wide orientation program varies among agencies and may last one or more days. Representatives from the organization's human resource or training and development departments often coordinate it. Nursing staff development educators may participate in some aspect of the program.

For nurses, a nursing department orientation program developed by staff development educators usually follows this organization-wide orientation program. The department orientation might be followed by an additional orientation that often focuses on a specialty area, such as critical care, oncology, or transplantation. The orientation process then concludes at the unit-based level.

Figure 4-4 illustrates a process that a newly hired nurse may experience in an organization, beginning with an organization-wide orientation upon hire and concluding with a unit-based orientation program. Each of these orientations will be discussed in the remaining section of this chapter, with an emphasis on developing a unit-based orientation program.

Figure 4-4.
An Example of the Orientation Process of a Newly Hired Nurse

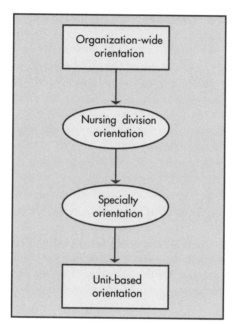

Nursing Department Orientation

Following the organization-wide orientation, new employees hired within the nursing department usually proceed to a general nursing orientation program sponsored by the centralized staff development department. Other new employees, such as social workers, housekeepers, and physical therapists, proceed to their respective departments or units for further orientation.

The nursing department orientation may include all nursing personnel together (RNs, GNs, LPNs, and AP) or may be provided separately to these subgroups. For example, the orientation for RNs and GNs may be separate from the programs provided for AP or NAs. In some organizations, these groups are combined for portions of the orientation in which they have common needs then continue in separate orientations designed specifically for their roles and responsibilities (Amerson, 2002). Combing these groups may save costs incurred with staff and time.

The nursing department orientation focuses on patient care activities and prepares nurses for their specific roles and responsibilities within the organization. It centers on the information that is needed by all nurses, regardless of their specialty, and reviews relevant policies and procedures related to patient care. Mandatory requirements that affect patient care are explained during this orientation, if not already covered in the organization-wide program. Figure 4-5 illustrates examples of content that may be included in a nursing department orientation.

The purpose of a nursing orientation program is to familiarize new nurses with the nursing department's philosophy, goals, and objectives and illustrate how these are congruent with those presented in the organization-wide orientation. Orientees are introduced to the structure and communication pathway of the nursing department and often have an opportunity to meet key leaders in the department.

This orientation program is often the time when nurses' general competencies may be assessed and validated, such as CPR, medication administration, and documentation. These competencies should be evaluated before the orientees begin the clinical portion of the orientation program (Abruzzese, 1996). Competencies specific to their clinical unit may reviewed later during the specialty and unit-based orientation programs.

Third, the nursing department orientation provides nurse orientees with an opportunity to socialize with other nurses hired to work on other clinical units and introduces them to how professional nursing is viewed by the organization. As mentioned previously, orientees have an opportunity to meet nurse leaders of the nursing department.

The nursing orientation may be the time when the employer verifies the nurses' credentials, if this not completed during the orientation at the organization level. This may include evidence of current RN license, CPR, and immunizations and other health requirements. The length of the nursing orientation may vary among organizations, lasting one day or longer.

• Welcome and introductions to key nursing department personnel • Mission statement of the nursing department • Philosophy of the nursing department • Goals and objectives • Departmental structure and communication lines • Tour of department and other areas of interest • Policies and procedures and rules and regulations • Strategic plan of the department (and fit with organization's plan) • Collaborative relationship with other departments • Review of job descriptions and performance standards • Performance appraisal system (evaluation process) • Nursing role in fire, safety, emergency, and disaster plans

• CPR training and verification and crash cart review • Medication administration • Charting and documentation • Confidentiality of patient and health information • Nutritional support • Promotions (clinical ladder) and transfers • Portfolio preparation • Infection control and isolation procedures • Patient's Bill of Rights • Advanced directives • Body mechanics and patient transfers • Ethical dilemmas • Restraint use • IV fluids and central lines • Blood product administration • Organ procurement • Oxygen therapy • Computer training

Figure 4-5.
Content That May Be Included in a Nursing Department Orientation

Specialty Orientations

Some healthcare organizations may require nurse orientees to attend a specialty orientation following the nursing department orientation, because nurses may be assigned to various specialty units that require different knowledge and skills to function safely and effectively. The purpose of specialty orientation programs is to prepare nurses with the competencies unique to their role in the clinical area to which they are assigned (e.g., oncology, critical care, dialysis, cardiac care, burn units).

For example, suppose a nurse was hired to work in a surgical ICU at your organization. That nurse would attend the scheduled organization-wide orientation program and then proceed to the nursing department orientation, followed by a critical care orientation and an arrhythmia course. The critical care orientation would include all nurses who were hired to work in any of the organization's six critical care units, and then the specific unit would be used to provide the nurse with clinical experience in this area.

Although specialty orientation programs differ in content and learning experiences, they often include classroom presentations and clinical experiences. Clinical experiences may be integrated with classes or scheduled after the orientee successfully completes the required course work.

As a unit-based educator for a surgical ICU, you may be involved in planning and implementing the critical care orientation program or coordinating the clinical portion of the orientation on your ICU unit. If you are responsible for presenting some of the classes, Chapter 7 will help you in developing a teaching plan and selecting teaching strategies. Chapter 10 will help you in developing a formal presentation.

Internships and Residency Programs

Some organizations offer internships or residency programs for new orientees. Intern programs often are designed for GNs and provide them with additional clinical experience under the direction of a preceptor, at which time they can develop their skills and work on the transition to the professional nursing role (Beecroft, Kunzman, & Krozek, 2001). These programs also are used as a recruitment and retention strategy for organizations. Both programs may focus on clinical specialty areas. Internships and residency programs often last several months, and GNs are paid for their services. The benefits of these programs need to be weighed against the costs associated with time and personnel, because the orientee and preceptor may not be contributing to the full staffing needs on the unit during this extended orientation period.

Beecroft et al. (2001) described the positive outcomes of a one-year RN internship pilot program in pediatrics. Nurses who participated in the internship over an eight-month period were assessed as being equal or stronger on all measures when compared with a control group of RNs who possessed up to two years of clinical experience. More than two-thirds of the interns remained in the organization following the pilot program.

Olson et al. (2001) described similar success with a 900-hour nursing student residency program that was developed through a collaborative effort among three educational programs and three hospitals. The nurses needed less orientation upon hire and stayed longer over a two-year period when compared with nurses who did not attend the program. The hospital also reported reduced costs associated with their recruitment of nurses.

DeSimone (1999) described a successful one-year nurse internship program that focused on developing both leadership and clinical skills in 10 GNs. This program was a collaborative effort among associate and baccalaureate degree faculty and nurse administrators at a community hospital and included portions of the hospital's orientation program. Nurse managers mentored the GNs, whereas faculty provided both theory and clinical experiences in leadership and clinical skills. Program evaluation revealed an increase in leadership competencies in both GNs and mentors.

Developing a Competency-Based Orientation Program for Your Clinical Unit

Now that you have a general understanding of the orientation programs that a nurse orientee needs to complete at your organization, focus on developing your unit-based CBO program. As mentioned earlier, clarify whether your unit-based orientation program is considered part of the nursing department or specialty orientations, or if it is a separate clinical experience that builds upon these orientations.

Conduct an Assessment of the Clinical Unit

Begin this process by gathering information about the learners and resources available on your clinical unit. Your assessment also should include the readiness of the staff on your unit to meet the learning needs of these orientees. This information will help you develop a detailed plan for your program. Each of these elements will be discussed in the following section.

Meet With the Nurse Manager

Begin your assessment by meeting with the nurse manager of the clinical unit and developing a good working relationship. The nurse manager, as administrator of the clinical unit, has the ultimate responsibility for ensuring that nursing staff provide safe, quality nursing care to patients on the unit (JCAHO, 2003). The nurse manager also has the authority to implement unit-based strategies and resources to make this happen.

Be sure that you have the understanding and support of the unit's nurse manager as it relates to your role as a unit-based educator. Develop a regular meeting schedule and communication system. Express your specific needs related to your role in the unit-based orientation program. Keep the manager informed of the orientees' progress toward program outcomes.

Assess the Learners

Talk with the staff development educator or nurse manager to obtain information about the number of orientees assigned to your unit. Also, obtain their names and credentials, including information about their past experience. If available, discover their particular strengths and areas that need improved. Review any documentation describing the orientees' performance to date.

Although you have a general idea of what their learning needs may be based on your past experience working with nurses who have attended orientation, gaining additional information about these particular learners can help you match them with preceptors and develop an orientation plan for each nurse.

Identify Outcomes Attained in Previous Orientations

If you are not familiar with the nursing and specialty orientations offered by your organization, then investigate these programs and the outcomes expected of orientees. If the specialty orientation includes the unit-based clinical experience, review the clinical competencies. If the specialty orientation does not include your unit-based experience, then you will need to develop these outcomes. Regardless of your approach, this information will help you build upon the orientees' prior experiences at your organization and plan appropriate clinical learning experiences before they arrive.

Clarify Designated Unit-Based Competencies

Clarify the unit-based competencies that you and the nursing staff have developed for the unit's CBO and make any needed changes. Strategies to develop these unit-specific competencies were discussed earlier in this chapter. Make sure that everyone on the unit is familiar with these competencies.

Select Qualified Preceptors

After you have information about the number of orientees and their skill levels, identify qualified staff from the unit who can serve as preceptors. Be sure that they have successfully completed a preceptor preparation program as described in Chapter 5 and are familiar with the CBO process. Discuss your selections with the nurse manager of your unit, and clarify any staffing or scheduling changes that need to be made for these preceptors while they are working with their orientees.

Consider matching less experienced preceptors with orientees who are GNs and teaming seasoned preceptors with more experienced orientees. More information about selecting and preparing nurses for the preceptor role is discussed in Chapter 5. Include these preceptors in planning the unit-based orientation, and keep them abreast of information regarding their orientees.

Confirm Resources Available on the Clinical Unit

In addition to the availability of qualified preceptors, determine other resources that are available to you for the unit-based orientation program. For example, check with the nurse manager or staff development educator to determine if the program is included in his or her budget, because you may incur expenses for duplication, supplies, equipment, typing services, and refreshments. Secure a private room that can be used by preceptors and orientees for clinical conferences and evaluation sessions. Assess the patient census on the unit to determine if it will be sufficient for appropriate type and number of clinical assignments. Inquire about access to a clinical skills laboratory to assist with competency testing, if needed.

In addition to these resources, consider inviting a team of staff nurses, such as experienced preceptors, to work with you in developing the unit-based orientation program. Successful outcomes were attained using a similar approach in planning a critical care nurse residency program (Williams, Sims, Burkhead, & Ward, 2002). A Preceptor Leadership Council, composed of preceptors and clinical educators, was created to develop, implement, and evaluate an orientation program. Outcomes revealed an increase in the nurses' satisfaction with the orientation program and a significant reduction in turnover rates in that area.

Assess the Learning Environment

Assess the environment on the unit, and determine if it is conducive to the learning of orientees. Discuss the orientation needs with staff, and assess their willingness to participate in the overall program. Ensure that nursing staff possess knowledge about the orientation process and are able to provide orientees with the proper guidance and direction. More information on ways to develop a learning environment will be discussed next in the planning section.

Assessing the learning environment is an important step, because interactions that occur between new orientees and nurses on the clinical unit during the orientation period can have a significant impact on the orientees' professional development and socialization. For example, Thomka (2001) studied the descriptions of 16 nurses who reflected on their past experiences as a new graduate during their first year of employment. These nurses reported various inconsistencies in the way they were assisted by other nurses related to learning about patient care.

Clarify the Outcomes of the Unit-Based Orientation Program

After carefully reviewing your assessment data, analyze it to determine the specific learning needs of the orientees assigned to your clinical unit. Clarify these learning needs with appropriate individuals at your organization, including the nurse manager of your unit and the staff development educator. If you have an opportunity to meet with orientees before they arrive on the unit, assist preceptors in reviewing these learning needs with them and obtain their input. If you do not have access to the orientees at this point, include this step when orientees begin the unit-based program.

Clarify the Purpose of the Unit-Based Competency-Based Orientation Program

After clarifying the orientees' learning needs, clarify the general purposes of the unit-based orientation program. As discussed earlier in this chapter, orientation programs introduce orientees to the healthcare organization and assist with their socialization (ANA, 2000). Orientations, similar to all staff development activities, focus on assessing the orientees' competencies and developing them (ANA, 2000). Therefore, your unit-based orientation program should include these purposes within the context of the clinical unit.

Develop Unit-Based Competencies for the Orientation Program

After identifying the purpose of your unit-based program, clarify that the unit-specific competencies are congruent with the purpose and principles of adult learning (ANA, 2000) that were discussed earlier in this chapter. Make sure that these competencies are realistic so that orientees will be able to attain these outcomes within a reasonable time frame. Discuss these competencies with the nurse manager, staff development educator, and preceptors for your unit, and gain their input.

Unit-based competencies also should be congruent with those included in the specialty and nursing department orientations and should build upon them. Because clinical competencies may be integrated within the competencies of the specialty orientation, check with appropriate individuals within your organization to determine this. As mentioned earlier in this chapter, your unit-based orientation efforts may be considered an integral part of the specialty orientation rather than as a separate entity.

Plan the Unit-Based Orientation

After you have determined the purpose and competencies for your unit-based orientation program, develop a detailed plan to implement it. Although planning takes time and energy, it will help you determine the work that needs to be completed before the orientees arrive on your clinical unit and will indicate who is responsible for completing these tasks. Planning also helps you determine the relative time frame for the orientation, clarify outcomes, identify appropriate clinical assignments, and determine the evaluation plan. Your plan also can help orientees successfully attain program outcomes and, ultimately, become productive members of the nursing staff on the clinical unit.

Recognize the Importance of Planning and Team Building

To understand the importance of developing a plan before you implement your unit-based orientation program, examine this analogy of planning a football game with you as the coach or quarterback. When planning for a football game, the ultimate goal for the team is to score points and win the game. The team starts with planning and discussing various plays or strategies that will help it win the game. Team members know their role in the game and what to do. Once the game is in play, all team members work together to implement the plan, attempting to score in the midst of activity, unexpected confusion, and time constraints.

During its plays, the team uses its resources wisely and makes the best use of the time. Each team player makes a significant contribution to the game, takes ownership of the game, and feels valued as a member of the football team. After the game, the coach and team debrief. They discuss what they did well during the game and consider upon which plays they could have improved. Finally, they start this process over again, planning for the next game. Without this careful planning, they may not have scored points and attained their goal of winning.

The planning process that you need to use in developing your unit-based orientation program is quite similar to the football example mentioned above. The goals of the program are to develop the clinical competencies of orientees, help them become socialized, and facilitate their role transition. Clinical nurses are expected to deliver safe, quality care to patients on your unit. The nursing staff on your unit, with you as the coach or quarterback, comprises the team that is responsible for helping orientees attain the outcomes of the orientation. The orientation team develops a plan to accomplish these goals, with each team member being aware of his or her roles and responsibilities.

When the orientee arrives on the clinical unit, you and the team members work together with the orientee to help the orientee reach these goals. This occurs in the midst of an often busy and chaotic clinical unit. The team uses its resources wisely, recruiting experienced nurses to serve as preceptors. The team makes good use of the time allotted for the orientation.

After orientees successfully complete the unit-based orientation program, they are able to provide competent nursing care to patients on the unit. These new employees feel they are valued members of the clinical unit and are more at ease in their role as a professional nurse. The unit staff debriefs, reviewing all aspects of the unit-based orientation program. The staff, along with you and the preceptors, feel that they have made a significant contribution to the orientees' learning and to patient care. They discuss ways to improve upon the orientation, and start planning for the next one. The unit-based orientation was successful because of your careful planning.

Develop a Plan Based on Each Orientee's Learning Needs and Goals

Use the unit-specific competencies to help you develop a plan for the nurses attending the unit-based orientation. Start with a teaching plan, like the one described in Chapter 7 for in-service education programs. Figure 4-6 lists examples of content that may be included in an orientation program.

Next, outline any content and teaching strategies that will help the orientee attain the expected outcomes. After determining whether your unit-based orientation stands alone from the specialty orientation, determine a need for including didactic content in addition to clinical assignments.

Be sure to include various active learning exercises that are congruent with each competency. Chapter 7 describes some examples of learning activities. Provide the orientees with a variety of learning options that they can complete at their own pace. Use learning activities, such as clinical simulations described earlier in this chapter, that resemble the actual clinical environment.

Preceptors need to observe the orientees as they demonstrate these competencies. As mentioned earlier, this assessment can be conducted by methods such as performance checklists or written examinations (Alspach, 1996).

Familiarize Unit Staff to Adult Learning Principles

Before the orientees arrive on the clinical unit, help the nursing staff develop an understanding of how adults learn, and provide them with practical strategies to use when interacting with the orientees. Although preceptors already should have an understanding of these principles as part of their preceptor preparation program described in

- Philosophy
- Goals and objectives
- Policies and procedures and rules and regulations
- Strategic plan (and fit with nursing department plan)
- Organizational structure of the unit personnel
- Tour of physical plan of the unit
- Patient documentation system
- Time sheets, schedule, requests for vacations, call-off procedures, etc.
- Breaks and meals, designated eating areas
- Patient assignments
- Use of communication systems
- Location of emergency numbers and equipment
- Ordering equipment and supplies
- Unit educational plan
- Committee structure and assignments
- Review of job description and performance appraisal process at unit level

Figure 4-6. Content That May Be Included in a Unit-Based Orientation Program

Chapter 5, it is important that all staff who will be interacting with the orientees understand how adults learn. Consider conducting a unit-based in-service for staff on adult learning principles, or develop a packet of information that they can review at their own pace.

When preparing staff for the orientation program, ask them to reflect on the emotions they experienced when they were new to the clinical unit. Explore staff behaviors that were most effective in making them feel welcomed. Ask nursing staff to recall specific teaching strategies and learning activities that were most effective in helping them develop their clinical competencies.

Create a Unit-Based Orientation Schedule With Target Dates

After developing your plan, create a schedule for the unit-based orientation and assign target dates when orientees are expected to complete particular competencies. Although there are usually no pre-established end dates for CBOs, target dates may keep orientees on track (Abruzzese, 1996). Orientees usually progress through a unit-based orientation at their own rate as they validate their competencies. It is likely that some orientees, such as experienced RNs, may complete the unit-based orientation before inexperienced GNs.

When developing a schedule for the unit-based program, include the day of the week, date, times, the learning activity, its location, and the guest speaker or person responsible to oversee this activity. Also include the names of the orientees and their respective preceptors.

Distribute the schedule to appropriate individuals in your organization, such as the nurse manager, staff development educator, orientees, and preceptors. Post a schedule on the unit's bulletin board so that all staff can view it. Save a copy of the schedule for your education files along with your plan.

Consider inviting staff from the clinical unit to serve as guest speakers for the orientation program, if this is part of your unit-based plan. Invite members of the interdisciplinary team, including the unit's social worker, physical therapist, and nutritionist, to participate.

Develop an Evaluation Plan for the Program

Develop an evaluation plan for the unit-based orientation program before the orientees arrive on the unit. This plan should include key individuals involved in the unit-based program, such as the orientees, preceptors, you as the unit-based educator, the nurse manager, and others, as appropriate. This plan should consider both formative and summative evaluations.

Formative Evaluation

Formative evaluation occurs on an ongoing basis during the unit-based orientation and provides learners with timely feedback regarding their progress toward program outcomes (Gaberson & Oermann, 1998). It also enables orientees to seek learning experiences that will strengthen their competencies. Formative evaluation helps to determine the orientees' learning needs and does not determine whether the orientee successfully completed the orientation program.

Preceptors can provide formative evaluation to orientees in a variety of ways. Because preceptors observe orientees as they provide direct patient care and understand the behaviors expected of orientees during their clinical experience, they are in a prime position to evaluate the orientees' performance. Preceptors should provide orientees with timely verbal and written feedback about their clinical performance and work closely with orientees to develop strategies to improve their performance.

A variety of methods can be used to evaluate the orientee's performance during the unit-based orientation program. First, preceptors can document the orientee's performance through daily, written anecdotes. Anecdotes are narrative descriptions of an orientee's performance, based on the preceptor's observations (Gaberson & Oermann, 1998). Anecdotes may or may not include the preceptor's interpretation of the observation (Gaberson & Oermann). These observations should be discussed privately with the orientees, providing them with immediate feedback about their behavior and an opportunity to clarify misconceptions. Together, the preceptor and orientee can develop a personal plan to strengthen any deficiencies.

Second, preceptors should assess and validate the orientee's performance related to unit-specific competencies. As mentioned earlier in this chapter, clinical competencies often are evaluated using performance checklists. These checklists include key competency statements and evaluation criteria. Figure 4-7 is an example of a competency validation tool that was developed for nurses employed on a critical care unit. The tool lists the competency, along with criteria that indicate successful completion of the competency. The method of validation used (documentation, observation, or testing) and selection criteria (high-risk, problem prone, or essential) are recorded. The preceptor indicates gender and age-specific information (neonate, pediatric, adolescent, adult, geriatric) and provides an opportunity for the preceptor to comment on the orientee's performance. Both the orientee and preceptor, as the validator, sign and date each competency. The nurse manager and orientee sign and date the checklist after it is completed.

Preceptors also may summarize the orientee's overall progress during the orientation program on a weekly basis, using the tool depicted in Figure 4-8. This tool includes a summary of the orientee's experiences, strengths, and areas for improvement. Daily anecdotes and the competency validation tool can be used to develop this evaluation. Specific goals for the orientee are developed based on these data. Both the orientee and the preceptor have an opportunity to provide comments. The orientee, preceptor, nurse manager, and educator sign this weekly evaluation.

Third, some organizations may include additional forms to document the progress of the orientee during orientation. Figure 4-9 is an example of a progress conference form in which the preceptor summarizes the orientee's accomplishments to date. The preceptor and orientee identify specific goals based on these accomplishments and provide comments, as needed. This evaluation may be used near the end of the orientation period, once the orientee has successfully completed the program, or at specific intervals, in the event that an orientee is not performing as expected. The nurse manager and educator may be present during this evaluation.

Summative Evaluation

In addition to formative evaluation, conduct a summative evaluation at the conclusion of the unit-based orientation to determine if the orientees have attained the expected competencies and if the program outcomes have been achieved (Oermann & Gaberson, 1998). The summative evaluation should include input

Figure 4-7.
Sample Employee
Competency Verifi-
cation Document

(Continued on
next page)

SUBURBAN GENERAL HOSPITAL
West Penn Allegheny Health System

Employee Competency Verification Document
Fiscal Year 2002

X Annual Evaluation
Initial Competency
Must be completed within 6 months

Name: _____   Employee Number: _____

Department: Critical Care Area   **Job Title:** Registered Nurse

Selection Criteria
HR = High Risk   PP = Problem Prone   ESS = Essential

Competency	Method of Validation	Selection Criteria	Successful Completion of Competency
1.) Meets all written and behavioral performance criteria for initiation for standing orders.	Documentation	HR	1. Successful completion of standing orders competency test.
	X Observation	PP	2. States appropriate interventions for given arrhythmias.
	X Test (Cognitive) Record Score	X ESS	

Age Category	Patient Age	Gender (M/F)	Anecdote	Validation Signature/Date
Neonate (birth - 28 days)				
Pediatric (29 days - 11 years)				
Adolescent (12 years - 18 years)				
Adult (19 years - 64 years)				
Geriatric (65 years +)				
Competency is not age related				

Figure 4-7.
Sample Employee Competency Verification Document
(*Continued*)

Criteria Selection
HR = High Risk
PP = Problem Prone
ESS = Essential

Competency	Method of Validation	Selection Criteria	Successful Completion of Competency
2.) Demonstrates skills necessary for safe use of a Defibrillator/Monitor for defibrillation, cardioversion, and external pacing.	Documentation	HR	1. Appropriately identifies situations in which defibrillation, cardioversion, or external pacing is indicated.
	X Observation	PP	2. Assembles necessary equipment.
	Test (Cognitive) Record Score	X ESS	3. Performs procedure correctly.

Age Category	Patient Age	Gender (M/F)	Anecdote	Validation Signature/Date
Neonate (birth - 28 days)				
Pediatric (29 days - 11 years)				
Adolescent (12 years - 18 years)				
Adult (19 years - 64 years)				
Geriatric (65 years +)				
Competency is not age related				

(Continued on next page)

Figure 4-7.
Sample Employee
Competency Verifi-
cation Document
(*Continued*)

Criteria Selection
HR = High Risk
PP = Problem Prone
ESS = Essential

Competency	Method of Validation	Selection Criteria	Successful Completion of Competency
3.) Meets all written and behavioral performance criteria for detection of arrhythmias.	Documentation X Observation X Test (Cognitive) Record Score	X HR PP X ESS	1. Demonstrates ability to correctly identify normal EKG pattern and arrhythmias. 2. Demonstrates ability to accurately measure PR intervals, QRS duration, QT intervals, and heart rate. 3. Documents rhythm strip correctly.

Age Category	Patient Age	Gender (M/F)	Anecdote	Validation Signature/Date
Neonate (birth - 28 days)				
Pediatric (29 days - 11 years)				
Adolescent (12 years - 18 years)				
Adult (19 years - 64 years)				
Geriatric (65 years +)				
Competency is not age related				

(Continued on next page)

Figure 4-7.
Sample Employee Competency Verification Document
(*Continued*)

Criteria Selection
HR = High Risk
PP = Problem Prone
ESS = Essential

Competency	Method of Validation	Selection Criteria	Successful Completion of Competency

4.) Demonstrates the skills necessary to operate the Microject Epidural pump.	Documentation	HR	1. Assembles equipment.
			2. Properly inserts tubing into epidural pump.
			3. Utilizes Microject Pump.
			  a. Programs pump to infuse correct medication dosage.
			  b. Changes dose infusing correctly.
			  c. Gives bolus dose via pump.
			  d. Discontinues infusion properly.

	X Observation	PP	
	Test (Cognitive) Record Score	X ESS	

Age Category	Patient Age	Gender (M/F)	Anecdote	Validation Signature/Date
Neonate (birth - 28 days)				
Pediatric (29 days - 11 years)				
Adolescent (12 years - 18 years)				
Adult (19 years - 64 years)				
Geriatric (65 years +)				
Competency is not age related				

(Continued on next page)

Figure 4-7.
Sample Employee
Competency Verifi-
cation Document
(Continued)

Note. Figure courtesy
of Suburban General
Hospital, West Penn
Allegheny Health Sys-
tem, Pittsburgh, PA.
Used with permission.

Criteria Selection
HR = High Risk
PP = Problem Prone
ESS = Essential

Competency	Method of Validation	Selection Criteria	Successful Completion of Competency
5.) Demonstrates skills necessary to work with a Swan-Ganz catheter.	Documentation	HR	1. Successfully completes Swan-Ganz migration test.
	X Observation	PP	2. Identifies indications for Swan-Ganz catheter.
			3. Accurately identifies waveforms.
	X Test (Cognitive) Record Score	X ESS	4. Correctly inflates balloon to obtain a wedge.
			5. States procedure if balloon is in wedge postion.

Age Category	Patient Age	Gender (M/F)	Anecdote	Validation Signature/Date
Neonate (birth - 28 days)				
Pediatric (29 days - 11 years)				
Adolescent (12 years - 18 years)				
Adult (19 years - 64 years)				
Geriatric (65 years +)				
Competency is not age related				

Employee Signature _____ Date _____

Manager Signature _____ Date _____

Name: _____

Date: _____

Week number: _____

SUBURBAN GENERAL HOSPITAL
Weekly Orientation Evaluation

Experiences:

Strengths:

Areas for improvement:

Goals:

Comments (Orientee):

Comments (Preceptor):

Preceptor's signature: _____

Orientee's signature: _____

Nurse manager: _____

Nurse educator: _____

Figure 4-8.
Sample Weekly Orientation Evaluation Document

Note. Figure courtesy of Suburban General Hospital, West Penn Allegheny Health System, Pittsburgh, PA. Used with permission.

Figure 4-9.
Sample Compe-
tency-Based
Orientation
Progress
Conference
Document

Note. Figure courtesy
of Suburban General
Hospital, West Penn
Allegheny Health Sys-
tem, Pittsburgh, PA.
Used with permission.

Name: _____

Date: _____

Week number: _____

SUBURBAN GENERAL HOSPITAL
CRITICAL CARE AREA
Competency-Based Orientation
Progress Conference Form

Summary of accomplishments:

Goals:

Comments:

Preceptor's signature: _____

Orientee's signature: _____

Nurse manager: _____

Nurse educator: _____

from all individuals who actively participated in the orientation program, including the orientees, their preceptors, you as the unit-based educator, and the nurse manager.

Table 4-1 illustrates the possible perspectives that you can obtain for this evaluation. The grid lists all the individuals mentioned previously across the top axis. The vertical axis indicates the various perspectives you may obtain. For example, you may wish to obtain the orientees' evaluations of themselves in a self-evaluation, as well as their feedback on the effectiveness of the preceptor, you as the unit-based educator, and the nurse manager. Repeat this process with the remaining individuals. The completed competency validation form mentioned previously in Figure 4-7 can serve as evidence of the orientee's performance related to unit-specific competencies.

In addition, obtain feedback from all individuals on the orientation program. This evaluation should include the orientees' feedback on the degree to which the program enabled them to attain their competencies and their overall satisfaction with the program. Ask participants for their ideas for future orientations. Figure 4-10 is an example of an orientation evaluation tool used by a healthcare organization that addresses many of these perspectives.

Establish a Documentation and Record-Keeping System

Determine the documents that you will need to maintain as part of the unit-based orientation program, along with a system to maintain these records. Start by meeting with the staff development educator responsible for the specialty orientation and the nurse manager to help you identify these items. Regardless of the system you choose, be sure that it offers privacy and allows records to be easily retrieved and accessed.

You will need to maintain certain documents related to the unit-based program. For example, each orientee's competency validation form should be maintained. Some organizations prefer to keep these forms in the nurse manager's office on the clinical unit, whereas others prefer that these files be kept in the orientee's personnel file located in the human resource department. Copies of the unit-based plan, schedules, and completed evaluations also should be maintained, most often in the staff development education files.

Determine Expenses

With careful planning, you should be able to determine the costs you anticipate incurring for the unit-based orientation program. Talk with the nurse man-

Table 4-1. Grid for Determining Unit-Based Orientation Program Evaluation				
	Orientee	**Preceptor**	**Unit-Based Educator**	**Nurse Manager**
Orientee	Self-evaluation	X	X	X
Preceptor	X	Self-evaluation	X	X
Unit-Based Educator	X	X	Self-evaluation	X
Nurse Manager	X	X	X	Self-evaluation

Figure 4-10.
Sample
Competency
Orientation
Evaluation
Document

SUBURBAN GENERAL HOSPITAL
CRITICAL CARE AREA
COMPETENCY ORIENTATION EVALUATION

Name: _____ Date: _____

Length of orientation: _____

1. Please rate how valuable the orientation program was in helping you to:
   Scale:
   4 = Very Valuable
   3 = Somewhat Valuable
   2 = Little Value
   1 = No Value

a. Become familiar with the organization and philosophy of the Critical Care Area and Suburban General Hospital	4	3	2	1
b. Become oriented to hospital policies and procedures and standards.	4	3	2	1
c. Develop competency in performing technical skills frequently done on your unit.	4	3	2	1
d. Develop organizational skills necessary for the delivery of patient care.	4	3	2	1
e. Utilize and communicate with other members of the healthcare team effectively.	4	3	2	1
f. Develop confidence in your ability to function as a professional nurse in the critical care setting.	4	3	2	1

2. Describe the support and direction received from the following and include any comments that may be helpful for program improvement.
   a. Preceptor:
   b. Charge nurse:
   c. Nurse manager:
   d. Clinical educator:
   e. Peers:

3. Please comment on the following areas concerning your preceptor.
   a. Providing instruction of technical skills:
   b. Providing discussions of patient pathophysiology, treatment modalities, and potential problems:
   c. Seeking out learning opportunities:
   d. Meeting your clinical needs:
   e. Presenting weekly performance evaluations:

(Continued on next page)

4. Please comment on the following educational programs.

   a. Basic arrhythmia course: _____

   b. Critical care course: _____

   c. Competency workshop day: _____

   d. IV therapy day:

5. Were your previous experiences and your competency assessment taken into account in the planning of your orientation? If not, please elaborate.

6. Please comment on the competency orientation book, program description, evaluation checklists, study guides, etc.

7. Were the expectations for your evaluation clearly stated? If not, please elaborate.

8. Did you receive frequent and timely feedback on your performance?

9. Were the Progress Evaluation Conferences beneficial?

10. Were educational resources available to assist with your development?

11. Rate your overall orientation on a scale of 1 to 10.

12. List any suggestions for improving the orientation experience in the critical care area.

13. Please write any additional comments.

Figure 4-10.
Sample Competency Orientation Evaluation Document *(Continued)*

Note. Figure courtesy of Suburban General Hospital, West Penn Allegheny Health System, Pittsburgh, PA. Used with permission.

ager and the staff development educator to clarify this procedure. It is important to plan a program that is cost-effective.

Implement the Unit-Based Orientation Program

Careful planning for your unit-based orientation program will help you get organized and keep you on track once the orientees arrive on the clinical unit. Spend this time welcoming the orientees to the clinical unit, orienting them to the CBO and his or her expectations, and pairing them with their preceptors. Preceptors can work with their respective orientees in developing individualized plans for meeting their learning needs.

Create an Environment Conducive to Learning on the Clinical Unit

Clinical units often can be very stressful, chaotic, and busy places, not only for patients but also for nursing staff who work on the unit. Attempt to transform the clinical unit into a place that is conducive to learning and a setting in which orientees feel comfortable and welcomed. This is especially important given the shortage of nurses and the personal and financial investment an organization makes during orientation. Although there are some elements in the work environment you may not be able to change, focus your energy on the things that you can positively influence.

Start by coordinating a welcoming reception on the unit when the orientees arrive. This will give them an opportunity to meet their preceptor and nurse manager, if they did not have this opportunity previously, and to interact with the nursing staff on the unit. Invite other individuals with whom they may interact on the unit, such as physicians, social workers, and therapists. Consider taking photographs of this event, with permission, and post them on the unit's bulletin board so that all nursing staff can feel involved in the program.

Provide orientees with an opportunity to share their past experiences and professional goals. Have preceptors build upon these experiences in developing individualized learning options for each of their orientees.

Introduce the Orientees to the Unit-Based Competency Orientation Program and Preceptors

Introduce the orientees to the goals of the unit-based CBO program and review the competencies they are expected to demonstrate and how they can successfully progress through the program. Clarify their specific roles and responsibilities and those of the preceptors, yourself as the unit-based educator, and the nurse manager. Inform them of the various learning options that are available to them. Explain the program's evaluation plan that was designed to provide orientees with ongoing feedback about their progress. Orient the new nurses to the physical layout of the unit, so they can locate supplies and equipment they need as they provide patient care.

Select Meaningful Clinical Assignments

Assist preceptors in designing learning experiences so that orientees can demonstrate or develop the unit-specific expected competencies. These competencies may be completed while providing patient care under the supervision of the preceptor or through available learning options. Assist preceptors in selecting appropriate patient care assignments, if needed. If the orientees require additional information and practice to attain these competencies, provide them with learning opportunities. Ensure that the preceptors' evaluation of the orientees' performance is objective and is consistent among all learners.

Provide Support and Guidance

Although it is vital that the orientees receive ongoing support and guidance from their preceptors during the orientation program, include this support for preceptors, as well. Consider scheduling private meetings with preceptors on a regular basis to determine their learning needs and to provide them with support and direction in their role. Be available to preceptors on a daily basis in the event that problems arise. Provide preceptors with feedback about their performance and develop ways to strengthen their behaviors.

Encourage preceptors to allow their orientees to progress through the orientation program at their own pace while keeping them on target. Remind preceptors that GNs may require more support than more experienced nurses. Alert them to nonverbal cues that may indicate that an orientee may be experiencing difficulties, in the event they do not verbalize this.

Document the Progress of the Orientees

Assist the preceptors as they document the progress of the orientees' performance during the orientation program, using the tools mentioned earlier in this chapter. Help them as they develop individualized action plans to strengthen the competencies of the orientees or in dealing with unique issues, such as attitude problems, lack of motivation, or an inability to meet performance expectations.

Evaluating Outcomes of the Unit-Based Orientation

Rely on the comprehensive plan you previously developed to evaluate key aspects of the orientation program, with a focus on the orientee's performance related to the unit-specific competencies. Consider scheduling a focus group with the nursing staff and preceptors to gain their input regarding the orientation program. Determine the cost of the program, and consider ways to streamline it. Use these evaluation data to revise future unit-based orientation programs. Finally, monitor the unit-based outcomes that may have been influenced by the orientation program, including staff satisfaction, recruitment, and retention rates.

Summary

The orientation component of nursing staff development, such as in-service educational activities and continuing education programs, focuses on assessing and developing the competencies of both new and experienced nurses in healthcare organizations. The ultimate goal of ensuring competency is to enable nurses to provide safe, quality care to patients. Although the primary responsibility for continuing competence belongs to individual nurses, others, including unit-based educators, play an important role in contributing to this goal.

Educators need to understand the orientation process at their organization and develop quality, cost-effective unit-based programs that will ensure competency of orientees and meet their educational needs as adult learners. These programs need to include a comprehensive evaluation program that can determine the outcome of these interventions on orientees, nursing staff, patient care, and the healthcare organization.

References

Abruzzese, R.S. (1996). *Nursing staff development: Strategies for success* (2nd ed.). St. Louis, MO: Mosby.

Alspach, J.G. (1996). *Designing competency assessment programs: A handbook for nursing and health-related professions.* Pensacola, FL: National Nursing Staff Development Organization.

American Nurses Association. (1998). *Standards of clinical nursing practice* (2nd ed.). Washington, DC: Author.

American Nurses Association. (2000). *Scope and standards of practice for nursing professional development.* Washington, DC: Author.

American Nurses Association & Oncology Nursing Society. (1996). *Statement on the scope and standards of oncology nursing practice.* Washington, DC: American Nurses Publishing.

Amerson, R. (2002). Orientation. In K.L. O'Shea (Ed.), *Staff development nursing secrets* (pp. 161–174). Philadelphia: Hanley and Belfus.

Beauman, S.S. (2001). Didactic components of a comprehensive pediatric competency program. *Journal of Infusion Nursing, 24,* 367–374.

Beecroft, P.C., Kunzman, L., & Krozek, C. (2001). RN internship: Outcomes of a one-year pilot program. *Journal of Nursing Administration, 31,* 575–582.

Benjamin, B.A. (1997). Level of literacy in the nurses aid population. *Journal for Nurses in Staff Development, 13,* 149–154.

Bloom, B.S., Englehart, M.D., & Furst, E.J. (1956). *Taxonomies for the cognitive and affective domains.* New York: David McKay.

Bumgarner, S.D., & Biggerstaff, G.H. (2000). A patient-centered approach to nurse orientation. *Journal for Nurses in Staff Development, 16,* 249–256.

Clutter, P. (2001). Nurse educator. An effective, fun annual emergency competency day/skills fair: St. John's two-year experience. *Journal of Emergency Nursing, 27,* 500–502.

Connelly, L.M. (1998). *A qualitative study of charge nurse competencies.* Bethesda, MD: TriService Nursing Research Program.

Cooper, D.C. (2002). The "C" word: Competency. In K.L. O'Shea (Ed.), *Staff development nursing secrets* (pp. 175–184). Philadelphia: Hanley and Belfus.

del Bueno, D.J. (1997). *Assuring continued competence: State of the science* (background paper at Nursing Futures and Regulation Conference). Retrieved July 1, 2003, from http://www.nursingworld/ojin/tpc3/tpc3_3.htm

del Bueno, D.J., Weeks, L., & Brown-Stewart, P. (1987). Clinical assessment centers: A cost-effective alternative for competency development. *Nursing Economics, 5*(1), 21–26.

DeSimone, B.B. (1999). Perceptions of leadership competence between interns and mentors in a cooperative nurse internship. *Nurse Educator, 24*(4), 21–25.

Eichelberger, L.W., & Hewlett, P.O. (1999). Competency model 101: The process of developing core competencies. *Nursing and Health Care Perspectives, 20,* 204–208.

Exstrom, S.M. (2001). The state board of nursing and its role in continued competency. *Journal of Continuing Education in Nursing, 32,* 118–125.

First hand. Developing an orientation brochure to make sure forensic staff get the information they need. (2002). *Joint Commission Benchmark, 4*(3), 6–7.

Francis, R.J., & Batsie, C. (1998). Critical pathways: Not for patients anymore. *Nursing Management, 29*(10), 46–48.

Gaberson, K.B., & Oermann, M.H. (1998). *Clinical teaching strategies in nursing.* New York: Springer Publishing.

Glass, J.C., Jr., & Todd-Atkinson, S. (1999). Continuing education needs of nurses employed in nursing facilities. *Journal of Continuing Education in Nursing, 30,* 219–228.

Godinez, G., Schweiger, J., Gruver, J., & Ryan, P. (1999). Role transition from graduate nurse to staff nurse: A qualitative analysis. *Journal for Nurses in Staff Development, 15,* 97–110.

Guin, P., Counsell, C.M., & Briggs, S. (2002). Round out your department: Increase staff members' learning opportunities with bedside clinical teaching rounds. *Nursing Management, 33*(5), 24.

Gurney, D. (2002). Developing a successful 16-week "transition ED nursing" program: One busy community hospital's experience. *Journal of Emergency Nursing, 28,* 505–514.

Hohler, S.E. (2003). Creating an environment conducive to adult learning [Electronic version]. *AORN Online, 77,* 833–835.

Jenkins, J. (2002). Genetics competency: New directions for nursing. *AACN Clinical Issues: Advanced Practice in Acute Critical Care, 13,* 486–491.

Johnson, R. (2001). For the love of nursing: Externs find their niche. *Nursing Spectrum, 14*(20), 15.

Johnson, T., Opfer, K., VanCura, B.J., & Williams, L. (2000). A comprehensive interactive competency program part II: Implementation, outcomes, and follow-up. *MEDSURG Nursing, 9,* 308–310.

Johnston, P.A., & Ferraro, C.A. (2001). Application of critical pathways in the maternity nursing orientation process. *Journal for Nurses in Staff Development, 17,* 61–66.

Joint Commission on Accreditation of Healthcare Organizations. (2003). *2003 hospital accreditation standards: Accreditation policies, standards, intent statements.* Oakbrook Terrace, IL: Author.

Jones, A.G., Jasperson, J., & Gusa, D. (2000). Cranial Nerve Wheel of Competencies. *Journal of Continuing Education in Nursing, 31,* 152–154.

Jones, T., Cason, C.L., & Mancini, M.E. (2002). Evaluating nurse competency: Evidence of validity for a skills recredentialing program. *Journal of Professional Nursing, 18*(1), 22–28.

Kanaskie, M.L., & Arnold, E. (1999). New ways to evaluate chemotherapy competencies. *Nursing Management, 30*(11), 41–43.

Knowles, M.S. (1980). *The modern practice of adult education: From pedagogy to andragogy* (revised and updated). Chicago: Follett Publishing.

Knowles, M.S. (1990). *The adult learner: A neglected species* (4th ed.). Houston, TX: Gulf Publishing.

Krozek, C., & Scoggins, A. (2000). *Ambulatory medicine department competencies: Registered nurse.* Glendale, CA: Cinahl Information Systems.

LaDuke, S.D. (2001). The role of staff development in assuring competence. *Journal for Nurses in Staff Development, 17,* 221–225.

Leonard, B.J., & Plotnikoff, G.A. (2000). Awareness: The heart of cultural competence. *AACN Clinical Issues: Advanced Practice in Acute Critical Care, 11,* 51–59.

Marrone, S.R. (1999). Designing a competency-based nursing practice model in a multicultural setting. *Journal for Nurses in Staff Development, 15,* 56–62.

McGuire, C.A., & Weisenbeck, S.M. (2001). Revolution or evolution: Competency validation in Kentucky. *Nursing Administration Quarterly, 25*(2), 31–37.

Miller, E., & Arquiza, E. (1999). Improving computer skills to support hospital restructuring. *Journal of Nursing Care Quality, 13*(5), 44–56.

Miller, E., Flynn, J.M., & Umadac, J. (1998). Assessing, developing, and maintaining staff's competency in times of restructuring. *Journal of Nursing Care Quality, 12*(6), 9–17.

Occupational Safety and Health Administration. (2003). *OSHA's mission statement.* Retrieved July 1, 2003, from http://www.osha.gov

Oermann, M.H., & Gaberson, K.B. (1998). *Evaluation and testing in nursing education.* New York: Springer Publishing.

Oermann, M.H., & Garvin, M.F. (2002). Stresses and challenges for new graduates in hospitals. *Nurse Education Today, 22,* 225–230.

Oermann, M.H., Truesdell, S., & Ziolkowski, L. (2000). Strategy to assess, develop, and evaluate critical thinking. *Journal of Continuing Education in Nursing, 31,* 155–160.

Olson, R.K., Nelson, M., Stuart, C., Young, L., Kleinsasser, A., Schroedermeier, R., et al. (2001). Nursing student residency program: A model for a seamless transition from nursing student to RN. *Journal of Nursing Administration, 31*(1), 40–48.

Oncology Nursing Society. (2003). *Statement on the scope and standards of advanced practice nursing in oncology.* Pittsburgh, PA: Author.

O'Shea, K.L., & Smith, L.S. (2002). The mandatories. In K.L. O'Shea (Ed.), *Staff development nursing secrets* (pp. 185–195). Philadelphia: Hanley and Belfus.

Poorman, S.G., Mastorovich, M.L., & Webb, C.A. (2002). When a GN doesn't become an RN: How the staff educator can help. *Journal for Nurses in Staff Development, 18,* 14–21.

Proehl, J.A. (2002). Developing emergency nursing competence. *Nursing Clinics of North America, 37*(1), 89–96.

Purnell, L.D., & Paulanka, B.J. (1998). *Transcultural health care: A culturally competent approach.* Philadelphia: F.A. Davis.

Rudzik, J. (1999). Establishing and maintaining competency. *Journal of Intravenous Nursing, 22*(2), 69–73.

Thomka, L.A. (2001). Graduate nurses' experiences of interactions with professional nursing staff during transition to professional role. *Journal of Continuing Education in Nursing, 32*(1), 15–19.

Williams, T., Sims, J., Burkhead, C., & Ward, P.M. (2002). The creation, implementation, and evaluation of a nurse residency program through a shared leadership model in the intensive care setting. *Dimensions of Critical Care Nursing, 21*(4), 154–161.

CHAPTER 5

Developing a Unit-Based Clinical Preceptorship Program

Nurses who work in clinical settings frequently are asked to share their expertise with less experienced nurses, nursing students and faculty, and other healthcare workers. One method of accomplishing this goal is through a preceptor program, a model of teaching used in clinical settings. In a preceptor program, an experienced nurse, referred to as a preceptor, is partnered with a less experienced nurse, called a preceptee. The preceptor guides the learning experience of the preceptee through supervision and clinical instruction. Detailed information about preceptor programs will be discussed throughout this chapter.

As a unit-based educator, you may be involved with preceptor programs in a variety of ways. First, you may be asked to develop a preceptor program for your clinical unit or to manage an already existing program. This responsibility may entail supervising nursing staff who currently serve as preceptors, selecting experienced nurses to become preceptors, developing these nurses for the preceptor role, and evaluating their performance. You may assist the staff development educator in developing the curriculum for a preceptor program, serving as faculty, and coordinating clinical experiences (Jackson, 2001). You also may serve as the liaison between your healthcare agency and faculty at affiliated schools of nursing who request preceptors for their nursing students.

Second, you may serve as a preceptor yourself, working on the clinical unit in a one-on-one arrangement with a new staff nurse. You also may partner with a nurse who recently assumed the role of unit-based educator for another clinical unit in your organization or an RN student who is enrolled in a leadership course.

Finally, you might assume the role of the learner in a preceptor program, working with an experienced staff development nurse educator. This arrangement can help you learn more about your role as a unit-based educator and develop the required competencies.

Regardless of the nature of your involvement, you will need to understand the key components of a successful preceptor program, how to manage this program for your clinical unit, and ways to coordinate your efforts within your own organization. Each of these roles will be discussed throughout this chapter.

Understanding Preceptor Programs

The idea of partnering an inexperienced nurse with a more experienced one in order to learn in the work setting has existed throughout the history of nursing.

The use of preceptors in clinical teaching has been evident in the nursing literature for nearly three decades. Despite its current popularity, the concept of clinical preceptors may assume different meanings depending on the healthcare setting.

In some organizations, the role of a preceptor is used interchangeably with that of a mentor or coach and associated with less formal teaching models that have been used during orientation. Regardless of the term used at your workplace, it is important for you to understand the meaning of a preceptorship, as well as the roles and responsibilities associated with being a preceptor and a preceptee.

A preceptorship is a formally planned arrangement in which an experienced nurse is paired with an inexperienced nurse to facilitate learning in a clinical setting (Gaberson & Oermann, 1999). The experienced nurse is employed by the healthcare organization in which the learning takes place. This arrangement lasts for a predetermined length of time, after which the inexperienced nurse may be "weaned" from the direct supervision of the preceptor (Gurney, 2002). The preceptor focuses on a specific period of learning and usually is not involved in long-term career guidance (Finger & Pape, 2002).

Preceptorships include two key individuals: an experienced preceptor who directs the learning process and a preceptee who is the learner. A variety of individuals can serve as a preceptee, such as a newly hired staff nurse, a student nurse or faculty member, or an experienced nurse who is unfamiliar with the work of the clinical unit.

Before you, as a unit-based educator, become involved in any aspect of a preceptor program, take time to thoroughly prepare yourself for this role. One way to learn more about preceptor programs is to reflect upon your own experience as a student nurse or as a graduate nurse (GN) in your first job. You were probably paired with an experienced nurse, but this arrangement may not have been formally referred to as a preceptorship. Regardless of the term that was used, the learning process you experienced during this partnership was probably very different than most of your experiences in which a faculty member directly supervised your nursing care.

Next, think about what happened during this encounter that made it a positive one. Although all of your experiences may not have been ideal, hopefully you learned from them. If you had a negative experience with your preceptor, think about what made it unsatisfactory. Try to relive your experience and determine what could have improved it. Reflect upon the relationship you had with your preceptor, focusing specifically on the professional goals that you were able to attain because of your preceptor. Figure 5-1 offers some questions to ask yourself when reflecting on your past experience with a preceptor. Consider these issues when developing yourself and other nurses for the preceptor role.

Figure 5-1. Sample Questions to Ask Yourself About Past Preceptors

- What did my preceptor do best to help me learn in the clinical setting?
- What could my preceptor have done differently that would have increased my learning?
- How did I learn new clinical skills and concepts best?
- How did I feel about learning with a preceptor versus instructor or alone?
- What did I like best about my relationship with my preceptor?
- What did I like the least about my preceptor?
- How did my preceptor provide me with feedback about my performance?
- What kind of learning environment did my preceptor create on the clinical unit?
- How did the attitude (mood) of my preceptor influence mine?
- Was my time with a preceptor sufficient? If not, how much more time did I need?

Reasons for Preceptor Programs

Preceptor programs are used in clinical settings for a variety of reasons, both within a healthcare organization and between a healthcare organization and school of nursing with which it is affiliated. Figure 5-2 illustrates some common reasons for using preceptors. These uses will be described further in this chapter.

Orientation in the Healthcare Organization

When used within a healthcare organization, a preceptor program is often an integral part of the orientation component of staff development. For example, individuals who require an orientation may not only include inexperienced GNs but experienced RNs who were either relocated to a new unit or who assumed a new position in the organization (ANA, 1994, 2000). Other individuals who may be involved in the orientation include faculty and students from affiliated schools of nursing, assistive personnel (AP), and healthcare workers from other professions.

When used during orientation, preceptor programs help new employees meet the goals of orientation, as mentioned earlier in Chapters 2 and 4. Through their expertise, experienced nurses serving as preceptors help introduce new nurses to information they need to know to function in their assigned roles on the clinical unit (ANA, 1994, 2000). Preceptors also play a role in helping new staff become socialized into the organization and clinical unit, gain an understanding of the work environment, and develop clinical competencies (ANA, 1994, 2000). Preceptors help GNs ease their transition from nursing students to professional nurses (Pfeil, 1999) and manage increasingly complex patient care assignments (Godinez, Schweiger, Gruver, & Ryan, 1999).

Nurses with some clinical experience also can benefit from a preceptored orientation. Gurney (2002) described a 16-week "transition ED nursing" program designed to recruit nurses with a minimum of six months medical-surgical experience and a telemetry course to the emergency room of a small community hospital. This 16-week competency-based orientation program included both classroom instruction and clinical experience with a seasoned preceptor.

Courses Offered by Schools of Nursing

In addition to orientation programs, preceptors are used with undergraduate and graduate nursing students enrolled in academic courses (Letizia & Jennrich, 1998). In this situation, preceptors work closely with nursing students on designated clinical units, helping them achieve clinical objectives, develop their knowledge and clinical skills (Letizia & Jennrich), and link theory with clinical practice (Gallo, 1999).

This preceptor arrangement usually is initiated by faculty who request a preceptor through the clinical agency's clinical coordinator, a nurse employed by the clinical agency who serves as a liaison between the healthcare organization and school of nursing. Unit-based educators may assume this role in some organiza-

---

Orientation of employees
- Experienced and inexperienced nurses
- Nurses being cross-trained, PRN, agency nurses
- Assistive personnel (nursing assistants)
- Unit secretaries
- Non-nursing staff (social workers, nutritionists)
- Nurses assuming a new role (leadership, educator)

Outside the healthcare organization
- Students participating in special programs (internships and externships)
- Faculty employed by affiliating schools of nursing
- Student nurses enrolled in academic courses (undergraduate and graduate)

Figure 5-2.
Reasons for Using Preceptors

tions. The clinical coordinator is responsible for identifying and recruiting qualified preceptors through discussions with various individuals, such as nurse managers, staff development educators, and nursing staff.

Preceptors and student nurses usually are partnered during the length of the clinical course. Although preceptors, students, and faculty participate in the evaluation process, faculty members maintain ultimate responsibility for the student's evaluation, with input from the preceptor (Gaberson & Oermann, 1999). Specific information about this type of preceptor program will be discussed later in this chapter.

Many undergraduate programs use preceptors as clinical instructors with nursing students enrolled in upper-level clinical courses. Many of these experiences occur in various clinical areas and help students with their transition from being a student nurse to a professional nurse (Bryant & Williams, 2002; Freiburger, 2002; Mills, Jenkins, & Waltz, 2000). Some experts claim that preceptored clinical experiences make nursing graduates more competitive in the job market (McGregor, 1999).

Some preceptored courses help nursing students develop competencies in specific areas of nursing, such as perioperative nursing (Finger & Pape, 2002), critical care (Johantgen, 2001), emergency departments (Gurney, 2002), public health nursing (Brehaut, Turik, & Wade, 1998), orthopedic nursing (Bashford, 2002), community nursing (Schneiderman, Askew, & Reed, 2002), and leadership and management (Johnson, 1999).

Other preceptored courses are designed to enable students to master a specific clinical skill. This was the case in a clinical practicum described by Frame and Chrystal (1999), in which senior nursing students were paired with IV therapy nurse specialists to gain expertise in IV therapy.

Although preceptored clinical experiences often occur in clinical settings within a reasonable distance of the student's school of nursing, Johnson (1999) described a successful preceptored clinical experience that involved RN students enrolled in a distance learning leadership and management course.

In addition to senior-level courses, preceptors have been used in clinical courses with select beginning nursing students (Nordgren, Richardson, & Laurella, 1998). Evaluations from students who participated in this pilot project were favorable and warranted the continued use of preceptors with this level of nursing students.

Graduate nursing programs also use preceptors in clinical courses to help students develop competencies in advanced nursing practice roles such as educator, administrator, clinical practitioner, and researcher. In these courses, graduate nursing students are partnered in clinical practicum with nurses who function in these leadership roles within healthcare organizations.

Internships Sponsored by Healthcare Organizations

Preceptor programs have been used in intern and extern programs targeted to students enrolled in schools of nursing and sponsored by healthcare organizations. Many of these programs are scheduled during the summer months when some students may not be enrolled in courses. These preceptored clinical programs help to minimize the impact of the nursing shortage, with hospitals recruiting these students to be employees upon graduation (Lawless, Demers, & Baker, 2002).

Trends Supporting Preceptors in Clinical Teaching

Recent trends in health care and the nursing profession support the need for creative and cost-effective strategies to help nurses provide competent care to patients. Preceptor programs are one way to meet this goal. The following section will discuss specific changes that support the need for preceptor programs now and in the future.

Nursing Shortage and Turnover of Nursing Staff

As mentioned in Chapter 1, healthcare organizations are facing a current and future shortage of nurses, compounded by a turnover of experienced nurses employed in their agencies. As a result, many organizations are actively recruiting nurses to fill their vacant positions by using unique strategies to not only attract them but to also retain them (Maes, 2000). This situation has forced healthcare organizations to hire GNs and RNs with limited experience (Jackson, 2001) and to cross-train or relocate experienced nurses to other patient care units. Some places have recruited foreign-educated nurses to fill their vacancies (Purnell & Paulanka, 1998). This trend poses potential issues related to culture and communication in the workplace and may increase the demand for experienced preceptors to assist with clinical teaching. Unfortunately, in some healthcare organizations, the nursing shortage has resulted in inexperienced nurses functioning in the preceptor role (Jackson).

Healthcare organizations also have developed innovative strategies to recruit new nurses and to retain experienced nurses they currently employ. Student internships are one approach that organizations have used to deal with the nursing shortage (Jackson, 2001). Unit-based preceptors are an important element in many of these initiatives.

Shift From Centralized to Unit-Based Education

As mentioned in Chapters 1 and 2, many nursing staff development departments in healthcare organizations were downsized over the past few years or, in some instances, totally eliminated. This change has resulted in fewer staff development educators and a shift of many education responsibilities, formerly assumed by staff educators, reassigned to nurses working on clinical units. These staff nurses, called unit-based educators, frequently assume responsibility for meeting the orientation needs of new employees and, along with other experienced nurses on the clinical units, serve as preceptors. Some healthcare agencies include serving as a preceptor as an expected behavior in job descriptions, clinical advancement programs, and clinical ladders. This shift in the centralized educator role to a decentralized approach suggests the need for experienced preceptors to help prepare other nurses to effectively function in this role.

Changes in Patient Acuity, Length of Stay, and the Demand for Competent Nursing Staff

Chapter 1 discussed healthcare changes that resulted in patients not only staying in the hospital a shorter period of time but also who were more acutely ill while they were hospitalized. Nurses who cared for these patients with complex needs had to strengthen their competencies to deliver safe, quality care. Agencies that accredit healthcare organizations, such as the Joint Commission on Accreditation of Healthcare Organizations (JCAHO), recognized this need in "assessing, maintaining, and improving staff competence" (JCAHO, 2000, p. HR-1). Unit-based preceptors and staff development educators play significant roles in this goal through verifying and developing the clinical competencies of both new and experienced nursing staff.

Collaboration Between Schools of Nursing and Clinical Agencies

In recent years, increased numbers of schools of nursing and healthcare organizations have collaborated on joint initiatives for students' clinical experiences that utilize preceptors (Frame & Chrystal, 1999; Laforet-Fliesser, Ward-Griffin, & Beynon, 1999). Conversely, the use of preceptors as clinical teachers for students also served to foster more partnerships between these academic and service organizations (McGregor, 1999).

A shortage of qualified nursing faculty, both now and anticipated for the future, supports the need for experienced preceptors to assist with the clinical learning of nursing students (Nordgren et al., 1998). As a unit-based educator, it is important for you to anticipate these increased demands for preceptor programs and to prepare the nursing staff in your organization to function effectively in the preceptor role.

Advantages and Disadvantages of Preceptor Programs

Preceptor programs pose a variety of benefits (Godinez et al., 1999) as well as challenges for the healthcare organizations and individuals actively involved in preceptorships (Letizia & Jennrich, 1998). These individuals include the preceptee, the preceptor, the unit-based educator, and faculty in schools of nursing. The healthcare organization, schools of nursing, and patients who are recipients of nursing care also experience these advantages and disadvantages. Tables 5-1 and 5-2 illustrate some examples of possible advantages and disadvantages posed by preceptor programs.

As a unit-based educator, it is important for you to carefully weigh these factors in determining if preceptorships are appropriate for your staff and clinical units. Develop a proactive approach in dealing with the disadvantages posed by preceptorships, while maximizing on the benefits. Strategies you can use to accomplish this task will be discussed throughout the remainder of this chapter.

Table 5-1. Potential Advantages of Preceptor Programs	
Participant	**Advantages**
Preceptor	Develop leadership, teaching, and clinical skills. Opportunity to mentor and develop new nurses Review previous learned concepts. Favorable status to serve as a preceptor Opportunity to network with school of nursing faculty
Preceptee	Helps with socialization to clinical unit Eases transition from student to staff role One-on-one teaching experience on the clinical unit Helps increase ability to function in organization
Unit-based educator	Source of staff leadership development for staff Assist with task of orienting new staff.
Patient	Receives care from competent nurses An experienced nurse supervises care.
Organization	Improves retention and recruitment Staff on unit contributes to learning of colleagues Encourages collaborative relationships between agency and school of nursing

Table 5-2. Potential Disadvantages of Preceptor Programs	
Participant	**Disadvantages**
Preceptor	Time consuming, especially with patient care assignment Requires preparation (education and practice) Difficult if unprepared in role, unclear objectives
Preceptee	Possible poor match with preceptor Difficult if unprepared in role, unclear objectives
Unit-based educator	Time-consuming process (selection, training, evaluation) Need to provide preparation and feedback
Patient	May perceive preceptor as care that requires supervision More nurses in contact with patient, role confusion
Organization	Direct patient care hours used for supervision of staff

Advantages of Preceptor Programs

Preceptor programs offer several advantages to key individuals who participate in the preceptor arrangement. Many experts agree that a preceptor program enables preceptees to grow professionally (Hill, Wolf, Bossetti, & Saddam, 1999) and helps them develop their clinical competencies (Freiburger, 2002) and critical thinking skills (Myrick, 2002; Myrick & Yonge, 2001, 2002a, 2002b). Preceptor programs also help nursing students in making their transition to the professional nurse role (Mills et al., 2000), enabling them to be competitive applicants for positions upon graduation (McGregor, 1999). Others view preceptorships as an effective mechanism to increase preceptees' self-confidence in their role (Freiburger, 2002). The one-on-one nature of preceptorships offers nursing students a learning experience that is not only intense but also consistent (Freiburger, 2001). Preceptees are able to validate their professional identity and gain an understanding of the organization's culture (McConnell & Dadich, 1999).

Nurses who serve as preceptors also can develop professionally from this partnership (McGregor, 1999). For example, having the opportunity to be a preceptor can be viewed as an incentive for both experienced and inexperienced nurses on the clinical unit. Preceptors may feel energized by the experience, be able to view their work from a different perspective, and become motivated to strengthen their own nursing skills (Lawless et al., 2002).

Experienced preceptors who assist with the educational needs of employees and nursing students can help healthcare organizations and unit-based educators attain their goal of employing competent nurses who provide safe, quality patient care. This outcome also can help organizations in meeting accreditation standards and in marketing their agency. Preceptor programs can improve an organization's recruitment and retention efforts (Lawless et al., 2002) and strengthen collaborative partnerships with schools of nursing (Haas et al., 2002; McGregor, 1999). Unit-based educators can strengthen their leadership and educator skills by planning and coordinating a preceptor program.

The use of preceptors in clinical courses enables faculty in schools of nursing to provide their students with realistic clinical experiences, individualized teaching, and role models. Preceptorships can minimize the impact of fewer faculty and clinical resources, providing faculty with time to concentrate on their requirements for scholarship (Nordgren et al., 1998).

Disadvantages of Preceptor Programs

Although preceptor programs offer a variety of advantages to key individuals involved in the experience, they also present some negative features. In fact, preceptorships can be a stressful experience for both preceptors (Yonge, Krahn, Trojan, Reid, & Haase, 2002) and preceptees (Yonge, Myrick, & Haase, 2002). Problems can arise if the personalities and teaching or learning styles of preceptees paired with preceptors differ (Gurney, 2002).

Nurses who assume the role of preceptor may feel overwhelmed in managing their teaching role in addition to their patient care role. Some preceptors may be expected to work various shifts to fulfill both roles (Jackson, 2001). Other preceptors may be disappointed if teamed with a preceptee who lacks the motivation to learn and who demonstrates poor professional and personal behaviors (Hill et al., 1999).

Organizations need to carefully examine the costs of their preceptor programs weighed against the benefits. Both unit-based educators and faculty may find planning and coordinating a preceptor experience to be an overwhelming task. They may have difficulty in recruiting experienced, qualified nurses to function in the capacity of preceptor, especially in light of the nursing shortage. Available candidates may be experienced nurses who are new to the preceptor role (Jackson, 2001).

Assessing the Need, Scope, and Direction for Preceptor Programs

Before implementing a formal preceptor program on your clinical unit, conduct a preliminary investigation on this endeavor within your organization, clinical units, and other healthcare agencies. This information will lay the groundwork for your preceptor program and help you determine the direction and extent of your unit-based efforts. Although healthcare and professional trends mentioned earlier in this chapter indicate the overall need for preceptor programs in clinical settings, only you as the unit-based educator can determine the unit-based efforts that are needed within your particular healthcare organization. Your input is essential to ensure the success of a preceptor program you plan on implementing at your work place.

Gaining an Organizational Perspective of Preceptor Programs

Start your investigation by meeting with nursing staff development educators in your organization's staff development department, if this option is available. The purpose of this meeting is to help you understand if this department already sponsors a preceptor program in your organization and, if so, to learn more about it.

If a preceptor program does exist, ask the educators to review any policies and procedures they have developed for this program. These documents may include topics such as reasons for using preceptors in the agency, ways to select preceptors and match them with preceptees, programs to prepare preceptors, methods to evaluate preceptor performance, and ways to recognize the contributions of preceptors.

Explore peak times of the year when preceptors may be needed, such as the dates scheduled for hiring and orienting new employees. Confirm the amount of time preceptors usually commit to an arrangement (e.g., a couple of weeks, several months). Ask about human and financial resources available to you at the unit level, along with the procedure to follow in requesting these resources. Uncover additional support that may be available to you for developing a unit-based preceptor program, such as secretarial services.

Use this opportunity to clarify how your unit-based efforts will blend with any centralized preceptor program or with informal preceptor programs sponsored by other clinical units within your organization. If a preceptor program does not exist on other units, meet with other unit-based educators in your organization to determine opportunities for collaborative efforts in developing one.

In addition to reviewing current information on preceptor programs with staff development educators, explore the need for preceptors they anticipate in the near future. This information will help you determine both the immediate and long-term preceptor needs for your unit and the resources you will need to implement them.

Obtaining a Unit-Based Viewpoint of Preceptor Programs

After meeting with key individuals in your organization at the departmental level, discuss your plans for a preceptor program with the nurse manager and nursing staff on your clinical unit. Meeting with the nurse manager will help you clarify unit goals and implications for future preceptor needs. For example, if future plans for your unit include its merger with another unit or increasing the number of patient beds, qualified preceptors will be needed to orient new staff that may be hired or cross-trained in this area.

Discuss the manager's expectations of a preceptor's clinical workload, especially patient care assignments the nurse must assume while serving as a preceptor. Determine what the preceptor's work schedule would be like while assigned to work with a preceptee, including specific shifts that may require staffing. Taking inventory of available unit-based resources can help you develop your preceptor program and determine anticipated costs of implementing a unit-based preceptor program.

Next, meet with unit staff to gain their perspective about the preceptor program. Providing staff with an opportunity to have input into the planning of a preceptor program may give them a sense of ownership and may influence the success of the project. Nurses who have served as preceptors in the past can provide you with personal insight into various aspects involved in developing a preceptor program, such as the learning needs of nurses for this role. These experienced nurses also can provide you with feedback regarding strategies to match preceptors with preceptees, the type of support preceptors require, and how to manage the overall preceptor program. It is important for unit staff to understand the roles and responsibilities of everyone involved in the preceptor program.

Seeking Information About Preceptor Programs Outside Your Workplace

In addition to resources within your healthcare organization, gain a perspective of existing preceptor programs from a regional and national perspective. One way is to search the nursing literature for recent articles that focus on preceptor programs. If your healthcare organization does not have a librarian to help you with a literature search, contact faculty at an affiliated school of nursing for help. Review the articles for unique approaches that may fit within your own organization. Many researchers have published personal accounts of preceptor programs from the perspective of preceptors and preceptees (Hill et al., 1999; Myrick & Yonge, 2002a, 2002b; Ohrling & Hallberg, 2000a, 2000b, 2001; Robbins, 1999; Sawin, Kissinger, Rowan, & Davis, 2001; Yonge, Krahn, et al., 2002) that may provide you with insight and factors to consider in developing your program.

Another way to obtain other perspectives about preceptor programs is to attend continuing education offerings on this topic at professional nursing conferences. Many organizations that sponsor these programs schedule roundtable sessions where clinical teaching topics, such as preceptor programs, are discussed among other nurses who face similar challenges. If a preceptor program is not a topic on the agenda for these programs, communicate this learning need to the conference planning committee of your professional nursing organization.

Finally, consult other unit-based educators who work at healthcare organizations in your vicinity and ask them to share information about their preceptor programs. Start by negotiating this request with an agency for which you recently shared your clinical expertise. Contact nursing faculty at an affiliated school of nursing for assistance with your preceptor program, and explore opportunities for sharing your expertise with students in their program in exchange.

Planning a Preceptor Program

After collecting information about preceptor programs from the various sources mentioned previously in this chapter, develop a detailed plan for your own unit-based preceptor program. Although designing such a plan may be a time-consuming task, this step will enable you to anticipate potential problems and to manage them before they pose barriers to the success of the program. Careful planning will help your preceptor program run more smoothly once it is implemented.

Recording this planning information in a personal notebook as you proceed through this process may be helpful for future reference, especially when you are ready to develop policies and procedures for your program. Tracking resources, including time spent on each step of the planning phase, will help you determine the cost-effectiveness of this endeavor in light of its benefits. The following section will review the essential features you should consider in developing your unit-based preceptor program. Figure 5-3 provides you with a checklist to use to track each step of the planning process.

Identify the Purpose and Objectives of the Preceptor Program

Start the planning process by developing the overall purpose and specific objectives for your preceptor program. This step is very important because it will help you develop a focus for your program and, more specifically, the outcomes you hope to accomplish by implementing your program (Freiburger, 2002). For example, a preceptorship program may focus on developing GNs' clinical competencies or increasing their self-confidence in their role as a professional nurse on the clinical unit. Developing the purpose and objectives of your program also will determine the way you will prepare preceptors and where you can obtain resources and support.

Planning a Preceptor Program	Check
1. Develop the purpose and objectives of your program.	
2. Clarify roles and responsibilities of key players.	
3. Develop criteria for preceptor selection.	
4. Prepare preceptors for their role.	
5. Provide support and incentives for preceptors.	
6. Develop key documents and a record-keeping system.	
7. Establish a communication system among players.	
8. Develop an evaluation plan.	
9. Clarify key steps in the process.	
10. Determine a time line.	

Figure 5-3.
Checklist for Planning a Unit-Based Preceptor Program

To develop the purpose of your preceptor program, decide if you will use preceptors with new or experienced nurses during the orientation phase of staff development or with nursing students enrolled in academic courses. Perhaps the preceptees will be faculty or other healthcare workers, such as AP or unit secretaries.

After you have identified the purpose of your program, develop specific objectives or outcomes based on this purpose. These objectives should be focused on the learner, measurable, and realistic. Ideas for developing objectives used in preceptor programs were mentioned earlier in this chapter. Chapters 6 and 7 will provide you with specific guidance in constructing your objectives.

After clarifying the purpose and objectives for your preceptor program, determine when this formal arrangement will begin and when it will conclude. Various factors in your organization may influence this time span. For example, you may decide to match newly hired nurses with experienced staff nurses on the first day of a five-week orientation and end this formal arrangement on the last day; or you may decide to continue this relationship on a more informal basis for an extended period of time after the formal five-week orientation is over. The length of time that preceptors are matched with nursing students may be easier to predict, because preceptorships usually end after a student fulfills the clinical objectives and credit hours required for the course.

If you serve as your agency's liaison for schools of nursing, communicate dates for clinical experiences with appropriate individuals in the staff development department and on your clinical unit. If you are not the liaison, obtain the information you will need to plan these preceptor arrangements from the individual who assumes this role. Determine the hiring dates for new employees at your organization so that you may anticipate preceptor placements needed during this time. Representatives in your human resource department or nursing staff development department may have this information. Finally, work with educators in staff development to coordinate scheduling nurses who need to participate in programs to prepare them for the preceptor role.

Clarify the Role and Responsibilities of Key Players

Collaboration is essential in planning effective preceptor programs (Freiburger, 2002; Letizia & Jennrich, 1998). After defining the goals and objectives of your preceptor program, identify key individuals who will be involved in this process. Although the preceptor and preceptee play key roles, be sure to consider others who function in supporting roles. These individuals include you as the unit-based educator or liaison, the nurse manager of the unit, unit staff, and educators in your nursing staff development department. If nursing students participate, involve course faculty from schools of nursing as key players in this process.

Clarify the roles and responsibilities of these individuals, and communicate these to everyone involved in the program. Make these duties explicit by developing written descriptions to include among your formal documents (e.g., policies, procedures, position [job] descriptions). Placing this information in writing will not only clarify roles but will help to maintain consistency in performance, minimize confusion, and help with performance evaluations. Realize that the roles and responsibilities of these individuals may vary, depending on your organization and the school of nursing. Figures 5-4 through 5-7 provide examples of some duties commonly assumed by preceptors, preceptees, unit-based educators, and faculty in schools of nursing.

Figure 5-4.
Responsibilities of Preceptors

- Assist with competency verification, socialization, and role transition.
- Provide psychosocial support for preceptee in role.
- Understand objectives and outcomes of the learning experience (e.g., orientation, course).
- Communicate learning needs regarding preceptor role to unit-based educator.
- Demonstrate self-direction in meeting learning needs related to role.
- Evaluate performance of preceptees.
- Provide ongoing (formative) and end-of-program (summative) feedback to preceptee.
- Contribute to a positive learning environment.

Nurses who precept undergraduate nursing students should meet with these students prior to the experience to discuss course objectives, clarify role expectations, and review the organization's policies (Zimmermann, 2002). Preceptors should meet with school of nursing faculty to discuss students' current competencies, specific learning needs, and organizational policies, such as charting and medication administration. Similar to new employees, students need to be oriented to the organization, including mandatory training such as emergency procedures, charting and medication policies, and reporting procedures (Zimmermann).

Figure 5-5.
Responsibilities of Preceptees

- Assume responsibility for self-learning needs.
- Understand clinical objectives and expected outcomes.
- Communicate learning needs to preceptor.
- Conduct a self-evaluation of performance.
- Provide feedback on preceptor process.
- Contribute to a positive learning environment.

In addition to clarifying the expectations and learning needs of the students, preceptors and faculty should clarify each other's roles and responsibilities (Zimmermann, 2002). Although faculty is responsible for the students' performance and patient care assignments, preceptors assume responsibility for patient care (Zimmermann).

Develop Criteria for Selection of Unit-Based Preceptors

After developing the program's purpose and objectives and clarifying the responsibilities of key players, develop criteria that you will use to select a cadre of potential preceptors from your clinical unit. In some organizations, nurse managers assume the responsibility for selecting preceptors (Jackson, 2001), so be sure to clarify what the practice is at your workplace. If criteria for selection of preceptors are not already available at your workplace, then develop a list of these qualities yourself using the resources you have obtained. For example, use the nursing literature on preceptors that you recently reviewed, and obtain input from experts at your workplace, such as staff development educators and nurse managers. If preceptors will be partnered with nursing students, contact faculty from affiliating schools of nursing.

- Coordinate the preceptor process.
- Prepare preceptors to assume their role.
- Provide support to preceptors in their role.
- Select preceptors and match with preceptees.
- Evaluate preceptor performance (or provide input).
- Evaluate preceptor process.
- Contribute to a positive learning environment.

Figure 5-6.
Responsibilities of Unit-Based Educator (Liaison)

Start this process by brainstorming a list of personal and professional characteristics and skills that you think a preceptor should ideally possess. Be sure to include specific knowledge, skills, attitudes, and behaviors that are needed to fulfill this role. Gurney (2002) recruited preceptors for an emergency department's transition program based on their knowledge of and commitment to a competency-based concept of learning and critical thinking.

- Assist with the preparation of preceptors to their role.
- Clarify the meaning of preceptors with students.
- Maintain constant communication with preceptors.
- Clarify clinical objectives and specific expectations of students.
- Communicate with unit-based educator (liaison).
- Meet preceptor needs in a timely manner.
- Assist with the selection and matching of preceptors with preceptees.
- Provide feedback on the preceptor process.
- Deal with issues that develop during the course.
- Facilitate the preceptor process.
- Evaluate preceptor performance (or provide input).
- Compile final evaluation of student.
- Evaluate overall preceptors program.

Figure 5-7.
Responsibilities of School of Nursing Faculty

After you have developed this list, prioritize these items along a continuum from "most essential qualities" to "least essential qualities." Keep in mind which characteristics and skills on your list can easily be developed in your preceptors through continuing education offerings. Figure 5-8 lists some commonly identified criteria used when selecting preceptors.

It is important to remember that criteria required of preceptors who orient staff nurses to the clinical unit may differ from the criteria required of preceptors who are teamed with nursing students. Preceptors who are partnered with nursing students often need to meet specific criteria established by schools of nursing in response to mandates by their regulatory and accreditation agencies. Preceptors who are teamed with nursing students often need to possess specific clinical skills and educational preparation based on the nursing course and level of students they precept. These preceptors who work with undergraduate nursing students often need to hold a minimum of a bachelor's degree (BSN), and those nurses precepting graduate students need to hold a minimum of a graduate degree in nursing (MSN). Some students enrolled in a leadership and management course may need to be matched with nursing staff who assume specific leadership positions in your organization, such as a charge nurse or staff educator.

Use your criteria to select the first group of nurses on the unit you plan to develop as preceptors. The process you use to select preceptors will depend on your

Figure 5-8.
Common Criteria
for Selection of
Preceptors

- Education background (BSN, MSN)
- Clinical expertise in area of focus
- Effective communication skills
- Good interpersonal skills (i.e., listener)
- Professional leadership qualities and role model
- Willingness to participate and interested in helping new nurses
- Past experience in teaching is helpful.
- Ability to create a positive learning environment

organization's policies and procedures. In some agencies, nurses volunteer to serve as preceptors, whereas other organizations require all nurses to serve as preceptors and include it as an expected behavior in their job description. Regardless of your agency's guidelines, begin your preceptor program using nurses who you predict will be most effective in the preceptor role. This will not only help your preceptor program to be successful but will also help you to gradually develop a group of experienced preceptors who can mentor other nurses on the unit in this role.

Prepare Preceptors for Their Role

Nurses who serve as preceptors for nursing staff and students assume multiple roles, including teacher, facilitator, mentor, colleague, role model, evaluator, coach, advisor, expert clinician, guide, consultant, tutor, and counselor. As a unit-based educator, you are instrumental in not only selecting potential preceptors but also in ensuring that they are prepared to function effectively in their role.

One way to prepare nurses as preceptors is to provide them with educational offerings designed to help them carry out their designated responsibilities. Envision a preceptor preparation program using a variety of contexts within the scope of nursing staff development, such as those described in Chapters 1 through 4.

One approach mentioned in Chapter 4 is to think of the preceptor preparation program as an orientation program geared to help experienced nurses assume the new role of preceptor on the clinical unit. You might think of a preceptor preparation program as a way to enhance the professional development of nurses through a series of unit-based in-service offerings, as described in Chapters 6 and 7, or as a continuing education program, as discussed in Chapter 14.

You may use various levels of preceptor preparation programs, each one providing participants with higher levels of knowledge and skills. For example, the first program can help nurses develop basic skills as a preceptor, and a second or third offering might present advanced preceptor skills. You might start with a basic continuing education course to provide nurses with a foundation for preparing for the role of preceptor, followed by a series of unit-based in-service offerings aimed at gradually introducing new and more complex topics.

Depending on your workplace, you as a unit-based educator may be responsible for developing this program for your unit, or you might be asked to participate in a program sponsored by your centralized nursing staff development department. In some settings, school of nursing faculty who request preceptors for their nursing students provide educational programs or information for nursing staff who work on a clinical unit to prepare them in this role. Faculty members also have the responsibility to prepare their students for their role in this preceptored clinical experience (Souers, 2002).

Regardless of who sponsors the preceptor preparation program, there are common skills that preceptors need to master. Several studies have identified characteristics and behaviors of preceptors that were judged by their preceptees as contributing to their learning (Finger & Pape, 2002; Jackson, 2001). Figure 5-9 lists examples of topics that can be included in preceptor development programs. Although a variety of topics are included in this list, it is important to recognize the impact of the interpersonal skills of preceptors in helping students with their transition to the role of staff nurse (Godinez et al., 1999). Gurney (2002) suggested the use of case studies to help novice preceptors learn how to effectively manage difficult situations that may arise in a preceptorship. Preceptors also should understand which responsibilities are appropriate to be delegated to nursing students who serve in a preceptored clinical experience (Zimmermann, 2002).

• Understanding the role and responsibilities of a unit-based preceptor • Understanding the job description (expectations) of the preceptee • How to teach effectively in the clinical setting (assessing learning needs) • How to work with healthcare professionals who are adult learners • How to understand and deal with various learning styles • Maintaining effective communication skills in a preceptor role (constructive feedback) • Evaluating clinical performance (validating clinical competencies)	• Documenting clinical performance (anecdotal notes, checklists) • Dealing with difficult situations (conflict) on the clinical unit • Maintaining confidentiality and ethics as a preceptor • Demonstrating an optimistic attitude in stressful situations • Role modeling professional behaviors in difficult circumstances • Understanding the impact of culture on learning • How to determine appropriate patient care assignments based on preceptee expertise

Figure 5-9. Common Content of Preceptor Development Programs

Preceptors need to develop a self-awareness of their verbal and nonverbal behaviors exhibited during the precepted experience. A recent study in which perioperative preceptees evaluated the behaviors of their preceptors revealed that preceptors illustrated both positive "inviting" behaviors and negative "disinviting" behaviors when sharing their knowledge and skills with preceptees (Finger & Pape, 2002). "Inviting" preceptorships can increase recruitment efforts and decrease retention issues. Preceptors should work with educators to develop strategies to improve "disinviting" behaviors.

When implementing your preceptor preparation program, use scheduling techniques that match the staffing needs for patient care on your clinical unit. The length of preceptor training may vary among organizations, with some programs lasting only one or two days (Jackson, 2001). Some programs consist of formal courses, whereas others employ a more informal approach with an experienced preceptor serving as a mentor (Jackson).

Because experienced preceptors have firsthand knowledge of the preceptor-preceptee relationship, be sure to include them in the planning and implementation phases of your program. They can be instrumental in role-playing difficult situations they may have encountered as preceptors and provide effective ways to respond to these issues. Finally, be creative and use a variety of active teaching strategies in your program, such as the examples described in Chapters 6 and 7.

Provide Support and Rewards for Preceptors

In addition to preparing nurses for the preceptor role, it is also important to provide them with both ongoing support (Pfeil, 1999) and rewards (Hill et al., 1999). Preceptors play an essential role in the learning process of new nurses and students and contribute to the quality of patient care on the clinical unit. There-fore, it is vital that you develop a work environment that values this role and re-gards it as an honor, privilege, and integral step in nursing professional development.

Support

In addition to the preceptor role, nurses often are expected to assume multiple roles on the clinical unit, such as the provider of direct patient care. Nurses who serve as preceptors constantly face multiple complex issues in an often hectic work environment. Because of this stress, it is important that preceptors have ongoing opportunities to share their concerns with you and have help in developing strat-egies to effectively deal with these issues.

Although there are several ways to provide preceptors with ongoing support in the work environment, be creative and develop unique strategies that are helpful to preceptors in your setting. One way is to pair new preceptors with experienced preceptors, such as yourself or other nurses within your organization, in a precep-tor network. A second approach is to develop a formal discussion group, where preceptors from one or more units gather to share their experiences with each other on an ongoing basis. If e-mail is available at your organization, think about extending the group's discussions using this technology. Including experienced preceptors as faculty in staff development programs to prepare preceptors also may serve as a source of support for nurses new to this role. Preceptors who work with nursing students may find ongoing communication and feedback from school of nursing faculty as sources of support for their role. Regardless of the strategies you choose, it is important for you as the unit-based educator to be available as a resource to preceptors.

Rewards

In addition to providing support for preceptors, investigate ways of providing these nurses who serve as preceptors with meaningful incentives or rewards. These rewards not only may motivate them to serve as preceptors in the future but also will publicly recognize the contribution they make to the success of the organiza-tion. Because this task may involve agency resources or policy changes, be sure to discuss available opportunities with appropriate individuals in your organization, such as your nurse manager or staff development educator.

Several types of rewards can be provided to nurses who serve as preceptors. Because you as a unit-based educator know the nursing staff on your unit, think about what types of incentives and rewards they may perceive as being important to them. Present this topic as a point of discussion at a unit-based staff meeting, or ask your unit manager to discuss this issue with other managers at an administra-tive meeting.

Ask preceptors for their comments regarding the rewards that they value for serving in this capacity. Stone and Rowles (2002) used this approach when they asked preceptors to complete a survey asking about rewards that were meaningful to them. Results were evaluated based on available resources within the context of the healthcare organization and school of nursing.

Many nurses find various rewards in serving as a preceptor. Some nurses find personal satisfaction in helping students develop their clinical skills and in ob-serving their growth as professional nurses (Hill et al., 1999). Other preceptors find pleasure in witnessing the benefits to patient care and team building that result on the clinical unit from developing a competent nursing staff. Conversely, some preceptors have been discouraged by preceptees who have been poorly motivated or who have displayed unprofessional behaviors in the clinical setting. Recent changes in healthcare organizations, such as restructuring, have decreased the internal rewards that some preceptors had previously experienced (Hill et al.).

In addition to these internal rewards offered through preceptorships, some nurses value the benefits that stem from external sources. For example, some healthcare organizations include participation as a preceptor as an expected behavior in the nurse's job description and consider it as part of his or her performance evaluation and clinical advancement program. Some settings offer preceptors a decreased patient care assignment (Yonge, Krahn, et al., 2002) or a daylight work schedule in order to accommodate preceptees. However, other units require preceptors to work rotating shifts in order to provide the preceptee with a realistic perspective of the work expectations (Jackson, 2001).

One hospital developed a successful Preceptor Incentive Program (PIP) to reward their nurses for serving as preceptors (Jackson, 2001). Nurses earned $1.25 of PIP education credit for each hour they spent as a preceptor. The PIP credits could be accumulated and applied toward approved educational programs within a designated period of time.

Some agencies acknowledge preceptors by providing them with thank you letters or certificates of recognition (Bryant & Williams, 2002), publishing their names in the organization's newsletter, or sponsoring recognition celebrations in their honor, such as luncheons or dinners. One school of nursing rewarded their preceptors with a "care" basket that included items to promote their personal pampering (Bryant & Williams).

Schools of nursing also acknowledge agency nurses who serve as preceptors for their students. In addition to sending letters thanking preceptors for their unique contributions to the learning of nursing students, some schools award preceptors with a signed certificate of recognition, invite them to a campus celebration for preceptors, or offer them a reduced or free registration to educational programs or courses sponsored by the school (Gaberson & Oermann, 1999). In exchange for preceptors, some schools offer organizations their assistance based on their expertise, such as with research projects or educational programs. Other schools of nursing confer titles, such as adjunct faculty on preceptors (Gaberson & Oermann), especially to preceptors who repeatedly work with students from their school. Finally, some schools present preceptors with small mementos imprinted with the school's name or logo, such as coffee mugs, mouse pads, or pens.

Develop Key Documents and a Record-Keeping System

Chapter 3 discussed the importance of developing key documents and a record-keeping system for the professional development activities you offer in staff development programs. Developing these items for your preceptor program will not only help it run smoothly but will also provide you with a system in which documents can be easily retrieved for accrediting agencies and other reviewers.

Before you attempt to develop documents and a system that will manage your records, discuss your plans with appropriate individuals in your agency. This will help you avoid duplicating documents that already exist or prevent you from excluding features in documents that are applicable on a unit-based level. Find out how policies and procedures are reviewed and approved within your workplace.

Clinical educators in the nursing staff development department, unit managers, and experienced unit-based educators and preceptors on other units can help guide you in this process. Nurses who are preceptors at other healthcare agencies also may be of some help.

In addition to designing course materials for your preceptor preparation program, such as the materials presented in Chapter 7, you will need to develop policies, procedures, and forms to use. Remember that these items should reflect the philosophy, purpose, and objectives of your preceptor program, the clinical unit, and nursing staff development department.

Policies and procedures are extremely important to the success of your preceptor program and need to be communicated to all staff. Policies are statements that guide individuals in your organization in making decisions (Marquis & Huston, 2000) and will affect your preceptor program. Because policies are based on goals, they also help staff focus their efforts in a specified direction. A policy about criteria for selection of preceptors for new nurses or nursing students will guide you and others in this process. Figure 5-10 lists examples of policies that you should consider developing for your program.

Procedures help nurses implement policies. They outline detailed steps included in the process and arrange them in sequence (Marquis & Huston, 2000). In reference to the example mentioned earlier, you might choose to develop a procedure for school of nursing faculty to follow when they are requesting preceptors from your organization for their nursing students. Figure 5-10 lists examples of procedures that may prove helpful for a unit-based preceptor program.

In addition to these policies and procedures, you will need to develop forms that will help to facilitate your work in the preceptor program. Figure 5-11 lists documents that you may consider. These documents can serve as templates for individuals who participate in the program and also can add consistency to your program. The following section of this chapter will review the steps to follow in developing your preceptor program. Use these ideas to determine what forms you may need for your program.

You may consider including the following documents as a start: assessment of learning needs in preceptees, preceptorship clinical schedule, daily clinical feedback form, final evaluation form, and daily preceptee logs. If this is your first preceptor program, develop drafts of these items before you begin the program, and revise them after you complete your first group of preceptors-preceptees. Be sure to keep your originals in a folder along with a computer disk, and note changes on the forms while the process is still fresh in your mind.

If you do not have an existing record-keeping system tailored to your preceptor program, develop one for your unit-based program. It is important to keep

Figure 5-10. Suggested Policies and Procedures for a Preceptor Program

Policies
- Criteria for Preceptors Paired With Agency Personnel
- Criteria for Preceptors Paired With Undergraduate Nursing Students
- Criteria for Preceptors Paired With Graduate Nursing Students
- Roles and Responsibilities of Preceptors
- Roles and Responsibilities of Preceptees
- Roles and Responsibilities of Unit-Based Educators (Liaison)
- Roles and Responsibilities of School of Nursing Faculty
- Clinical Workload of Nurses Serving as Preceptors

Procedures
- Requesting Preceptors for Agency Personnel
- Requesting Preceptors for Nursing Students From Schools of Nursing
- Evaluation of Preceptee Performance
- Evaluation of Preceptors

records related to your program for several reasons. First, you need to document the progress in performance for the preceptee and preceptor. Second, having a record system allows you to critically evaluate the effectiveness of your unit-based efforts based on program goals. Finally, records provide you with evidence that may be shared with accreditation agencies, such as JCAHO.

- Preceptor-preceptee assignment
- Unit-based schedule
- Unit-based orientation plan and objectives
- Needs assessment
- Competency validation reports
- Daily anecdotes and checklists
- Summary evaluation of preceptee
- Summary evaluation of preceptor
- Self-evaluations

Figure 5-11.
Sample Documents and Forms for a Unit-Based Preceptor Program

Develop your record-keeping system using a variety of methods, ranging from a box of file folders to a more sophisticated computerized program. Before you start, investigate resources available to you within your agency to see how you can add your program files to a system that already exists.

In most instances, you will need to organize three sets of documents: (a) policies and procedures, (b) original templates of documents used in the program, and (c) actual documentation about the progress and performance of each preceptee and preceptor. The following section of this chapter is intended to provide you with suggestions on ways to maintain these records. Your preference may differ, depending on the resources and needs of your particular healthcare organization. Regardless of your approach, develop a system that is easily accessible and requires little energy to use and maintain. Documents such as policies and procedures can be kept in a three-ring notebook for easy reference by staff on your clinical unit. This same system can be used to maintain original templates of documents you frequently use during the preceptor program. Protecting each form in a plastic cover not only makes it easy to locate but also preserves it for duplication purposes. Label separate file folders with the name and start date of each preceptee, and file completed documentation about the preceptee in it. Include a copy of the preceptee's schedule in this folder. Repeat this process for collecting feedback such as evaluations and anecdotal notes regarding the performance of preceptors on the unit. You can use the same approach for nursing students who are preceptored on your unit, and also include a copy of the course profile and clinical objectives in the folder.

Be sure to keep personalized documents about employees or students in a secured location (e.g., locked file cabinet). Determine who is permitted to access these confidential files and how long these files need to be maintained. Finally, talk with your unit's nurse manager to determine when and if any of these documents, such as summary evaluations, should be forwarded to the employee's permanent personnel file.

Establish Communication Among Key Players in the Program

Before you implement your preceptor program, establish communication pathways among key individuals involved in the program. This feature was discussed earlier in Chapter 3. Communication is essential for the goals of the preceptor program to be accomplished and facilitates collaboration among all individuals involved. Schedule regular meetings with individuals involved in the preceptor program (Gurney, 2002).

Start creating a communication system by identifying the key players. In addition to the preceptor and preceptee, include yourself as the unit-based educator, the centralized staff development educator for your unit, your nurse manager, and nursing staff on the clinical unit. You also may choose to include the human resource department that processes information on new employees and other unit-based educators in your organization. When dealing with preceptors for nursing students, you will need to include faculty assigned to the course and other contacts within both the school of nursing and your organization.

Next, investigate potential communication methods within your organization that you can use to accomplish this goal. In addition to using traditional communication methods, such as telephone calls, announcements at meetings, a unit communication book, or memos that are mailed or posted on unit bulletin boards, consider other strategies. For example, e-mail, a unit newsletter, or the agency's newsletter may be helpful ways to convey information to others within your organization. Schedule a "welcome reception" for new preceptees and their preceptors on the unit during the first week of orientation, and invite staff. Post photographs (with permission) of new nursing staff and their preceptors on the unit to enable staff who work other shifts to recognize them. Encourage existing staff to send a small note to welcome preceptees to the clinical unit. Strategies such as these help contribute to the goals of orientation by allowing preceptees to feel welcomed on the unit and perceived as individuals valued by the organization.

Determine what information about the preceptor program should be shared, with whom, and when. One way to accomplish this task is to review the key steps of the preceptor program that is described in the section that follows. Determine which individuals on your list of key players need to have this information to effectively contribute to the preceptor program. Decide at which point in this process this individual needs this information.

Two steps that occur early in most preceptor programs are obtaining a list of new employees with their start date and matching them with specific nurses who will be their unit-based preceptors. This information would be of value to all people involved in the preceptor program before the new nurses arrive on the clinical unit. Think about the most effective way that this information can be communicated.

Develop an Evaluation Plan for the Preceptor Program

Before you implement a unit-based preceptor program, develop a plan to evaluate key aspects of the program. This evaluation plan should be a comprehensive one that enables you to determine the effectiveness of your approach in attaining the outcomes previously identified, such as the performance of preceptees and preceptors. This plan also will provide you with objective data to implement changes needed to improve your preceptor program.

An evaluation plan should provide you with feedback about two perspectives: (a) the performance or behaviors of key individuals involved in the preceptorship program (e.g., preceptee, preceptor, unit-based educator, school of nursing faculty, nurse manager) and (b) their overall satisfaction with the process and content of the preceptorship program (e.g., objectives, content, clinical teaching strategies, evaluation methods). Additional information on evaluation is discussed later in Chapters 6 and 7.

Although you are responsible for collecting evaluation data on preceptor programs sponsored by your organization, schools of nursing often utilize their own procedures and documents when evaluating preceptors paired with their nursing students at your clinical agency. Faculties often ask preceptors to provide documentation regarding a student's daily performance on the clinical unit and to offer their input in a final summary evaluation of the student at the end of the course. Course faculty are ultimately responsible for the student's evaluation and for determining if the student satisfactorily met the clinical objectives of the course (Gaberson & Oermann, 1999). Preceptors often are asked by faculty to provide feedback about the clinical course and the coordination efforts of faculty. Figure 5-12 is an example of a tool used by a school of nursing in which preceptors evaluate both the management of the course (Part 1) and the performance of the student (Part 2) in a preceptored leadership-management course for RN students.

In addition to the preceptor's role in evaluation, nursing students as preceptees should be asked to evaluate their experience. These elements include their own clinical performance, the effectiveness of their preceptor in helping them attain clinical objectives, the clinical site, the coordination efforts of faculty, and the clinical course. Figure 5-13 is an example of a tool used by nursing students to evaluate both the clinical site and preceptor in a preceptored leadership-management course for RN students.

Figures 5-14 and 5-15 provide examples of clinical evaluation tools used by preceptors and faculty in a prepared clinical course targeted to senior undergraduate nursing students.

A recent study supported the reliability of a tool–the invitational operating room teaching survey (IORTS)–in measuring the attitudes of perioperative nurse preceptees toward their preceptors and in defining characteristics of effective preceptors (Finger & Pape, 2002). Findings support the use of IORTS as an assessment tool for educators to use prior to the start of a preceptorship.

Because you, as a unit-based educator, select and develop unit-based preceptors, it is important for you to obtain feedback from faculty regarding your performance and the effectiveness of the clinical setting for learning. This information can help you develop strategies to assist preceptors on your unit and to make improvements.

Performance of Key Individuals

Because the evaluation process may be an overwhelming task, conceptualize this process using smaller components. Compare this approach to the evaluation process used for in-service education offerings described in Chapters 6 and 7.

First, decide which individuals in your program will need to be evaluated. Start by listing these individuals and names into a table, as illustrated in Table 5-3. Based on this matrix, decide what aspects should be evaluated within your organization and mark the appropriate block with an X. For example, preceptors should not only have an opportunity to evaluate their own performance but also a chance to evaluate the behaviors of their preceptees and the unit-based educator as the facilitator of the program. Likewise, preceptees should evaluate their own performance, along with the performances of their preceptor and unit-based educator. Finally, the unit-based educator should have input into the evaluation of both the preceptor and preceptee, along with themselves. Depending on your situation, you may choose to include the nurse manager and faculty in this process.

Preceptees should receive feedback from their preceptors about their performance on a daily basis and at the conclusion of the clinical experience. Daily evaluation of the preceptee's performance, called formative evaluation, provides learners with feedback needed to help them shape their behaviors or competen-

Figure 5-12.
Evaluation of
Course and Stu-
dent (completed
by preceptor)

Note. Figure courtesy
of Duquesne Univer-
sity School of Nurs-
ing. Used with per-
mission.

**Duquesne University School of Nursing
Evaluation of Course and Student by Preceptor
N455 Leadership and Management of Clinical Care**

Directions: The clinical experience for this course was designed to provide the RN/BSN student with an opportunity to observe the role of the nurse as leader and manager. An integral part of this experience is the evaluation process. Your comments would be appreciated with regard to your role as preceptor for this experience. Please review your comments with your student, and then forward them to me via the student, fax, or e-mail.

Part 1—Course Evaluation
1. How well do you think the basic purpose of the clinical experience was made clear to you? What would have helped?
   _____
   _____

2. How well do you think the time requirement for the clinical experience enabled the student to fulfill the course objectives? What other arrangements would you suggest?
   _____
   _____

3. What other comments or recommendations would you like to make regarding this clinical experience?
   _____
   _____

Part 2—Student Evaluation
1. Has the student successfully completed the objectives of the course and articulated them into weekly activities within your organization? ____Yes____No
   Please comment on the student's strengths and weaknesses:
   _____
   _____

2. Has the student met all other obligations that were agreed upon at the beginning of the semester? ____Yes____No
   Please comment:
   _____
   _____

3. How would you rate the student with regards to punctuality, attendance, self-direction, and general ease in following the requirements for the clinical experience?
   _____
   _____

4. Please provide any additional comments that will help with the student's evaluation.
   _____
   _____
   _____
   _____
   _____
   _____

Student's name: _____ Preceptor's signature: _____
Date: _____

Duquesne University School of Nursing
Evaluation of Clinical Preceptor and Clinical Site by Student
N455 Leadership and Management of Clinical Care

Student's name: _____

Preceptor's name: _____

Clinical agency and unit: _____ Date: _____

Please rate the following aspects of your clinical experience in the course by placing the appropriate number after each sentence:

5 = Excellent
4 = Above average
3 = Average
2 = Below average
1 = Unsatisfactory
NA = Not applicable

Evaluation of Clinical Site

1. Overall quality of this clinical learning experience.

2. Clinical facility's provision of suitable opportunities to meet learning goals.

3. Nursing staff's ability and willingness to serve as resource persons in the clinical setting.

4. Overall physical condition of the clinical setting in being conducive to the learning process.

Evaluation of Preceptor

5. Preceptor's ability to guide student in thinking through problems in the clinical setting.

6. Preceptor's ability to relate the clinical experience with classroom activities.

7. Overall evaluation of the preceptor's ability to promote growth and learning.

8. Preceptor's ability to serve as a resource person in the clinical setting.

9. Preceptor's ability to facilitate student's recognition of own learning needs.

10. Preceptor's ability to provide constructive feedback that fosters learning.

11. Preceptor's provision for adequate orientation to the unique aspects of the clinical experience.

12. Preceptor's ability to stimulate questions and discussion in the clinical setting.

13. What was most helpful about this clinical experience? _____
_____
_____

14. What was least helpful about this clinical experience? _____
_____
_____

15. Suggestions for improvement: _____
_____
_____
_____
_____
_____
_____
_____

Figure 5-13.
Evaluation of Clinical Site and Preceptor (completed by student)

Note. Figure courtesy of Duquesne University School of Nursing. Used with permission.

Figure 5-14.
Clinical Progress
Tool Guidelines

Duquesne University School of Nursing
Clinical Progress Tool Guidelines

Please indicate your rating of the student's performance on the Clinical Progress Tool, using the learning indicator below. (Students **must** achieve a rating of at least an "S" level on these behaviors to pass the course.)

1. Promotes health regardless of the person's condition.

   Examples of behaviors that indicate achievement of this outcome:
   - Awareness of primary health care.
   - Health teaching.
   - Used current research findings when caring for clients and families

2. Provides safe, organized, holistic, and effective care within a caring context, based on a synthesis of knowledge, for persons with a range of health problems.

   Examples of behaviors that indicate achievement of this outcome:
   - Accurately prepared for and safely administer medications.
   - Includes family in the planning for and in the care of the client.
   - Identifies components of safe practice.
   - Utilizes standards of care and knowledge of professional role in practice situations.

3. Uses nursing process effectively while caring for persons with complex health needs and/or problems.

   Examples of behaviors that indicate achievement of this outcome:
   - Continually assesses client for changes in status.
   - Continually evaluates nursing care for effectiveness.
   - Plans for the implementation of nursing care of groups of clients.
   - Organizes nursing care for a small group.
   - Directs outcomes of client care.

4. Provides rationale for nursing decisions using relevant knowledge, principles, and theories.

   Examples of behaviors that indicate achievement of this outcome:
   - Prepared for all clinical experiences.
   - Incorporates pathophysiology in the care of the client and family.
   - Demonstrates the ability to make decisions by using appropriate critical thinking skills.
   - Seeks appropriate literature to enhance knowledge of professional growth.
   - Utilizes appropriate literature to enhance knowledge and skill.

5. Demonstrates cultural caring in the practice of nursing.

   Examples of behaviors that indicate achievement of this outcome:
   - Exhibits sensitivity to clients and families.
   - Identifies cultural and religious backgrounds which are important in the plan of care.
   - Promotes the cultural beliefs of clients and families.

6. Employs critical thinking and creative approaches to all healthcare situations.

   Examples of behaviors that indicate achievement of this outcome:
   - Utilizes critical thinking in making decisions for goal attainment.
   - Identifies the value of role theory in exploring a professional identity.

(Continued on next page)

7. Communicates/collaborates effectively with persons in various health states.
Examples of behaviors that indicate achievement of this outcome: - Uses appropriate communication skills with clients and families. - Acknowledges the presence of stress in the client and family. - Communicates effectively with families in stressful situations. - Utilizes principles of formal and informal communication skills.
8. Communicates/collaborates effectively with healthcare providers to ensure quality care.
Examples of behaviors that indicate achievement of this outcome: - Uses interpersonal communication skills to achieve effective group process. - Interacts appropriately with other members of the healthcare team. - Communicates relevant information verbally and in written documentation. - Encourages open communication within the work group. - Analyzes group process. - Delegates responsibility for assigned activity appropriately. - Participates in the reporting process within the assigned nursing unit.
9. Acts as an advocate for the person.
Examples of behaviors that indicate achievement of this outcome: - Uses opportunities to advocate for the client and family during new and stressful situations.
10. Is accountable for own nursing practice and professional growth.
Examples of behaviors that indicate achievement of this outcome: - Consistently presents self in a professional and accountable manner. - Aware of hospital policies/procedures regarding standards of care. - Takes responsibility for knowledge to provide safe care for the client. - Evaluates self in relation to professional growth. - Examines factors affecting the transition from a student role to a professional nursing role. - Seeks opportunities to participate in new experiences. - Applies leadership concepts in the development of the role of the professional nurse. - Identifies the management functions of the professional nurse in working with groups of clients.

Figure 5-14.
Clinical Progress
Tool Guidelines
(*Continued*)

Note. Figure courtesy of Duquesne University School of Nursing. Used with permission. Adapted with permission from "The Clinical Evaluation Tool: A Measure of the Quality of Clinical Performance of Baccalaureate Nursing Students," by K. Krichbaum, M. Rowan, L. Duckett, M.B. Ryden, and K. Savik, 1994, *Journal of Nursing Education, 33*, p. 398. Copyright 1994 by Slack, Inc.

cies related to the objectives of the program or course (Oermann & Gaberson, 1998).

To provide accurate feedback to preceptees regarding their performance, preceptors should consider recording daily notes that document the preceptee's learning activities and performance (Godinez et al., 1999). This documentation also can help determine what learning experiences the preceptee will need in the future.

Evaluation that occurs at the conclusion of a clinical program, referred to as summative evaluation, helps determine if the preceptee attained the clinical objectives (Oermann & Gaberson, 1998). This evaluation provides learners with a summary regarding their behaviors compared to the clinical objectives for the program or course.

Program Satisfaction

As mentioned earlier, it is important that all individuals involved in the preceptor program have an opportunity to evaluate various aspects of their clinical experience. Although evaluation of program satisfaction often occurs at the con-

Figure 5-15.
Final Clinical
Evaluation

Duquesne University School of Nursing Final Clinical Evaluation UPNSG 405 Clinical Integration in Complex Settings

Agency _____   ❒ Faculty

Date _____   ❒ Preceptor

Name _____   ❒ Student

Rating Scale: I - Independent   S - Satisfactory   A - Assisted   M - Marginal   D - Dependent
(Rating of "S" is needed to be considered passing grade for this course.)

1. Promotes health regardless of the person's condition. (Program Outcomes 1, 8)

Rating:	Comments:
I	
S	
A	
M	
D	

2. Provides safe, organized, holistic and effective care within a caring context, based on a synthesis of knowledge, for persons with a range of health problems. (Program Outcomes 2, 4, 8)

Rating:	Comments:
I	
S	
A	
M	
D	

3. Uses nursing process effectively while caring for persons with complex health needs and/ or problems. (Program Outcome 1)

Rating:	Comments:
I	
S	
A	
M	
D	

4. Provides rationale for nursing decisions using relevant knowledge, principles, and theories. (Program Outcomes 1, 9)

Rating:	Comments:
I	
S	
A	
M	
D	

5. Demonstrates cultural caring in the practice of nursing. (Program Outcome 3)

Rating:	Comments:
I	
S	
A	
M	
D	

(Continued on next page)

6. Employs critical thinking and creative approaches to all healthcare situations. (Program Outcomes 2, 9)	
Rating: I S A M D	Comments:

7. Communicates/collaborates effectively with persons in various health states. (Program Outcomes 1, 8)	
Rating: I S A M D	Comments:

8. Communicates/collaborates effectively with healthcare providers to ensure quality care. (Program Outcomes 5, 8)	
Rating: I S A M D	Comments:

9. Acts as an advocate for the person. (Program Outcomes 7, 10, 11)	
Rating: I S A M D	Comments:

10. Is accountable for own nursing practice and professional growth. (Program Outcomes 6, 11)	
Rating: I S A M D	Comments:

Figure 5-15.
Final Clinical
Evaluation
(Continued)

Note. Figure courtesy of Duquesne University School of Nursing. Used with permission. Adapted with permission from "The Clinical Evaluation Tool: A Measure of the Quality of Clinical Performance of Baccalaureate Nursing Students," by K. Krichbaum, M. Rowan, L. Duckett, M.B. Ryden, and K. Savik, 1994, *Journal of Nursing Education, 33,* p. 398. Copyright 1994 by Slack, Inc.

Table 5-3. Evaluation Map for the Unit-Based Preceptor Program				
	Preceptor	**Preceptee**	**Unit-Based Educator**	**Nurse Manager**
Preceptor	Self-evaluation	X	X	X
Preceptee	X	Self-evaluation	X	X
Unit-Based Educator	X	X	Self-evaluation	X
Nurse Manager	X	X	X	Self-evaluation

clusion of the program or course, it also should be conducted informally on a daily basis to allow for changes in the original plan. Because of their active involvement in preceptor programs, preceptees and preceptors are prime candidates to determine the effectiveness of the program.

In addition to written reports, a variety of other methods can be used to conduct evaluations during your preceptor program. For example, consider conducting focus groups to obtain feedback about the preceptor program from preceptors and preceptees either during or at the conclusion of the program. Feedback obtained while the preceptor program is still in progress can be used to make immediate changes, if needed.

Clarify the Preceptor Program Process

Before you implement your first preceptor program, outline the individual steps you will need to follow in this process. This process should begin from the time you first realized the need for preceptors to the final evaluation and revision of the program. When outlining your steps, include requests for preceptors that are made both by you and by faculty in affiliated schools of nursing.

The following section of this chapter will review the tasks you need to complete for the preceptor program. Prepare nurses on your unit as preceptors well in advance of the preceptees arriving on the clinical unit. Check if faculty and nursing students need to attend an orientation to the organization before the preceptored experience begins. You can find this information in the affiliation agreement between your organization and the school of nursing.

Match Preceptees With Appropriate Preceptors

The process involved in a preceptor program begins when you, as the unit-based educator, receive notification that new nursing staff have been hired, or staff previously employed on other units will need to be cross-trained and oriented to the clinical unit. This information, depending on your organization, can be obtained from your human resource department, the nursing staff development department, or nurse manager of your clinical unit. In addition to needing preceptors for new employees, faculty at affiliating schools of nursing may send you a request for preceptors to guide their nursing students on your clinical unit.

The earlier that you know when new nursing staff will begin on your unit, the more time you will have to plan an effective clinical preceptor experience. If your human resource department does not already have preset start dates for new nursing staff, then suggest this practice. These suggestions also apply to faculties who need preceptors. Discuss reasonable dates by which faculty need to notify you of a preceptor request.

After you know the names of incoming nursing staff and their arrival dates, think about the preceptors who are already prepared and available to work with these new nurses. If you need more preceptors than you have formally prepared, consider other strategies. For example, try working informally on preceptor skills with a staff nurse who shows promise in being a preceptor. Other approaches include pairing novice preceptors with more experienced preceptors who can guide them as they work with a preceptee on the clinical unit, or assign two new employees to one experienced preceptor who is able to handle multiple preceptees.

Before you match these preceptees with your available cadre of unit-based preceptors, obtain some background information about each preceptee. Start by reviewing each preceptee's resume, if appropriate, and note his or her formal and informal educational background, prior work experience, and professional contributions. If you have no opportunity to meet with the new hires, then schedule some time to talk with each preceptee within the first couple of days after he or she begins to obtain this information.

During your interview with the preceptees, ask them questions that will help you in pairing them with available preceptors on the clinical unit. For example, ask them how they best learn on the clinical unit, what they feel their strengths are, and what skills they hope to improve. Another approach you can use is to ask the preceptees to recall a positive experience they have had with a preceptor or clinical instructor. Listen to how they describe the characteristics or behaviors of the individual who facilitated their learning. This interview approach also may be helpful to implement with preceptors, especially if these nurses are unfamiliar to you.

Obtaining this information from preceptees will help you not only in matching them with preceptors but also in designing learning experiences that will strengthen their clinical competencies. Knowing more about your preceptees may help you realize contributions that new staff can make to the unit through in-service education offerings.

You may discover that a new staff nurse has expertise in caring for patients with a new IV catheter that will be introduced to the staff on your clinical unit next month. Asking this nurse to help with a future unit-based in-service offering on this topic may contribute to his or her self-confidence and perception as a valued staff member of the unit.

A similar strategy can be used to match nursing students with preceptors on your clinical unit. School of nursing faculty should provide you with the criteria they require of preceptors who will be paired with their students for a designated clinical course. Faculty can provide you with insight into the background and special learning needs of students so that you can match them with the most appropriate preceptor. For example, differences in preceptor, student, and faculty perceptions of ideal and actual learning outcomes were significant in a study conducted by Robbins (1999). Be sure to ask faculty if they prefer to use graduates of their school of nursing as preceptors to graduates of other schools.

Information regarding effective ways to match preceptors with preceptees is limited (Lockwood-Rayermann, 2003). However, organizations have used strategies to pair preceptors with preceptees to ensure that the experience is a positive one. Some agencies match preceptors with preceptees according to their teaching or learning styles (Chase, 2001), leadership styles (Lockwood-Rayermann), and personality characteristics (Anderson, 1998). Anderson supported the positive impact of matching preceptors and preceptees based on learning styles assessed through personality type. Orientees who matched their preceptors on the personality preferences of introversion or extroversion had significantly higher levels of satisfaction with the experience than those dyads who were not matched.

Some schools of nursing expect their students to seek their own preceptors. Other organizations consider demographic factors in this partnering. Regardless of the approach used in matching preceptees with preceptors, the primary focus should be on developing a team that can communicate and understand each other so that learning can occur.

Develop a Plan for the Preceptored Clinical Experience

After you have a tentative idea of how you plan to match preceptees with preceptors, develop a lesson plan for the preceptored clinical experience. The process used to develop a lesson plan is described later in Chapter 7. You may accomplish this in a variety of ways, depending on your organization.

One option is to integrate the preceptored clinical with the classroom teaching in an orientation program. Another approach is to combine both classroom teaching with clinical experience using a more informal unit-based approach. Ask your staff development educator which approach is used at your agency. Information on orientation programs in Chapter 4 also will help you in developing your method.

Regardless of your approach, be sure to include learning objectives in the lesson plan that are relevant to each preceptee (Pfeil, 1999), along with objectives designated by their job description. Be sure to review the plan with appropriate individuals on your unit, especially the preceptees and preceptors, and provide them with copies.

Lesson plans for preceptored experiences with nursing students may differ from those plans with new employees. When working with nursing students, ask faculty for a copy of the course profile or syllabus, evaluation forms, and a course schedule. The course profile/syllabus will provide you and preceptors with a general overview of the course, along with specific clinical objectives and expected competencies that nursing students need to demonstrate before the course ends. Clinical objectives will differ among courses and schools of nursing. Some students may be enrolled in specially designed courses, called directed studies, and may develop a personalized learning contract for this clinical experience. Be sure to keep a copy of these items in your files.

Finally, develop a schedule for your lesson plan. This schedule should include the date, hours, clinical focus (objective) for each day, and classes. Help preceptors select patient assignments that will enable preceptees to attain their learning objectives. Similar to the lesson plan, the schedule may be integrated into a unit-based orientation program, or it may be separate. In addition to allotting time designated to direct patient care, schedule tranquil times away from the activities during which preceptees and preceptors can reflect either alone or together (Ohrling & Hallberg, 2000a, 2000b) and evaluate performance. Include time for you to meet with preceptors and provide support and guidance.

Implement the Preceptor Program

Now that you have matched preceptees with preceptors and developed a lesson plan for the clinical experience, implement the program. If you are implementing your plan for the first time, be sure to note its positive features and those areas that need improvement.

Depending on the needs of your organization, consider pilot testing your preceptor program on a small scale before you implement a full-scale program. Piloting your program will enable you to determine the effectiveness of its components such as policies, procedures, and documentation forms. It also will help you determine if preceptors need additional preparation. Evaluation comments received during pilot testing can help you revise the program for its next implementation.

Pilot testing your preceptor program also can provide you with data to calculate its cost in light of its benefits. Do this by tracking all expenses incurred in the program, such as time, materials, supplies, services, duplication costs, and staffing changes made to manage patient care. Ask your nurse manager for suggestions on how to best estimate these costs in your organization.

Use your "star" preceptors for this first cohort of preceptees to maximize its success. Consider serving as a preceptor yourself during its first implementation to experience first-hand how the process works. Encourage a friendly, nonjudgmental learning environment on the clinical unit during the implementation of the program. Although some staff may experience a bad day now and then, encourage them to be professional and discuss their concerns in a private setting.

Use Evaluation Data to Make Program Revisions

After the first pilot preceptor program is completed, collect and analyze evaluation data, using the methods you selected that were described earlier in this chapter. Discuss how the program progressed with unit staff and preceptors, and decide what changes need to be implemented before the next program is conducted. Obtain feedback about the preceptor program from the preceptees' perspective immediately following the program and at a later time, possibly six months and one year after their experience. Consider designing and implementing a research study to validate the effectiveness of your preceptor program on learning outcomes.

Summary

Preceptor programs are used as a clinical teaching method by both healthcare organizations and schools of nursing. Nurses who assume the role of preceptor require appropriate preparation and support in order to function effectively. The unit-based educator plays a pivotal role in coordinating unit-based preceptor programs and in evaluating their overall effectiveness related to safe, quality patient care and cost-effectiveness.

References

American Nurses Association. (1994). *Standards for nursing professional development: Continuing education and staff development.* Washington, DC: Author.

American Nurses Association. (2000). *Scope and standards of practice for nursing professional development.* Washington, DC: Author.

Anderson, J.K. (1998). Orientation with style: Matching teaching/learning style. *Journal for Nurses in Staff Development, 14,* 192–197.

Bashford, C.W. (2002). Breaking into orthopaedic nursing: Preceptorship for novice nurses. *Orthopaedic Nursing, 21*(3), 14–20.

Brehaut, C.J., Turik, L.J., & Wade, K.E. (1998). A pilot study to compare the effectiveness of preceptored and nonpreceptored models of clinical education in promoting baccalaureate students' competence in public health nursing. *Journal of Nursing Education, 37,* 376–380.

Bryant, S.C., & Williams, D. (2002). The senior practicum. *Nurse Educator, 27*(4), 174–177.

Chase, C.R. (2001). Learning style theories: Matching preceptors, learners, and teaching strategies in the perioperative setting. *Seminars in Perioperative Nursing, 10*(4), 184–187.

Finger, S.D., & Pape, T.M. (2002). Invitational theory and perioperative nursing preceptorships. *AORN Online, 76,* 630–642.

Frame, K.B., & Chrystal, C. (1999). Faculty and clinicians collaborate to teach basic intravenous skills to senior baccalaureate nursing students. *Journal of Intravenous Nursing, 22,* 253–256.

Freiburger, O.A. (2001). A tribute to clinical preceptors: Developing a preceptor program for nursing students. *Journal for Nurses in Staff Development, 17,* 320–327.

Freiburger, O.A. (2002). Preceptor programs: Increasing student self-confidence and competency. *Nurse Educator, 27*(2), 58–60.

Gaberson, K.B., & Oermann, M.H. (1999). *Clinical teaching strategies in nursing.* New York: Springer Publishing.

Gallo, A. (1999). So, you've been paired with a student nurse. *American Journal of Nursing, 99*(12), 24B, 24D.

Godinez, G., Schweiger, J., Gruver, J., & Ryan, P. (1999). Role transition from graduate to staff nurse: A qualitative analysis. *Journal for Nurses in Staff Development, 15,* 97–110.

Gurney, D. (2002). Developing a successful 16-week "transition ED nursing" program: One busy community hospital's experience. *Journal of Emergency Nursing, 28,* 505–514.

Haas, B.K., Deardorff, K.U., Klotz, L., Baker, B., Coleman, J., & DeWitt, A. (2002). Creating a collaborative partnership between academia and service. *Journal of Nursing Education, 41,* 518–523.

Hill, N., Wolf, K.N., Bossetti, B., & Saddam, A. (1999). Preceptor appraisals of rewards and student preparedness in the clinical setting. *Journal of Allied Health, 28*(2), 86–90.

Jackson, M. (2001). A preceptor incentive program: Rewarding staff nurses for mentorship. *American Journal of Nursing, 101*(6), 24A–24E.

Johantgen, M.A. (2001). Orientation to the critical care unit. The value of preceptor programs. *Critical Care Nursing Clinics of North America, 13*(1), 131–136.

Johnson, C.G. (1999). Evaluating preceptorship experiences in a distance learning program. *Journal of the National Black Nurses Association, 10*(2), 65–78.

Joint Commission on Accreditation of Healthcare Organizations. (2000). *Comprehensive accreditation manual for hospitals: The official handbook.* Oakbrook Terrace, IL: Author.

Laforet-Fliesser, Y., Ward-Griffin, C., & Beynon, C. (1999). Self-efficacy of preceptors in the community: A partnership between service and education. *Nurse Education Today, 19*(1), 41–52.

Lawless, R.P., Demers, K.A., & Baker, L. (2002). Preceptor program boosts recruitment and retention. *Caring, 21*(9), 10–12.

Letizia, M., & Jennrich, J. (1998). A review of preceptorship in undergraduate nursing education: Implications for staff development. *Journal of Continuing Education in Nursing, 29*(5), 211–216.

Lockwood-Rayermann, S. (2003). Preceptor leadership style and the nursing practicum. *Journal of Professional Nursing, 19*(1), 32–37.

Maes, S. (2000). Where have all the nurses gone? *ONS News, 15*(5), 1, 4–5.

Marquis, B.L., & Huston, C.J. (2000). *Leadership roles and management functions in nursing: Theory and application* (3rd ed.). Philadelphia: Lippincott.

McConnell, E.A., & Dadich, K.A. (1999). Crystallization of the professional self: A concentrated, senior clinical experience. *Nursing Connections, 12*(1), 5–13.

McGregor, R.J. (1999). A precepted experience for senior nursing students. *Nurse Educator, 24*(3), 13–16.

Mills, M.E., Jenkins, L.S., & Waltz, C.F. (2000). Emphasis courses: Preparing baccalaureate students for transition to the workforce. *Journal of Professional Nursing, 16,* 300–306.

Myrick, F. (2002). Preceptorship and critical thinking in nursing education. *Journal of Nursing Education, 41,* 154–164.

Myrick, F., & Yonge, O. (2001). Creating a climate for critical thinking in the preceptorship experience. *Nurse Education Today, 21,* 461–467.

Myrick, F., & Yonge, O. (2002a). Preceptor behaviors integral to the promotion of student critical thinking. *Journal for Nurses in Staff Development, 18,* 127–135.

Myrick, F., & Yonge, O. (2002b). Preceptor questioning and student critical thinking. *Journal of Professional Nursing, 18,* 176–181.

Nordgren, J., Richardson, S.J., & Laurella, V.B. (1998). A collaborative preceptor model for clinical teaching of beginning nursing students. *Nurse Educator, 23*(3), 27–32.

Oermann, M.H., & Gaberson, K.B. (1998). *Evaluation and testing in nursing education.* New York: Springer Publishing.

Ohrling, K., & Hallberg, I.R. (2000a). Nurses' lived experience of being a preceptor. *Journal of Professional Nursing, 16,* 228–239.

Ohrling, K., & Hallberg, I.R. (2000b). Student nurses' experiences of preceptorship. Part 2–the preceptor-preceptee relationship. *International Journal of Nursing Studies, 37*(1), 25–36.

Ohrling, K., & Hallberg, I.R. (2001). The meaning of preceptorship: Nurses lived experience of being a preceptor. *Journal of Advanced Nursing, 33,* 530–540.

Pfeil, M. (1999). Preceptorship: The progression from student to staff nurse. *Journal of Child Health Care, 3*(3), 13–18.

Purnell, L.D., & Paulanka, B.J. (1998). *Transcultural health care: A culturally competent approach.* Philadelphia: F.A. Davis.

Robbins, L.B. (1999). Learning outcomes of integrative preceptorships. *Nursing Connections, 12*(3), 19–34.

Sawin, K.J., Kissinger, J., Rowan, K.J., & Davis, M. (2001). Teaching strategies used by experienced preceptors. *Issues in Interdisciplinary Care, 3*(3), 197–206.

Schneiderman, J.U., Askew, L.M., & Reed, T.M. (2002). A clinical experience with foster families. *Nurse Educator, 27*(4), 178–181.

Souers, C. (2002). Teaching strategies. Comprehensive performance review: Preparing students for a preceptor experience. *Nurse Educator, 27*(1), 9–12.

Stone, C.L., & Rowles, C.J. (2002). What rewards do clinical preceptors in nursing think are important? *Journal for Nurses in Staff Development, 18,* 162–166.

Yonge, O., Krahn, H., Trojan, L., Reid, D., & Hasse, M. (2002). Being a preceptor is stressful! *Journal for Nurses in Staff Development, 18,* 22–27.

Yonge, O., Myrick, F., & Haase, M. (2002). Student nurse stress in the preceptorship experience. *Nurse Educator, 27*(2), 84–88.

Zimmermann, P.G. (2002). So you're going to precept nursing students: One instructor's suggestions. *Journal of Emergency Nursing, 28,* 589–592.

UNIT 3

Developing Unit-Based Educational Programs

CHAPTER

Creating an Educational Plan That Meets the Learning Needs of Nursing Staff

As mentioned in Chapters 1 and 3, many healthcare organizations have responded to recent healthcare trends by shifting the responsibility for staff education from nurse educators based in centralized nursing staff development departments to unit-based nursing staff (Leslie & Churilla, 1998; Lockhart & Bryce, 1996). As a result, some of the responsibility for staff development has been assumed by clinical staff nurses, who also provide direct care to patients, or nurses who coordinate patient care activities.

As mentioned in Chapter 2, staff development is defined as the "systematic process of assessment, development, and evaluation that enhances the performance or professional development of healthcare providers and their continuing competence" (National Nursing Staff Development Organization, 1999, p. 1). The American Nurses Association (ANA) described staff development activities as those that often are sponsored by healthcare organizations that employ healthcare workers, such as nurses, and "focus on competence assessment and development" (ANA, 2000, p. 5). These staff development activities consist of three components: orientation, in-service educational activities, and continuing education (CE) (ANA). Orientation was discussed in Chapter 4. In-service education and CE will be described later in Chapters 7 and 14, respectively.

This need for carefully planned staff education also is supported by the standards set forth by the Joint Commission on Accreditation of Healthcare Organizations (JCAHO, 2003). The mission of JCAHO was discussed in Chapter 3. The Occupational Safety and Health Administration (OSHA) also supports this need for planned staff education aimed at promoting a safe and healthy work environment (OSHA, 2003).

Unit-Based Education

Although clinical nurses possess expertise as direct care providers, their experience in assessing, planning, directing, and evaluating the education needs of other staff often is limited. Although most RNs received formal instruction in and experience with the teaching-learning process in their initial preparation as an RN, this educational content often focused on learners such as patients and groups of lay people in the community. It is likely that clinical nurses, therefore, will need additional instruction and guidance to effectively assume the role of a unit-based staff educator.

with any new endeavor, it is advantageous to seek the assistance of an experi-ed educator who can serve as a mentor. Because of their credentials, experi-and job responsibilities, nurses such as staff development educators, advanced ice nurses, and faculty at schools of nursing possess expertise in this area.

he responsibilities associated with assuming the role of a unit-based educator y among healthcare organizations. For example, in some workplaces, a desig-ed nurse or a group of nurses on a clinical unit may assume staff education activities. Some agencies rotate responsibility for educational duties among all staff nurses on the clinical unit. Regardless of the approach, it is important to understand that the primary expectations of the unit-based educator role may in-clude the following activities: determining the learning needs of the staff, coordi-nating and developing an overall education plan for the unit, implementing this plan, and evaluating its effectiveness.

Assuming this staff development responsibility requires that unit-based educa-tors rethink their role as an "educator" to include other roles assumed by staff development educators. As mentioned in Chapter 2, these roles include facilita-tor, change agent, consultant, researcher, and leader (ANA, 2000). Focus on these multiple roles when developing a unit's educational plan.

This chapter will explain a process that you, as a unit-based educator, can use to develop a unit-based educational plan to meet the learning needs of clinical staff nurses at your healthcare organization. Figure 6-1 provides an overview of these essential steps. An example of how this process was implemented will be presented later in this chapter.

Understanding the Educational Needs of Clinical Staff

Before developing a unit-based educational plan, talk with your manager to clarify the boundaries and dimensions of your new educational role. Ask if your responsibility is confined to your clinical unit or if it extends to other clinical units within your organization. Check if you are responsible for developing the educational plan for programs offered at an organizational level. Regardless of the extent of your responsibilities, make sure that they are clearly defined, reduc-ing role confusion or misinterpretation of your performance by others.

Discuss the time commitment associated with your new role. Determine if you possess 24-hour accountability for staff development on your unit or if your re-sponsibilities are limited to your as-signed shift. Check if educational du-ties are shared with other nursing staff on your unit. This information can be especially useful as you determine the resources available to you to implement the educational plan for the unit.

Although developing an educational plan may take time, it provides a solid foundation from which you can base your educational offerings for the clini-cal unit. The educational plan also can serve as a communication tool to clini-cal staff and maximize the success of your overall educational plan.

Figure 6-1.
Key Steps for Developing a Unit-Based Educational Plan

- Assess the learning needs of staff.
  - Define the learners.
  - Conduct a needs assessment.
- Analyze the needs assessment data.
- Develop a master education plan for the unit.
  - Seek available resources.
  - Suggest a variety of teaching resources.
- Implement the education plan.
  - Gain support from staff and adminis-tration.
  - Encourage staff input and participation.
  - Develop a support system for presenters.
  - Monitor program implementation and effectiveness.
- Evaluate the overall unit-based education plan.

Begin developing a unit-based educational plan by defining the learners. Then, determine their specific learning needs. This second step involves collecting pertinent information from the staff on your clinical unit and a variety of other sources. Each of these two steps will be discussed in the section that follows.

Defining the Learners

Clarify the learners for whom you assume responsibility. For instance, find out if you are expected to meet the staff development needs of only licensed nursing staff, such as RNs or licensed practical and licensed vocational nurses, or if your responsibilities extend to assistive personnel (AP) and unit secretaries. Investigate if other unit-based employees, such as social workers, nutritionists, or physical therapists, are considered among your learners.

Once you have identified the learners, collect information that may help you understand their learning needs, and gather information that can help you anticipate their participation in developing and implementing the educational plan, such as their strengths and clinical interests. Information about their educational background, both formal and informal, as well as prior clinical experience can help you tailor the level of educational activities.

For example, suppose that all the RNs on your unit are certified in oncology. Because these nurses have already demonstrated their knowledge in oncology at a certain level, they may request unit-based educational programs prepared at a more advanced level than staff who are unfamiliar with this content. This approach also holds true for AP whose educational background and experiences may vary from each other's.

If you are the unit-based staff educator assigned to your own clinical unit, then you probably have some experience working with the staff. For example, you may be familiar with their learning style and preferred teaching-learning strategy. The information that you have gained from working with the nursing staff can help you develop and implement the educational plan. However, if you are the educator for a unit unfamiliar to you, meet with the unit's nurse manager to gain this insight about the staff. Consider informal discussions with staff members to obtain this information.

Conduct a Needs Assessment

Once you have determined who the learners are, conduct a thorough assessment of their learning needs that relate to their work on the clinical unit (ANA, 2000). Because assessing the learning needs of nursing staff should be a continuous, ongoing process (ANA), develop an approach that will help you accomplish this goal. For example, consider conducting a systematic needs assessment on your unit each year, allowing for additional learning needs to be added to this list as they arise.

Use a variety of direct and indirect sources to gather data regarding the learning needs of staff (ANA, 2000). Suggestions for sources to use when developing a needs assessment will be described in the following section of this chapter. Finally, use a method to assess learning needs that will allow you to easily track and access these data in the future (ANA).

Needs Identified by Learners

Be creative in assessing the learning needs of staff, and consider using both quantitative and qualitative approaches. One strategy frequently used by staff educators is to ask each learner to respond in writing to a preprinted needs assessment questionnaire developed by the unit-based educator. Figure 6-2 is a sample questionnaire that can be used with staff.

In this example, staff are asked to focus on learning needs that are specific to their role at the healthcare agency. Then, they rank the importance of each learning need using descriptors ranging from "essential to know" to "nice to know." Asking staff to rank each learning need will help you organize and prioritize the identified learning needs.

Francke, Garssen, Abu-Saad, and Grypdonck (1996) used several qualitative strategies to assess the learning needs of surgical oncology nurses regarding pain management. Data obtained from observations conducted on the clinical unit and interviews with patients and nurses on the unit were used to develop a CE program on pain management for these nurses.

Hopkins (2002) developed a tool designed to assess the learning needs of nurses responsible for supervising nursing assistants using a different approach. This strategy focused on issues related to delegation and obtained input regarding nurses' cognitive deficits. Results obtained through this process were used to design educational programs aimed at remedying these deficits.

Consider implementing successful approaches used by other organizations to assess learning needs in your setting. For example, the education committee of the local chapter of a national professional nursing organization used e-mail to assess the learning needs of its members (L. Worrall, personal communication, July 2, 2003). In an attempt to avoid overwhelming its members, the committee divided the needs assessment questionnaire into smaller sections that were transmitted at various times to members via e-mail. An incentive was provided to the first member who responded.

In addition to questionnaires, consider conducting focus group sessions with unit staff to explore their learning needs. Focus groups are meetings in which individuals gather to answer questions on a particular topic (Polit & Beck, 2004). For example, schedule a focus group session with staff nurses from your unit. Ask them to respond to a series of open-ended questions you developed that will help you identify their learning needs. This approach allows staff an opportunity to discuss their learning needs with you personally and may help you clarify the learning needs they identify.

Another approach is to ask the nurse manager on the unit to have staff discuss their learning needs following their annual performance appraisal meeting. This approach can help staff focus on learning needs based on their projected goals for the following year.

In addition to conducting a needs assessment, review feedback obtained from participants who attended past educational programs (ANA, 2000). Evaluation forms used in CE programs often include a question in which participants are asked to identify their future learning needs that may or may not be related to the CE program they attended. Include these data, if appropriate, in your needs assessment results.

Whatever method you choose, be sure that the learning needs of each staff member on the unit are equally represented. Avoid letting the unit education needs be determined by a few vocal or assertive staff members. It is important to obtain feedback from each learner so that your educational plan represents the needs of all staff.

When collecting information about learning needs, consider asking staff to identify their preferred method of learning unit-based programs. Figure 6-2 illus-

Figure 6-2.
Sample Needs
Assessment Form

Unit 6B Staff Needs Assessment

Instructions: In order to assist you in providing quality care to patients on your unit, we would like you to identify your learning needs. Using the form below, please list your personal top 10 learning needs for the upcoming year. Next, rank them from 1 (essential to know) to 5 (nice to know). Return your completed needs assessment form to the staff development box located in your conference room by October 1, 2004. Thank you for your input.

Learning need topic	1 (essential to know)	2	3	4	5 (nice to know)
1.					
2.					
3.					
4.					
5.					
6.					
7.					
8.					
9.					
10.					

Place an X next to your preferred learning method(s):
_____ Lecture and discussion
_____ Case presentations
_____ Posters
_____ Displays
_____ Self-learning modules
_____ Journal article review (journal club)
_____ Audiovisuals (video, slides)
_____ Written materials (pamphlets, books)
_____ Games and simulations
_____ Computer-assisted instruction
_____ Other (describe) _____

Name: _____   Date: _____

trates how this feature can be added to a needs assessment questionnaire. For example, ask staff if they favor learning by teaching strategies such as posters, unit-based lectures with discussions, self-learning modules, or other strategies. Provide staff with a list of teaching-learning strategies from which to choose. Also consider asking them to identify the best day(s) and time(s) for scheduling face-to-face sessions, such as a unit-based in-service session on their unit.

Ensure that all staff have an opportunity to share their learning needs. One approach is to enclose the needs assessment questionnaire in their payroll envelope or to attach the form to their annual performance appraisal evaluation.

Carefully schedule the date when staff need to return their completed needs assessments. Give yourself enough time, perhaps as much as one or two months, to organize the data, conduct an analysis, and develop the educational plan.

Needs Determined by Other Sources

In addition to capturing the learning needs as perceived by the staff themselves, consider other valuable sources that will help you identify other needs. Talk with nurse managers, supervisors, physicians, and other interdisciplinary healthcare workers who interact on a daily basis with the nursing staff. They can provide you with suggestions that can be incorporated into the unit's educational plan. These individuals also may have information regarding future plans for the unit that may necessitate other unit-based programs.

For example, the unit's nurse manager may know that a group of physicians plans to admit ventilator-dependent patients to your unit next year. This information can help you be proactive in meeting the learning needs of staff regarding the care of these patients. The unit's nutritionist may ask for your help in solving a problem associated with the incorrect administration of enteral feedings to patients on the unit. Although not all suggestions may warrant educational programs for staff, input from a variety of sources can help the unit's educational plan to be as comprehensive as possible.

Indications about the learning needs of staff also can be uncovered through research investigations conducted in your organization. For example, a retrospective review of hospital records was conducted to explore factors related to early readmission of elderly patients (Timms, Parker, Fallat, & Johnson, 2002). Findings revealed insufficient documentation in these records. Staff development educators addressed this learning need.

Feedback from your organization's committee reports and documents, such as incident reports, quality assurance reports, or patient satisfaction surveys, may be extremely useful in confirming the learning needs of staff. For instance, an increase in medication errors associated with IV medication administration may suggest the need for review of this material. Similarly, an increased number of patient falls following their surgery may warrant a review of safety precautions for staff.

Some learning needs for nursing staff are mandated not only by healthcare organizations but also by their regulatory and accreditation agencies, such as JCAHO and OSHA. For example, JCAHO requires staff to demonstrate ongoing competence on critical issues, such as providing cardiopulmonary resuscitation; emergency, fire, and safety policies; proper disposal of hazardous materials and wastes; and infection control policies. These topics should be included in each unit's educational plan.

As mentioned in Chapter 4, many healthcare organizations conduct annual unit-based clinical competency testing sessions in which staff verify their knowledge and skills in prescribed areas related to patient care. These sessions should be an integral part of the educational plan.

In addition to assessing the current learning needs of staff, anticipate any future learning requirements that may stem from changes in unit goals and affiliations, patient care needs, technology, and documentation. For example, suppose your clinical unit has just been designated as a clinical site to be used by undergraduate and graduate students enrolled in a nearby school of nursing. It will be necessary to help staff understand the expectations of these students and to prepare staff nurses for their role as preceptors.

Perhaps you learned that physicians will start admitting international patients to your clinical unit next year. Obviously, you will need to help staff understand the needs of these patients related to cultural diversity. If new discharge procedures are developed for your organization, provide a mechanism to orient staff on these changes before the procedure begins.

Finally, consider initiatives communicated by professional nursing organizations or healthcare trends (ANA, 2000), such as the recent emphasis on strengthening palliative care skills of clinical nursing staff.

Analyze the Needs Assessment Data

Once you have collected the learning needs of staff from all possible sources, then you can organize these requests. One way to start this process is to sort these requests according to similar topics. Record each topic, along with its assigned priority rank from 1 to 10 as indicated by staff, on a separate sheet of paper, or use an appropriate computer program. Rather than eliminating redundant suggestions, record their frequency as an indication of need. Multiple requests for meeting the same learning need indicate a priority need perceived by staff on your unit.

Next, attempt to group smaller topics under the umbrella headings of larger groups. For example, if staff cited topics such as breath sounds, heart sounds, and bowel sounds, group these topics under the heading "physical assessment skills." This technique makes the needs list more manageable, minimizes duplication of content, and helps in designing educational programs.

If you are surveying the learning needs for staff located on more than one unit, it may be helpful to sort results on a unit-specific basis. Compare identified learning needs across all the units for common topics. Anticipate requests for similar topics that are shared by more than one unit.

After you have organized and tallied these needs, prioritize them by their frequency of occurrence. For instance, if "proper use of a pulse oximeter" was cited 15 times, and "review of tracheostomy tube care" was cited 25 times, you would assign the latter request a higher priority number or score. This approach helps you meet the learning needs expressed (as the top 10) by the greatest number of staff members. This process also should result in a smaller and more manageable learning needs list for the unit.

Reexamine this list based on their priority related to unit goals and patient care outcomes. Reorganize the list based on their frequency of occurrence on the clinical unit and their criticality. For example, assign a high rank of urgency to learning needs that have a direct impact on the quality and safety of patient care. This would include critical care skills for nurses who care for patients immediately postoperatively on a head and neck surgical unit. Place mandatory learning needs, such as those required by JCAHO and OSHA, early in the unit's educational plan to ensure their inclusion.

Consider discussing the results of the analysis with the nurse manager of the clinical unit, if appropriate. The manager can help you validate the needs you identified. Meet with staff to discuss the results and clarify their suggestions, if necessary.

Develop a Master Education Plan for the Unit

Once you have organized and prioritized the learning needs of staff, sequence them within a reasonable time frame. For example, arrange topics by month, based on a one-year time period. Depending on your unit's needs, organize the plan by either a calendar year (January through December) or fiscal year (July through June). Although you essentially have planned many of the learning needs for the entire year, divide your plan into two or more smaller pieces, each piece reflecting a plan for a four- or six-month time period. This approach will make the plan seem more manageable and will allow you to focus your efforts. When designing your annual plan, be sure to adjust the schedule based on unit patterns or trends, such as holidays, vacations, or changes in patient census.

Development of a Matrix

Once the educational needs are prioritized by month, develop a matrix that aids in the conceptualization of the plan. One approach, first depicted by Siegel (1991) and later expanded upon by Lockhart and Bryce (1996), is presented in Table 6-1. This six-month educational plan was designed by staff development educators for meeting the specialty unit-based education needs of nursing staff on a head and neck surgical unit in an academic medical center. In addition to listing in-service and CE topics arranged by month, they also identified possible resources, such as individuals who could serve as presenters, and a variety of traditional and nontraditional teaching strategies. Mandatory education and competency verification programs also were scheduled into this plan for the unit.

This model offers several advantages for helping staff become involved in planning a unit's education needs (Lockhart & Bryce, 1996). Sharing this plan with staff on the unit is a convenient way to communicate projected educational offerings in advance. Although a unit-based educator developed the plan, staff provided their input. Staff members not only have an opportunity to view the entire educational needs of staff on the unit but also can see where their particular learning needs fall within this plan. Staff can choose to present on a topic with which they are familiar and select a date and time that will give them sufficient opportunity to prepare. Suggestions for teaching strategies supplied on the grid also provide staff with a head start in designing their unit-based projects.

Another advantage of this model is that it permits the unit-based educator to accommodate new learning needs assessed after implementation of the plan (Lockhart & Bryce, 1996). Learning needs, such as the introduction of new equipment, medications, and procedures mentioned earlier in this chapter, can be easily satisfied, especially if the scheduling of content is kept to a reasonable level.

Although the educational plan is intended to serve as a guide in helping the unit-based educator meet the learning needs of staff, its ultimate outcome is to help nursing staff provide safe, quality patient care (Lockhart & Bryce, 1996).

Table 6-1. Six-Month Unit-Based Educational Plan								
Assessed Needs	JAN	FEB	MAR	APR	MAY	JUN	Resource	Teaching Strategy
Critical care clinical skill	x Monitor awareness		x Spinal drain		x PA catheters		Staff nurse	Unit-based in-service
Care of the patient's family		x					Social service	Unit-based in-service
Care of cranial base patients			x				Clinical instructor Staff nurse	Specialty orientation Unit-based in-service
Ethical issues	x	x	x	x	x	x	Center for medical ethics	Ethics for Lunch
Documentation		x		x			Staff nurse	Demonstration
Skin care	x						Clinical instructor	Flow chart
ENT emergencies			x	x		x	Clinical instructor Staff nurse	Specialty orientation Unit-based in-service
Surgical oncology update					x		Clinical nurse specialist	Unit-based in-service
Care of the alcoholic or abusive patient							Clinical specialist Social worker	Conference
Discharge teaching	x			x			Case manager	Poster
Physical assessment		x Respiratory	x Neuro		x Cardiac		Staff nurse	Unit-based in-service
Pharmacology update		x					Staff nurse	Poster
Tube feedings			x				Staff nurse	Unit-based in-service
CPR		x					Clinical instructor	Demonstration
Mandatory recertifications				x			Clinical instructor	Self-learning module
Competency verification						x	Clinical instructor	Peer review and testing

Note. Based on information from Lockhart & Bryce, 1996.

Because of this patient-focused priority, the educational plan should be flexible and not perceived as a mandate for staff learning.

Choosing a Staff Development Component

When developing your educational plan, determine which staff development component (orientation, in-service education, or CE) would be the best approach in meeting each learning need. For example, you may decide that a brief, unit-based in-service may be the best approach for helping current staff update their skills on a new medication protocol. You decide to add this information to your existing orientation program so new employees will be familiar with it before they work on the clinical units. Perhaps staff identified learning needs on physical assessment that could be met through a series of separate in-service sessions or as a one-day CE program.

Although staff may prefer unit-based in-service presentations as a format for educational offerings, consider other creative, less structured approaches that are not only cost-effective but can be easily incorporated into the nursing staff's work schedule. Track these informal educational activities, and include them in the unit's educational plan. The professional development of nurses involves a mixture of approaches (Incalcattera, 1999).

For example, an integrated educational approach to staff development was described by Arbour (2003), who needed to improve the administration and monitoring practices of surgical intensive care nurses related to sedatives, analgesics, and neuromuscular blocking agents. A combination of in-service education, bedside instruction, competency-based education modules, and orientation were used as quality improvement strategies. These methods were effective in meeting the learning needs of these nurses and in improving their nursing practice.

Seek Available Resources

Before seeking available resources for meeting these assessed learning needs, clarify your role in this educational plan. Although you may choose to present some of the educational sessions, you need to be available and mentor staff. Because of the diversity of learning needs in the educational plan, you will need to rely on others for assistance and support. You are not expected to be an expert on the various learning needs in the plan (Lockhart & Bryce, 1996). In fact, attempting to fulfill this unreasonable expectation has the potential to decrease your credibility. Rather, develop a strategy to deliver educational programs that not only maximize existing resources but also promote the professional development of staff. This approach requires you to focus on your other staff development roles: being a "leader" or "facilitator" of educational planning, being a "change agent" in developing a new approach to implementing the plan, and acting as a "consultant" to nursing staff who need to learn how to present these programs.

Once the learning needs of staff and projected times for meeting these needs are communicated, conduct a brainstorming session with staff to identify resources that exist within the workplace to meet these needs. Although some organizations allocate money in a clinical unit's budget for staff education purposes, these funds often are limited and restricted to CE programs rather than unit-based efforts. However, it is realistic to expect quality yet cost-effective unit-based in-service programs.

Start by thinking how some of the learning needs can be met through content that already exists within ongoing educational offerings at your workplace. As illustrated in Table 6-1, Lockhart and Bryce (1996) identified topics such as "ENT

Emergencies" and "Care of Cranial Base Patients" as content presented in an ongoing specialty orientation for staff. Therefore, they invited experienced nurses from the clinical unit to attend these sessions at their regularly scheduled times along with new orientees. Another learning need on ethical issues was addressed by communicating the dates and location of a series of monthly hospital-wide ethics sessions conducted during lunchtime.

Various individuals from your agency, such as staff nurses, clinical nurse specialists, clinical instructors, and other members of the interdisciplinary healthcare team, can be targeted as potential presenters. If nursing students use your unit for their clinical practicum, remember to include both faculty and students as potential speakers. Students, along with their colleagues in other classes, often need to conduct an education session as a course requirement. Nursing faculty can help update staff on topics pertaining to teaching, research, or publishing. Investigate education services available from representatives of pharmaceutical and supply companies. Many purchasing agreements include these services as well as provide printed materials and samples free of charge. Consider contacting your vendors for teaching materials and supplies for these programs.

Maximize available resources by collaborating with staff from other clinical units within your organization. For example, because some of the education needs identified in Table 6-1 were similar to those needs cited by nursing staff working on an adjacent clinical unit, Lockhart and Bryce (1996) scheduled joint unit-based programs, inviting staff from both units. Because another limited resource cited was sufficient space in which to conduct programs on the unit, try to share conference rooms and displays for in-service presentations that are of interest to more than one unit. For example, Lockhart and Bryce displayed a drug update bulletin board that was used by two patient care units on a rotating basis.

Suggest a Variety of Teaching Strategies

Encourage presenters to use a variety of teaching strategies in their educational programs. Inform them of staff preferences. Specific factors that educators should consider when selecting a teaching strategy for an educational activity will be discussed later in Chapter 7.

The positive impact of multiple teaching strategies on learning outcomes was demonstrated in a recent study conducted by Zapp (2001). Two staff development classes were implemented, one in which the educator used only lecture as the teaching strategy and another class in which learners were exposed to a variety of teaching strategies. Learners in the latter group attained significantly higher scores of knowledge acquisition and satisfaction than the learners who received the lecture-only class.

A variety of teaching strategies have been effective in enabling learners to attain the objectives of education programs in staff development. Figure 6-3 illustrates various teaching strategies that can be used to meet the learning needs of staff on a clinical unit.

- Lecture and discussion
- Case presentations
- Posters and bulletin boards
- Education fairs
- Clinical unit and clinical simulations
- Self-learning packets and modules
- Journal article review (journal club)
- Audiovisuals (video, Microsoft® PowerPoint®, slides, overhead transparencies)
- Written materials (pamphlets, books)
- Games and simulations
- Computer-assisted instruction, CD-ROMs, Internet

Figure 6-3. Teaching Strategies Available for Unit-Based Staff Development Programs

s

cational information presented in poster formats, including interactive
boards (Flournoy, Turner, & Combs, 2000) and storyboards (Hayes &
ss, 1999), can be effective teaching strategies for nursing staff to attain
outcomes. Various experts have supported the benefits of posters in their
ations through educational research and other investigations.

Doyle and Klein (2001) supported the benefits of using a poster session format
(PSF) compared with a traditional film discussion format (FDF) on post-test scores
of a knowledge test that dealt with violence in the workplace for hospital staff.
Participants who learned the program content by walking through a PSF at their
own pace had greater improved test scores than the FDF learners.

Thurber and Asselin (1999), who included posters in a three-day educational
fair designed to meet hospital-wide mandatory education requirements, also expressed the positive impact of poster presentations. Interactive stations on fire safety
and body mechanics allowed staff to actively participate in the learning process.
The authors concluded that poster sessions were a cost-effective teaching strategy
that resulted in positive learning outcomes.

Self-Learning Packets

Self-learning packets or modules are cost-effective educational tools used in
staff development (O'Very, 1999). These packets can be easily designed and consist of objectives, content, handouts, and audiovisuals, if appropriate. Learners
review these materials at their own pace, then complete an evaluation, which is
included in the packet. Other media can be used to deliver self-learning modules,
such as computer software or Web-based programs.

Clinical Unit and Laboratory Simulations

The clinical unit also can serve as a resource for teaching strategies. Segal and
Mason (1998) described their success in using teaching rounds focused on pain
management with nurses on a medical-surgical unit. This interactive clinical teaching strategy offered staff nurses an opportunity to strengthen their pain assessment skills as well as their interpersonal skills with patients and staff.

The patient care setting can be replicated using a clinical simulation laboratory where nurses can strengthen their practice skills. If this facility is not available at your organization, gain entry into one through an affiliated school of nursing. If budget constraints limit your access to teaching models, consider developing your own low-cost clinical teaching tools (Ross, 2000).

Games and Simulations

Various games and simulations, such as role-play, have been effective teaching
strategies with nursing staff employed in healthcare settings. In fact, some staff
educators have used games as a strategy to determine the learning styles of participants (Shaubach, 2000).

For example, Henry (1997) used a game format with staff nurses to enhance
their learning during an Infection Control Week, a mandatory in-service education program. Results supported this as an effective, stimulating teaching strategy
that allowed learners to receive immediate feedback on performance and application of principles within a realistic clinical setting.

Card games, word games (Stringer, 1997), and reproductions of game shows such as Jeopardy!^{SM} ("Tips," 1998) also have been used successfully in staff development. For example, educators used the card game Recall Rummy to reinforce clinical skills in nurses (Youseffi, Caldwell, Hadnot, & Blake, 2000).

Computer Technology and Multimedia

Consider using various audiovisual equipment to help staff learn in the clinical setting. If computers are available to staff in your setting, consider including various multimedia software, such as CD-ROMs (Backonja, 2001), or the Internet (Girotti, 1998; Hayes, Huckstadt, & Gibson, 2000) in your instruction. Be proactive in developing strategies to help nurses who are new to computers overcome possible barriers they may experience (Mamary & Charles, 2000).

Implement the Education Plan

After sharing the unit's education plan with staff, focus on strategies to successfully implement it. This involves gaining support from those affected by the plan, encouraging ongoing staff input and participation, and developing a support system for presenters. In addition, be sure to monitor the program's implementation and overall effectiveness. Chapter 7 will illustrate one method for helping nurses learn how to develop and present a unit-based in-service program. Practical suggestions are provided.

Gaining Support From Staff and Administration

Obtaining support from both staff and administration on the unit can help maximize the success of the education plan. Be sure to communicate the plan to everyone involved and ask for their input. Lockhart and Bryce (1996) acknowledged the support of the unit's clinical nurse manager as instrumental to the success of their unit-based education plan.

Encouraging Staff Input and Participation

Having staff provide input and participate in the education plan can foster a sense of ownership in the plan and maximize its success. As suggested earlier in this chapter, ask staff to identify their individual learning needs and respond to the initial draft of the plan. Then post the final matrix on the unit, asking staff to participate in approving the plan. As illustrated in Table 6-1, identify specific topics that can be assumed by staff nurses. The actual number of topics staff may be asked to present depends on a variety of factors, such as the size and mix of nursing staff, available resources, and the teaching experience and comfort level of the staff. It may be advantageous to begin the process with an experienced staff nurse who can serve as a positive role model.

Ask staff for their input in determining the best times and location for these unit-based efforts. For example, decide if it is best to schedule a program in the early morning, at lunch, or at change of shift. If the unit has 12-hour shifts, then determine the best time to accommodate the evening staff. Consider the number of times to repeat the program to ensure that all staff have an opportunity to attend. Decide where the programs will be conducted, such as the unit's conference room or in a place away from the unit. Many of these details need to be discussed and finalized before the overall education program for the unit is implemented.

In their unit-based staff development program, Lockhart and Bryce (1996) found that a hospital-wide clinical advancement program for staff nurses provided an incentive for staff to pursue professional activities. Presenting unit-based programs was part of the performance appraisal system for staff nurses and a criterion for promotion. The authors timed this requirement with an ongoing unit-based teaching project designed to help staff learn how to present a unit-based in-service program. This provided staff with the necessary information that empowered them to succeed in their new role. This project will be described in more detail in Chapter 7.

Developing a Support System for Presenters

It is essential to provide a support system for staff if they are expected to serve as presenters of unit-based education programs. Some nurses may be experienced in preparing and presenting educational programs, but this endeavor may be a new and uncomfortable one for others. Even though some staff may be at ease in giving presentations at regional or national conferences, they may fear sharing their expertise with peers at work. Therefore, it is important to determine the individual needs of each staff member and develop ways to create a nonthreatening environment on the unit. Remind staff to view this experience as part of the learning process related to professional development. Most likely, their comfort level will increase with repeated practice. Emphasize the added marketability of having effective presentation skills.

Create a nonthreatening environment when scheduling staff to present unit-based programs. For example, rather than presenting a program alone at first, some nurses may prefer to work on projects as a group or in pairs. Advise staff to start with a teaching strategy with which they are most comfortable. For example, rather than an oral presentation, a poster or the demonstration of a clinical skill may place a staff nurse more at ease when conducting an in-service offering for the first time. Suggest that the staff present on topics with which they possess clinical expertise. If possible, try videotaping the unit-based sessions. This approach not only provides staff with an opportunity to review their own presentation skills, but it also is a convenient way to give staff who are unable to attend the program a chance to benefit from it. Be sure to provide guidance and constructive feedback for staff during this entire learning process.

Monitor Program Implementation and Effectiveness

Develop a way to monitor the daily activities and progress of the unit's education plan. The manner in which you accomplish this depends on the existing structures within your healthcare organization and available resources. You may elect to track the overall plan yourself or decide to create a unit-based committee of staff members to help you accomplish this.

In addition to overseeing the operations of the program, it is essential to have a structure to judge the effectiveness of the overall education plan. This function will be addressed in greater detail in the evaluation section that follows.

Evaluate the Overall Unit-Based Education Plan

Along with implementing the unit-based education plan, attempt to determine both its effectiveness and efficiency in meeting the learning needs of clinical staff.

This evaluation process should be an ongoing one (ANA, 2000). It is important to focus on the overall plan itself, in addition to the impact of specific unit-based programs on learners' competencies. Information about evaluating specific program outcomes will be discussed in greater detail in Chapters 7 and 14. Although you may be able to evaluate the overall education plan yourself as the staff educator, it is valuable to invite input from clinical staff affected by the overall plan. Evaluation of the education plan is an ongoing process, and it is extremely helpful to formally evaluate the plan at least six months and one year following its implementation. You can use the results from the evaluation to refine the approach you will take in developing the following year's unit-based education plan.

Be sure to use a comprehensive approach when evaluating each unit's education plan. Start by identifying the main components of the process used in developing the plan, as described throughout this chapter: assessing the learning needs of staff, analyzing the data, developing a master education plan, and implementing the education plan. Figure 6-4 provides examples of questions that can be included in the evaluation process. Other questions may be added based upon your specific concerns. Note the overall strengths and weaknesses of the education plan, and focus upon both its degrees of effectiveness and its efficiency in providing quality, cost-effective education. Remember that the ultimate goal of this evaluation is to improve upon the approach you use to meet the unit-based education needs of clinical staff in strengthening their clinical competencies.

While evaluating the overall education plan, be sure to monitor for changes in quality indicators collected and monitored by the clinical units. These include measures such as patient and staff satisfaction surveys, quality assurance outcomes, competency testing of nursing staff, and employee performance appraisals. Although these measures can reflect a variety of changes that occur on the clinical unit, they can be used to understand the impact of the unit's education plan. Regardless of the indices you use, it is important that you obtain a complete picture of the process.

Assessing the learning needs of staff
- Were the learning needs of staff captured accurately?
- Were the data representative of all staff?
- Were data collected in an efficient and timely manner?

Analyzing the data
- Did the data analysis results reflect the overall learning needs of staff?
- How could the data analysis process be expedited?
- How can this process be facilitated in the future?

Developing a master education plan
- Was limiting the plan to a six-month time period manageable?
- Did the staff feel actively involved in the development process?
- Was the plan realistic?

- Were the plan flexible enough to permit the inclusion of new needs or changes?

Implementing the education plan
- Were staff prepared adequately to present unit-based programs?
- What teaching strategies did presenters use?
- Was the approach used cost-effective?
- What was the response of clinical staff involved?
- Did the process go smoothly?
- How did staff respond to their new role as providers of education?
- Did the staff feel prepared to present unit-based in-service programs?
- Could some programs be marketed to the community?
- How much individual assistance did staff need to present programs?

Figure 6-4.
Evaluating the Overall Education Plan: Key Components

Summary

Many clinical nurses have taken on unit-based education responsibilities previously assumed by clinical instructors in centralized staff development departments. This chapter provides information on how to assess the learning needs of clinical staff, design a comprehensive unit-based educational plan, implement the plan, and evaluate its overall effectiveness.

References

American Nurses Association. (2000). *Scope and standards of practice for nursing professional development.* Washington, DC: Author.

Arbour, R. (2003). A continuous quality improvement approach to improving clinical practice in the areas of sedation, analgesia, and neuromuscular blockade. *Journal of Continuing Education in Nursing, 34*(2), 64–71.

Backonja, M. (2001). Media reviews: CD-ROM for clinical staff development. *Journal of Pain and Symptom Management, 21*(1), 83.

Doyle, L.M., & Klein, M.C. (2001). Comparison of two methods of instruction for the prevention of workplace violence. *Journal for Nurses in Staff Development, 17,* 281–293.

Flournoy, E., Turner, G., & Combs, D. (2000). Staff development. Innovative teaching: Read the writing on the wall. *Dimensions of Critical Care Nursing, 19*(4), 36–37.

Francke, A.L., Garssen, B., Abu-Saad, H.H., & Grypdonck, M. (1996). Qualitative needs assessment prior to conducting a continuing education program. *Journal of Continuing Education in Nursing, 27*(1), 34–41.

Girotti, R.B. (1998). Developing an Internet in-service. *Nursing Spectrum, 2*(23), 7.

Hayes, K., Huckstadt, A., & Gibson, R. (2000). Developing interactive continuing education on the Web. *Journal of Continuing Education in Nursing, 31*(5), 199–203.

Hayes, S.K., & Childress, D.M. (1999). Fairy tales of storyboarding. *Journal for Nurses in Staff Development, 15,* 260–262.

Henry, J.M. (1997). Gaming: A teaching strategy to enhance adult learning. *Journal of Continuing Education in Nursing, 28*(5), 231–234.

Hopkins, D.L. (2002). Evaluating the knowledge deficits of registered nurses responsible for supervising nursing assistants: A learning needs assessment tool. *Journal for Nurses in Staff Development, 18,* 152–156.

Incalcattera, E. (1999). Is it continuing education or is it in-service? *New Jersey Nurse, 29*(6), 11.

Joint Commission on Accreditation of Healthcare Organizations. (2003). *Who is the Joint Commission?* Retrieved July 1, 2003, from http://www.jcaho.org

Leslie, M.L., & Churilla, P.G. (1998). Unit-based education: Meeting the needs of staff nurses in the 90's. *ORL-Head and Neck Nursing, 16*(2), 12–14.

Lockhart, J.S., & Bryce, J. (1996). A comprehensive plan to meet the unit-based education needs of nurses from several specialty units. *Journal for Nurses in Staff Development, 12,* 135–138.

Mamary, E.M., & Charles, P. (2000). On-site to on-line: Barriers to the use of computers for continuing education. *Journal of Continuing Education in the Health Care Professions, 20*(3), 171–175.

National Nursing Staff Development Organization. (1999). *Strategic plan 2000.* Pensacola, FL: Author.

Occupational Safety and Health Administration. (2003). *OSHA's mission.* Retrieved January 11, 2004, from http://www.osha.gov/oshinfo/mission.html

O'Very, D.I. (1999). Self-paced: The right place for staff development. *Journal of Continuing Education in Nursing, 30*(4), 182–187.

Polit, D.F., & Beck, C.T. (2004). *Nursing research: Principles and methods* (7th ed.). Philadelphia: Lippincott Williams & Wilkins.

Ross, C.A. (2000). Teaching tools: Developing low-cost clinical teaching tools. *Nurse Educator, 25*(3), 116.

Segal, S., & Mason, D.J. (1998). The art and science of teaching rounds: A strategy for staff development. *Journal for Nurses in Staff Development, 14,* 127–136.

Shaubach, K.C. (2000). Staff development stories. Using games to determine learning styles. *Journal for Nurses in Staff Development, 16,* 293–295.

Siegel, H. (1991). Innovative approaches to in-service education. *Journal for Nurses in Staff Development, 22,* 147–151.

Stringer, E.C. (1997). Focus. Word games as a cost-effective and innovative in-service method. *Journal for Nurses in Staff Development, 13*(3), 155–160.

Thurber, R.F., & Asselin, M.E. (1999). An educational fair and poster approach to organization-wide mandatory education. *Journal of Continuing Education in Nursing, 30*(1), 25–29.

Timms, J., Parker, V.G., Fallat, E.H., & Johnson, W.H. (2002). Documentation of characteristics of early hospital readmission of elderly patients: A challenge for in-service educators. *Journal for Nurse in Staff Development, 18,* 136–145.

Tips from the field. Lighten up April in-service with a "Jeopardy!" game. (1998). *Homecare Education Management, 3*(4), 62–65.

Youseffi, F., Caldwell, R., Hadnot, P., & Blake, B.J. (2000). Recall Rummy: Learning can be fun . . . a card game to reinforce proper skill techniques. *Journal of Continuing Education in Nursing, 31*(4), 161–162.

Zapp, L. (2001). Use of multiple teaching strategies in the staff development setting. *Journal for Nurses in Staff Development, 17,* 206–212.

CHAPTER

Helping Staff Present a Unit-Based In-Service Educational Program

After you, as a unit-based educator, have developed the education plan for your clinical unit as described in Chapter 6, consider strategies that will enable staff nurses to actively participate in this plan. Although some of these learning needs can be integrated into your unit's orientation program, as discussed in Chapter 4, probably most of them will be managed through either in-service education activities on your clinical unit or through continuing education (CE) programs. CE programs will be discussed later in Chapter 14. Nurses play an important role in all three of these components of staff development.

As mentioned in Chapter 2, in-service education activities are "learning experiences designed to help nurses acquire, maintain, or increase their competence in fulfilling their responsibility to deliver quality health care" American Nurses Association [ANA], 2000, p. 6). Similar to orientation and CE programs, in-service education activities focus on competence assessment and development (ANA, 2000).

As mentioned in Chapter 2, in-service educational activities are brief, usually less than 50 minutes long, and include topics that apply to the healthcare organization (Incalcattera, 1999). In-service education programs often focus on equipment updates, reviews of policies and procedures, documentation changes, and mandatory topics such as fire safety and infection control. The programs can be presented using any of the teaching strategies discussed earlier in Chapter 6.

Clinical nurses are expected to participate as learners in educational activities in an attempt to acquire and sustain their current knowledge and competency in nursing practice (ANA, 1998). Nurses also are expected to share their clinical expertise with other nurses and student nurses and contribute to a work environment that promotes clinical learning (ANA, 1998). In-service program activities offer clinical nurses an opportunity to meet these expectations of both learner and educator. Unit-based educators can play a significant role in mentoring nurses to develop their skills as an educator.

A Model for Helping Nurses Develop an In-Service Program

A model that was effective in helping staff nurses learn how to develop and present in-service educational activities was described by nursing staff development educators who worked in a large, university-affiliated medical center (Lockhart & Bryce, 1996). This model included a 30-minute instructional session called "How to Develop a Unit-Based In-Service Offering (UBIO)." The primary purpose of the UBIO was to help staff nurses learn how to plan, implement, and evaluate an in-service program on their clinical unit. Content focused on the entire educational process, from assessing learning needs to evaluating learning outcomes. The UBIO will be described and referred to throughout this chapter.

Unit-based clinical nurses completed the UBIO several months prior to the implementation of the unit's educational plan (Lockhart & Bryce, 1996). This timing gave staff nurses an opportunity to use the information they learned in the UBIO when developing their own in-service education program and to minimize any anxiety they experienced about presenting to their peers. In addition to providing nurses with this instructional session, the authors mentored them on an individual basis to help them develop their in-service educational programs. The UBIO was repeated at various times on several clinical units.

Handouts describing the key points of the UBIO, distributed during the session, were instrumental in contributing to the model's success and learning outcomes (Lockhart & Bryce, 1996). For example, providing information in print form enabled the learners to focus on the content of the UBIO session. They could spend more time listening and interacting with other nurses who attended the session, rather than concentrating on taking notes.

Second, because the majority of nurses who attended the session were scheduled to present their in-service education programs at a later date, these handouts served as a useful resource. Staff could refer to the handouts when they were preparing their in-service offering or when they needed to refresh their memory concerning the details.

Finally, printed handouts enabled Lockhart and Bryce (1996) to include a large amount of material within the 30-minute time constraint allotted for the UBIO. The educators could spend more time answering questions or discussing staff concerns.

In addition to an outline that detailed the content of the instructional session, nurses who attended the UBIO received the following materials: (a) the tool, a *10-Step Checklist for Conducting a Unit-Based In-Service Offering* (Figure 7-1), (b) a teaching plan for the UBIO, (c) a template of a blank teaching plan that staff nurses could duplicate when preparing their own in-service educational offering (Figure 7-2), (d) a list of action verbs they could use when writing objectives for their in-service program (Figure 7-3), and (e) a learning activity, *Choosing the Correct Educational Objective,* which participants completed together during the UBIO (Figure 7-4). Each of these items will be discussed in the section that follows.

10-Step Checklist for Conducting a Unit-Based In-Service Offering

The *10-Step Checklist for Conducting a Unit-Based In-Service Offering* guided the instructional session and is depicted in Figure 7-1. This educational tool designed by Lockhart and Bryce (1996) was intended to serve as a worksheet for nurses as they developed their in-service educational offerings. They limited the *number* of steps to 10 so staff nurses would perceive this new endeavor as a manageable one at which they could succeed. Although a few of the steps, such as "Step 3: Clarify mutual goals," were complex and required more understanding and preparation time, other steps, such as "Step 4: Schedule the date, time, place, and speaker," were simple and easy to accomplish in a brief time.

The unit-based educators began each UBIO by asking participants to explain, in their own words, the meaning of the term "in-service educational offerings"

	1. Assess learning needs.	
	2. Select your topic.	
	3. Clarify mutual goals.	
	4. Schedule the following: Date Time Place Speaker(s) if needed	
	5. Advertise the program.	
	6. Develop a teaching plan. Develop objectives. Outline content and allot time. Choose teaching strategies. Design audiovisuals and handouts. Develop evaluation form.	
	7. Conduct the in-service education offering. Obtain audiovisuals and equipment. Ask participants to sign attendance sheet. Introduce yourself and participants. Share objectives. Present program using lesson plan as a guide. Allow time for questions and participation	
	8. Evaluate the in-service offering. Participants Program Speaker(s)	
	9. Provide feedback to participants and speaker(s).	
	10. Revise in-service program for future presentations.	

Figure 7-1.
A 10-Step Checklist for Conducting a Unit-Based In-Service Offering

Note: From "A Comprehensive Plan to Meet the Unit-Based Education Needs of Nurses From Several Specialty Units," by J.S. Lockhart and J. Bryce, 1996, *Journal of Nursing Staff Development, 12*, p. 136. Copyright 1996 by Lippincott-Raven Publishers. Reprinted with permission.

(Lockhart & Bryce, 1996). This activity was used to help participants obtain a holistic perspective of staff development within the Framework for Nursing Professional Development (ANA, 2000) described earlier in Chapter 2. Participants also were asked to compare in-service educational activities to the other components of nursing staff development, such as orientation and CE programs.

Next, participants were asked to brainstorm and recall examples of nursing education programs they attended, both at work and in the community, over the past year (Lockhart & Bryce, 1996). This strategy enabled them to compile a list of several educational offerings. Participants were asked to compare these offerings and designate each learning experience as an orientation, in-service education, or CE component of staff development.

Participants benefited from this exercise in several ways. First, defining the boundaries of an in-service program helped them to understand their charge. Second, this activity helped them clarify the presenter's role, as well as the role of the unit-based educator. Third, this exercise helped participants understand the multiple dimensions of nursing staff development within the context of nursing professional development.

Figure 7-2.
Sample Teaching
Plan Form

Title: _____

Objectives	Content (time allotted)	Teaching Strategies	Audiovisuals and Handouts	Evaluation

Figure 7-3.
Behavioral Verbs
Appropriate for
Each Level of the
Three Taxonomies

I. Cognitive
    C1.0 Knowledge (Information)
          define   name
          identify   recall
          list   recognize
    C2.0 Comprehension
          C2.1 Translation level
                cite examples of   give in own words
          C2.2 Interpretation level
                choose   discriminate
                demonstrate use of   explain
                describe   interpret
                differentiate   select
          C2.3 Exploration level
                conclude   estimate
                detect   infer
                determine   predict
                draw conclusions
    C3.0 Application
          apply   generalize
          develop   relate
          employ   use
    C4.0 Analysis
          appraise   detect
          compare   distinguish
          contrast   evaluate
          criticize   identify
          deduce   problem solve
                                              think critically

    C5.0 Synthesis
          classify   produce
          create   reconstruct
          design   restructure
          develop   synthesize
          modify   systematize
          organize
    C6.0 Evaluation
          appraise   evaluate
          assess   judge
          critique   validate
II. Affective
    A1.0 Receiving
          acknowledge   show awareness of
          share
    A2.0 Responding
          act willingly   practice
          discuss willingly   respond
          express satisfaction in   seek opportunities
          is willing to support   select
          listen to   show interest
    A3.0 Valuing
          accept   cooperate with
          acclaim   help
          agree   participate in
          assist   respect
          assume responsibility   support
    A4.0 Organization of Values
          argue   formulate a position

(Continued on
next page)

Figure 7-3.
Behavioral Verbs
Appropriate for
Each Level of the
Three Taxonomies
(Continued)

Note. From *Behavioral Objectives: Evaluation in Nursing* (3rd ed., pp. 85–86) by D.E. Reilly and M.H. Oermann, 1990, New York: National League for Nursing. Copyright 1990 by National League for Nursing Publishers. Reprinted with permission.

A4.0	Organization of Values *(cont.)*		
	debate	is consistent	
	declare	take a stand	
	defend		
A5.0	Characterization by Value		
	act consistently	stand for	
	is accountable		
III.	Psychomotor		
P1.0	Imitation		
	follow example of		
	follow lead of		
P2.0	Manipulation		
	carry out according to procedure	follow procedure practice	
P3.0	Precision		
	demonstrate skill in using		
P4.0	Articulation		
	carry out	use	
	is skillful in using		
P5.0	Naturalization		
	is competent	carry out competently	
	is skilled		

Many of the nurses claimed that, prior to this exercise, they had not understood what in-service educational offerings were (Lockhart & Bryce, 1996). Only a few participants were familiar with the components of staff development and their relationship with each other. The nurses expressed feeling less anxious after learning the brief nature and core components of an in-service educational offering.

The 10 steps included in the checklist guided the content and sequence of the remaining portion of the UBIO (Lockhart & Bryce, 1996). To illustrate these 10 steps, the unit-based educators asked participants to identify a learning need (topic) that could be used as an example. Many nurses suggested the learning need that was identified as a priority in their unit's educational plan. For example, nurses who worked on a head and neck oncology unit suggested "How to conduct a neurological assessment" as an example to use during the session (Lockhart & Bryce). Nursing staff from other clinical units selected topics that were of interest to them, such as "Caring for central lines," "How to apply electrocardiogram (EKG) leads properly," and "Maintaining chest tubes."

Step 1: Assess Learning Needs

The first step in the *10-Step Checklist for Conducting a Unit-Based In-Service Offering* involves assessing the learning needs of staff on the clinical unit (Lockhart & Bryce, 1996). Assessing the learning needs and incorporating them into a unit's educational plan were described previously in Chapter 6. In this instance, Lockhart and Bryce already had identified the learning needs of clinical staff, analyzed the data, and prioritized the needs. However, it was still important to remind staff to conduct a needs assessment before developing an in-service education offering.

Step 2: Select Your Topic

For the second step of the checklist, participants were asked to select a topic from the list of learning needs identified in the unit's educational plan. As mentioned earlier in Chapter 6, some of the topics may be familiar to the staff nurses, but other new topics might pose a challenge. Each staff member was asked to sign his or her name next to the topic selected by writing directly on the educational plan posted on the clinical unit.

Step 3: Clarify Mutual Goals

The third step of the checklist required each presenter to validate that the learning need identified by unit staff and the participant's understanding of this need were congruent with each other (Lockhart & Bryce, 1996). For example, a learning need identified by staff was "How to change a laryngectomy tube." The nurse who chose this topic to develop as an in-service education program discussed this learning need with unit staff prior to developing the lesson plan and clarified specific objectives that the staff had in mind concerning this need.

The nurse also determined the staff's current knowledge and skills related to the topic. This included what the staff already knew about a total laryngectomy, the anatomical changes that result following this surgical procedure, and components of a laryngectomy tube. The nurse used this information to tailor the content of the in-service education program to the learning needs of staff.

Because in-service education sessions usually last a short time, knowing this information in advance of planning it is helpful. For instance, if the staff had little prior knowledge on this topic, the nurse might develop two separate in-service education offerings. The nurse may develop a poster that reviewed the parts of a laryngectomy tube prior to the scheduled in-service.

Step 4: Schedule the Date, Time, Place, and Speaker(s)

Step 4 in the checklist reminded participants to schedule the date, time, place, and speaker(s) for the presentation (Lockhart & Bryce, 1996). Scheduling the in-service education program should be completed well in advance so that all staff on the unit have an opportunity to attend. Ask your nurse manager or staff develop-

---

Figure 7-4.
Sample Exercise in Writing Educational Objectives

Directions: Circle the correctly worded objective from each of the following pairs of objectives.

1. A. After the in-service program on lung sounds, the nurse will understand the difference between wheezes and rhonchi.

   B. After the in-service program on lung sounds, the learner will use a stethoscope to correctly identify wheezes from rhonchi in a patient chosen by the presenter.

2. A. Following the CPR class, the instructor will use an adult mannequin to emphasize the correct position for chest compressions.

   B. Following the CPR class, the learner will use an adult mannequin to demonstrate the correct hand position for chest compressions.

3. **A. After the demonstration, the nurse will describe the proper procedure used to change a central line dressing.**

   B. After the demonstration, the nurse will develop an appreciation for the proper procedure to change a central line dressing.

Note. Correct answers are bolded.

ment educator for other strategies that have worked (e.g., refreshments) on your clinical unit to increase staff's attendance at in-service programs. Although some clinical staff prefer to have their unit-based in-service programs scheduled as early as four to six weeks in advance, others may only require one or two weeks notice. Clarify the exact time for the in-service offering, as well as the need for repeating the program to accommodate staff who rotate shifts. Remind staff that they can bring lunch or dinner, if appropriate, especially if you are presenting your in-service as "brown bag" sessions during mealtimes.

Reserve a room for the program. If you are not familiar with the location, visit the room before the scheduled date of the in-service offering to check its features, such as the design of the room, seating capacity, audiovisual accommodations, and lighting. It is much easier to plan and adapt your program around a physical environment if you have this information in advance. Regardless of your preference for the time and location of unit-based in-service offerings, check with the unit manager for these details.

If you are planning an in-service education program in which you will need a clinical laboratory setting, check the feasibility of using a clinical skills laboratory at a nearby school of nursing. This setting is ideal for practicing psychomotor skills, such as cardiopulmonary resuscitation, or for videotaping performance during a mock emergency code. If this option is not available, consider conducting the in-service education session in a vacant patient room.

If you are inviting a guest speaker to present the in-service education program, such as faculty from an affiliating school of nursing or a vendor, confirm the date and time with them. Check with your nurse manager to determine if there is a procedure you need to follow for allowing guests from outside organizations into your institution, especially commercial vendors. These individuals may need to obtain your organization's clearance before they visit a clinical unit.

Finally, reserve any equipment that you may need for your program well in advance. This may include items such as an overhead projector, screen, flip chart, or laptop and LCD. Clarify the procedure and time lines that need to be followed to duplicate program handouts.

Step 5: Advertise the Program

After you have completed Steps 1 through 4 on the checklist, you can begin to market your program to staff. Consider a communication method that is effective at your institution. This may involve posting a printed flier on the unit or advertising the program through e-mail, staff mailboxes, or closed-circuit television.

Submit information about the program to your organization's newsletter, if appropriate. Be creative in preparing an attention-getting colored flier. Include the title of the program, the speaker's name and credentials, and the date, time, and location of the program. Consider adding the program's objectives and eye-catching graphics. Post this information in a location on the unit that all staff will be sure to view it. Remind staff about the program the day before and shortly before the program.

Step 6: Develop a Teaching Plan

Step 6 comprised a major portion of the UBIO session that Lockhart and Bryce (1996) implemented. This step focused on the process used to develop a teaching plan that serves as a "blueprint" for an in-service education program.

Because most participants were not familiar with a teaching plan, Lockhart and Bryce (1996) used an analogy between this plan and a nursing care plan. A sample of a teaching plan was distributed, along with templates that participants could duplicate, as needed (see Figure 7-2). Participants were advised to limit their teaching plan to one or two pages, and use it as a "blueprint" for themselves to guide them during their presentation.

Because this organization had a clinical advancement program, participants planned on including their teaching plans in their professional portfolios (Lockhart & Bryce, 1996). Portfolios will be discussed later in Chapter 11. The participants commented that these written plans accurately reflected the content, organization, and depth of their unit-based in-service programs.

The teaching plan portion of the UBIO session focused on the following five topics: developing objectives, outlining specific content, choosing appropriate teaching strategies, designing audiovisuals and handouts, and developing an evaluation form (Lockhart & Bryce, 1996). These five topics were headings for each column included in the teaching plan. The sample teaching plan that was distributed to participants served as a guide.

Develop Objectives

Learning how to write realistic learner-centered objectives is an important step in designing a teaching plan for a unit-based in-service education program (Lockhart & Bryce, 1996). Most nurses already have experience in writing patient-centered objectives for a care plan. Building upon similarities that exist between these two plans helped these participants to develop their objectives.

Purpose of objectives. Briefly review the process used to develop educational objectives. Discuss the purpose that objectives play when preparing an in-service education offering. Objectives serve several purposes that benefit both the presenter and the learner. For example, objectives can help presenters focus on the specific learning needs identified by learners (Reilly & Oermann, 1990) when developing an in-service program. This is especially helpful for presenters who have a tendency to include more content than can logically be reviewed within the time allotted for an in-service program. Focusing on two or three key objectives when developing a program prevents presenters from covering "everything you ever wanted to know" during an in-service program.

Because objectives denote the learning outcomes of an educational program (Oermann & Gaberson, 1998), they help learners understand the specific behaviors the presenter will expect them to demonstrate following the in-service education offering. Therefore, share objectives with learners prior to the start of an educational program so those learners can concentrate on its purpose (Reilly & Oermann, 1990). Presenters need to review the program's objectives with learners in advance of the program so that they will understand what behaviors are expected of them.

Objectives guide the presenter in designing the educational program's content, in selecting teaching strategies and audiovisuals that will enable learners to attain the intended outcomes, and in determining a method of evaluation (Reilly & Oermann, 1990). Objectives help the presenter keep the program succinct and focused on its purpose.

Clearly stated objectives help the presenter determine if the learners were able to demonstrate the expected outcomes of the program (Reilly & Oermann, 1990). Because objectives are instrumental in evaluating the performance of learners, they need to be clearly written, measurable, and observable (Reilly & Oermann).

Main elements of objectives. According to Reilly and Oermann (1990), objectives, such as those included in a teaching plan for an in-service education offering, should contain four main elements: (a) a description of the *learner*, (b) a description of the *behavior* the learner will exhibit to demonstrate that competence has been attained, (c) a description of *conditions* under which the learner will demonstrate competence, and (d) a statement of *standard of performance* expected to indicate excellence.

Table 7-1 illustrates an example of how these four elements can be used to develop an objective for an in-service education program about the nursing care for patients following a total laryngectomy. Each of these four elements will be discussed further in the following section.

Learner. When developing objectives, first focus on the learners who will comprise the participants for your in-service education session. Determine their knowledge, skills, and attitudes regarding the topic. Keep these factors in mind when developing realistic outcomes for learners.

Defining who the learners are for an educational program is often an easy task for presenters. However, objectives may vary based on the knowledge and skill level of the learners. For example, you may need to develop different objectives for an in-service education program when presenting it to novice nurses as compared with more experienced nurses. Also, adapt your objectives appropriately when teaching a group of learners whose knowledge and skill levels are diverse, such as a group consisting of RNs, licensed practical/licensed vocational nurses, and assistive personnel. In the example provided in Table 7-1, the learners are RNs new to a head and neck oncology unit.

Behavior. The second step in developing objectives focuses on what the learner can perform as a result of attending an educational program (Mager, 1984). State exactly what you will expect the learner to do during or following the program. Use action verbs to describe this performance, such as those used in developing patient-centered objectives. Some examples of action-oriented verbs are included in Figure 7-3, listed according to their domain and level. Remember to make the learner's behavior specific, objective, and measurable. Limit each objective to only one behavior (Reilly & Oermann, 1990). In the example provided in Table 7-1, you are asking the staff nurse to demonstrate changing a laryngectomy tube.

Conditions. The third step included in developing objectives requires you, as the presenter, to describe the conditions or circumstances that you will impose upon the learner as he or she performs the outcome (Mager, 1984). In the example

Table 7-1. Sample Objective Depicting Main Elements	
After the in-service program on laryngectomy care, the staff nurse will follow hospital nursing standards when changing a laryngectomy tube on a five-day postoperative total laryngectomy patient.	
Element	**Content of Sample Objective**
Learner	Staff nurse
Behavior	Change a laryngectomy tube on a five-day postoperative total laryngectomy patient
Conditions	After the in-service program on laryngectomy care
Standard	Will follow hospital-nursing standards

provided in Table 7-1, you are asking learners to demonstrate the behavior (changing a laryngectomy tube) after they attended the in-service education program on laryngectomy care. You also asked them to change the laryngectomy tube on an actual patient who underwent a total laryngectomy five days prior. Instead, you could have asked the learner to change the tube on a mannequin in a clinical skills laboratory.

Standard of performance. Finally, the fourth step in developing objectives requires you to determine how well the learner must perform for you to consider it acceptable (Mager, 1984). This step requires you to think about how you will evaluate or judge the learner's performance based on each objective of the in-service education session. In Table 7-1, you asked the nurse to change the laryngectomy tube according to the procedure approved by your healthcare organization. This procedure would contain a list of critical behaviors that the nurse needed to demonstrate when changing the tube.

As mentioned in Chapter 4, this skill (changing a laryngectomy tube) may be one of your unit's competency requirements. New nurses would demonstrate changing a laryngectomy tube during their orientation, whereas experienced nurses could perform this skill during the unit's annual competency review.

Domains and levels of objectives. Just like objectives that are used in clinical practice, those developed for educational programs are categorized according to the type of behavior they reflect: cognitive, psychomotor, or affective (Reilly & Oermann, 1990).

An objective written in the cognitive domain focuses on outcomes that deal with the learner's knowledge or intellectual ability (Oermann & Gaberson, 1998). For example, in the objective illustrated in Table 7-1, you could have asked the staff nurse to verbally explain the procedure for changing a laryngectomy tube or to describe it in writing. However, in the first situation, you would know if the nurse actually could perform the tube change on a patient.

Psychomotor objectives relate to a learner's motor skills and competency using equipment or technology (Oermann & Gaberson, 1998). In reference to the objective presented in Table 7-1, you are asking nurses to demonstrate their psychomotor skills by changing a laryngectomy tube. You will be able to observe their coordination in performing this motor skill and to assess or validate this competency.

Finally, objectives written in the affective domain will focus on the learner's values, attitudes, or beliefs as a professional nurse (Oermann & Gaberson, 1998). In Table 7-1, the objective could have focused on the attitude or reaction that nurses experienced when changing the laryngectomy tube. The nurse may have had uncomfortable feelings if this was the first time he or she viewed a laryngectomee's stoma.

Regardless of the objective's domain, it is important that you match the domain of each objective with the intended purpose of the in-service education program. You also need to use teaching strategies that are appropriate for the objective's domain. For example, the objective provided in Table 7-1 is in the psychomotor domain because the learner is asked to demonstrate manual skills. Your teaching strategies during the in-service program may include practice in changing a tube on a mannequin. Matching teaching strategies with the domain of objectives will be discussed later in this chapter.

Objectives also can vary based on their complexity levels within each of the three domains mentioned earlier in this section (Reilly & Oermann, 1990). Figure 7-3 illustrates the various levels that exist with each of the three domains. Consider including objectives written at an appropriate level of difficulty in your program. For example, when developing objectives in the cognitive domain, ask learners to apply or relate the concepts they learned in a case study during the in-service program rather than merely having them verbally recite what you presented.

When developing a UBIO, match the teaching strategy you use in your in-service program with characteristics of your objective (Alspach, 1995; DeYoung, 1990). Therefore, when you ask the learner to perform a complex behavior, you will use teaching strategies that appropriately match. For example, if your goal is to have learners evaluate the effectiveness of interventions used to relieve pain in a postoperative patient, your teaching strategy may include the use of an actual case study and group discussion.

Lockhart and Bryce (1996) used a learning activity like the one depicted in Figure 7-4 in their UBIO to help participants learn more about developing objectives. In this exercise, they asked nurses who were given a pair of objectives to select the correctly written one.

You can use this approach with a group of learners to help them develop their objectives. Ask them to test their knowledge in identifying the domain in which the objective belongs. Active learning exercises such as this one can help nurses increase not only their understanding of objectives but also their confidence in developing and refining them.

Outline Content and Allot Time

After identifying the key objectives for your in-service education program, outline the content to be addressed in the program that will help learners meet the objectives and attain the outcomes. Contact the librarian at your organization or nearby school of nursing to help you locate resources for developing the content of your program. Familiarize yourself with the services offered at the library, such as locating healthcare resources or learning how to conduct a computerized literature search. Think about organizing group visits to the library so that other nursing staff can learn these skills.

Your content outline should be brief, consistent, and relate directly to the objectives you have identified. Organize your outline using a standard format (I., A., 1., a., b.). This outline approach should be one with which all nursing staff is familiar.

Once you have drafted the content outline, approximate the amount of time that you plan on dedicating to each of the major sections of the outline during your presentation. Because keeping on schedule is vital during a unit-based in-service program, estimating small segments of time will help you determine a realistic amount of content. Avoid overwhelming learners with vast amounts of information within a short period of time.

Allow sufficient time during the in-service program for questions, discussion, and demonstrations or return demonstrations of manual skills. As mentioned earlier, keep your in-service program within the prescribed allotted time, so those nurses can deal with patient care needs.

Choose Teaching Strategies

After you have developed the objectives and content for your in-service education program, choose teaching strategies that will best communicate this information to your learners. View teaching strategies as methods to help learners understand the content of the program and, therefore, meet the objectives.

When choosing a teaching strategy for your educational program, consider factors such as the objectives and content of your program, characteristics of the participants, your own preferences as a presenter, and resources available at your workplace (Alspach, 1995; DeYoung, 1990).

Objectives and content. As mentioned earlier in this chapter, choose teaching strategies that match the objectives and content of your in-service education offering (Alspach, 1995; DeYoung, 1990). Table 7-2 suggests teaching strategies matched with the domain of the program's objective. Many of these teaching strategies were discussed in Chapter 6.

For example, suppose you are planning an in-service education program on how to provide safe, quality nursing care for patients with a central IV line. One of your objectives for this session is, "Following the in-service session, the learner will change a central line dressing on a patient according to hospital procedure." Because this objective reflects behaviors from the psychomotor domain (changing a dressing), you dedicate a portion of your program for learners to practice this skill on a mannequin.

If you used an objective from a cognitive domain for the same in-service session, it might look like this: "Following the in-service education session, the learner will correctly state the steps used in applying a central line dressing based on hospital procedure." In this case, you may choose discussion as a teaching strategy, allowing time for learners to verbally state the steps they would follow in applying a central line dressing rather than actually having them perform the procedure. You also could have learners complete a written post-test that focused on these steps.

Finally, if your goal is to explore and possibly change the attitudes of nurses toward caring for patients from diverse cultural backgrounds, your teaching method might include the use of experiential approaches, such as role-play or game strategies. These options provide learners with an opportunity to experience a situation firsthand within a traditional teaching-learning setting.

For example, to simulate the culture shock often experienced by individuals who are placed in an environment different from their own, Lockhart and Resick (1997) used the cultural awareness simulation called BaFa BaFa (Shirts, 1977) with nursing students. This teaching strategy helped learners experience what it is like to interact with individuals from a different culture and what it feels like when visiting with others from a culture that is unfamiliar. These goals were accomplished within the confines of a traditional classroom setting.

Characteristics of the learner. Another element to consider when choosing a teaching strategy for your educational program is the characteristics of the learner

Table 7-2. Suggested Teaching Strategies Based on Objective Domain for In-Service Education Programs	
Objective Domain	**Suggested Teaching Strategies**
Cognitive	Lecture, group discussion, nursing rounds, self-learning modules, case studies, critical incidents
Psychomotor	Demonstration, return demonstration, simulation, checklists
Affective	Role-play, debate, games, simulations, role modeling

(Alspach, 1995; DeYoung, 1990). Some of this information is available to you in the data obtained from the needs assessment completed by clinical staff and described in Chapter 6. Use this information to help you determine characteristics of learners, such as their preferred teaching-learning strategies and their degree of competency regarding particular topics.

Consider both the number of learners who will attend your program and their clinical experience (DeYoung, 1990). Be ready to adjust your teaching method if the number of participants is larger than you originally had expected. Consider scheduling multiple sessions of your program if it involves a "hands-on" learning exercise.

If your group of learners is composed of nurses who vary in clinical expertise, consider presenting two separate sessions: one designed for new graduates at a beginning level and another session targeted at a more complex level for the experienced nurse. Utilize the clinical strength of the expert nurses to assist you with educating the novice nurses. This strategy can foster a mentor-mentee relationship among the nursing staff on a clinical unit.

Regardless of the approach you use, it is important that you can control for various learner characteristics, and if not, modify your program accordingly. Careful assessment of the learners can help you make the necessary changes in your in-service education session that can maximize the learning experience.

Preferences and strengths of the presenter. Third, reflect upon your own preferences and abilities as a presenter when choosing a teaching strategy for your program (Alspach, 1995; DeYoung, 1990). If you are new at conducting an in-service session, select a teaching method that matches the program's objectives and learners, but ensure it is one that you feel comfortable in using. As you gain more experience in presenting programs, experiment with other teaching strategies. Ask an experienced educator at your workplace to help you master these skills, or attend CE programs on this topic. Be creative when developing teaching strategies for your in-service education offering. Many of the teaching strategies (e.g., posters, self-learning packets, games) discussed in Chapter 6 can be used for these programs.

Resources available in the workplace. Finally, be realistic by selecting teaching strategies that are available to you in your work setting (Alspach, 1995; DeYoung, 1990). Consider issues such as the conference room and laboratory space, available equipment and supplies, financial support, and allotted time for in-service sessions. All of these things are mentioned in greater detail throughout this chapter.

Design Audiovisuals and Handouts

After you developed the objectives and content for your in-service education program, consider audiovisuals and handouts that will help you convey your message to learners. Written handouts, when added to your verbal presentation, can increase both the retention and learning of material by participants (Alspach, 1995).

Select your audiovisuals like teaching strategies, based on your objectives and their domains. Table 7-3 provides some examples of audiovisuals that vary in style, preparation, and cost.

Be cost-conscious when supplementing your presentation with printed handouts, and try to keep them at a minimum. Consider posting a copy of your handouts on the bulletin board of each unit's conference room for staff to duplicate, as

Table 7-3. Audiovisuals Appropriate for In-Service Educational Programs	
Category	**Examples**
Audiotapes	Audiotapes of breath sounds, heart sounds
Writing surfaces	Chalkboard, white board with dry markers, flip chart
Poster (handmade or commercially produced)	Diagram of venous access in the arm for IV use
Overhead transparencies	Main points of presentation, graphics, tables, figures
Slides (35 mm, Microsoft® PowerPoint®)	Main points of presentation, graphics, tables, figures, photographs
Print	Books, chapters, journal articles, printed handout (case study, chart form), pamphlets, commercially produced literature on drugs and products
Models	Mannequin, torso mannequin for CPR, selected body parts (eye, ear, larynx, kidney), arms equipped with veins for IV insertion practice, breasts with lumps used for palpation, medical equipment such as nasogastric tubes, suction catheters
Films	Videotapes, strip film, 16 mm film of surgical and patient care procedures, reenactments of situations
Computer software (computer-assisted instruction, compact discs, Internet)	Audio and/or visual reenactments of clinical scenarios that focus on decision making for nurses, review of core curriculum, Web pages of specialty nursing organizations, databases used to conduct literature searches
Television	Live broadcasts of surgery, conferences
Live subjects	Volunteer patient or clinical staff upon which to demonstrate clinical procedures such as proper application of EKG leads, central line dressings, and obtaining pulse and blood pressure readings

needed. You also could include a copy of your handouts in a three-ring notebook labeled "In-Service Education Program Handouts" so that staff can refer to them at their leisure.

Develop an Evaluation Form

As you design the objectives, content, teaching strategies, and audiovisuals for your in-service, remember to develop a way to evaluate the impact of your efforts on learners. Decide who should be involved in this evaluation process, what components of the program should be evaluated, and both how and when this evaluation should occur. Feedback obtained through the evaluation process can strengthen the educational plan and promote the professional development of staff nurses who serve as presenters.

Who should evaluate? Both you as the presenter of the in-service session and the learners should be involved in the evaluation process. To provide additional feedback on your performance as a speaker, you may choose to obtain input from your supervisor or mentor.

What should be evaluated? Several key components of your in-service offering should be included in the evaluation process. Include information about the learners' performance, the overall quality of the in-service education offering, the ability of the presenter, and feedback about the teaching-learning experience.

Ask learners about their ability to meet the stated objectives of the in-service session. Include responses about the quality of the content presented and teaching strategies and audiovisuals used in the session. Seek their feedback about your effectiveness and skill as a presenter. Finally, ask learners to evaluate the learning environment, such as space and accommodations. Determine if each learner met the objectives of the session. As mentioned earlier in this chapter, this task is facilitated with detailed and objectively stated goals.

How and when should evaluation be conducted? An example of a short evaluation form that can be adapted for any in-service education session is illustrated in Figure 7-5. Your organization already may have an evaluation form for this purpose. Include space at the end of the evaluation for participants' suggestions for future education programs.

Step 7: Conduct the In-Service Education Offering

Now that you have completed the first six steps of the checklist, you are ready to actually present your program. Use the *10-Step Checklist for Conducting a Unit-Based In-Service Offering* to keep track of the things you need to complete. Arrive earlier than the scheduled start time of the in-service session. This will not only give you time to deal with last-minute changes but will also minimize a rushed appearance on your part.

Obtain audiovisuals and equipment. Prior to the start of the program, either obtain the audiovisuals yourself or have them delivered by someone else. Take time to make the room conducive to learning. For example, if you are using a conference room, be sure that it is fairly clean and presentable. Adjust the temperature and lighting, as needed.

Ask participants to sign an attendance sheet. Ask all participants to sign an attendance sheet to verify their presence. Placing this form on a clipboard will avoid its getting lost during the session. If your institution does not have a standardized form, then adapt the form presented in Figure 7-6.

Introduce yourself and participants. Before you start your presentation, take a few minutes to introduce yourself. Share with the participants the reasons why you are presenting this in-service session and the benefits it offers to them. If you have not done so earlier, obtain information about the participants, such as their names, assigned unit, and previous experience with the topic. All of these things will help to create a more relaxed learning environment, placing both you and the learners at ease. This is especially important because in-service education programs usually are scheduled during work time. It often takes participants a while to shift their thinking from the caregiver role in a hurried clinical atmosphere to that of a learner in a classroom setting. Give the participants time to focus on the session.

Share objectives. As mentioned earlier in this chapter, explain the program objectives with the learners. Do this at the start of the session so those learners will understand what will be expected of them.

Present the program, using your teaching plan as a guide. Present your in-service educational program as you planned. Using your teaching plan as a blueprint for your presentation may be helpful, or rely on note cards or other cues to keep you on track. Consider assigning a colleague as a timekeeper so that you

HEALTHCARE-UNIVERSITY MEDICAL CENTER HOSPITAL
In-Service Offering Evaluation

Name (Optional): _____

Program: _____ Speaker: _____

Date and time: _____ Location: _____

<u>Directions:</u> Please provide us with your feedback regarding this in-service session. Circle the number that best represents your response. Provide comments if desired.

5 = Excellent; 4 = Above Average; 3 = Average; 2 = Below Average; 1 = Poor

1. Your ability to meet the stated objectives   5 4 3 2 1
    Comments: _____
    _____
    _____

2. The quality and relevance of the content presented   5 4 3 2 1
    Comments: _____
    _____
    _____

3. The overall effectiveness of the speaker   5 4 3 2 1
    Comments: _____
    _____
    _____

4. The teaching strategies used by the speaker   5 4 3 2 1
    Comments: _____
    _____
    _____

5. Audiovisuals/handouts used in this session   5 4 3 2 1
    Comments: _____
    _____
    _____

6. The teaching-learning environment   5 4 3 2 1
    Comments: _____
    _____
    _____

7. Your overall rating of the in-service offering   5 4 3 2 1
    Comments: _____
    _____
    _____

Please provide suggestions for future programs and speakers:
_____
_____
_____
_____
_____
_____

Figure 7-5.
Sample Evaluation Form

Figure 7-6.
Sample Atten-
dance Record

HEALTHCARE-UNIVERSITY MEDICAL CENTER HOSPITAL
Program Attendance Record

Program: _____

Speaker: _____

Date and time: _____

Location: _____

Name (Print first and last name)	Position (RN, LPN, AP, US)	Identification Number	Unit	Shift
1.				
2.				
3.				
4.				
5.				
6.				
7.				
8.				
9.				
10.				
11.				
12.				
13.				
14.				
15.				

can stay on schedule. Although you have carefully planned your program, be attentive to learners' needs and flexible to changes that may occur during the presentation. Observe both verbal and nonverbal cues from your learners.

Allow time for questions and participation. Inform learners in advance when you welcome questions from them. You may decide to entertain questions during your session, at the conclusion of the session, or both. Allow for this additional time when planning your session. If you run out of time or encounter an unusual number of questions, consider scheduling an additional session where you can continue this discussion.

Welcome, rather than fear, questions posed by participants. Although you have researched your topic, you are not expected to have all the answers. Rely on other learners who may be able to answer questions, or tell the participants that you will investigate their questions and get back to them. Be sure to thank the participants for their questions.

If your plan included learner participation during the program, such as demonstration of psychomotor skills, then allot time for this activity. Be flexible if you need to adjust your plan at the last minute.

Step 8: Evaluate the In-Service Education Offering

Evaluation is an essential component of any educational offering. Use the strategies discussed earlier in this chapter to evaluate learners and speakers.

Step 9: Provide Feedback to Participants and Speakers

Provide both learners and speakers, if appropriate, with feedback regarding their performance. You can provide learners with feedback during the program while observing them perform a dressing change or as they verbally discuss the steps involved in changing a sterile dressing. You can conduct the evaluation following the program. Use the objectives to evaluate learners' performances, and include both formal and informal feedback.

Step 10: Revise the In-Service Program for Future Presentations

While your in-service session is still fresh in your mind, note possible ways you could improve upon your presentation. Use evaluation comments provided by learners and your own personal insight. Determine if learners were able to meet the objectives. Consider changing your teaching plan when you repeat this presentation, such as sequencing the content in a different order or developing additional handouts to expedite the session. Each time you present your program, you will see areas for making it more effective. Regardless of the revisions, be sure to congratulate yourself on a job well done!

Summary

This chapter describes a model designed to assist nursing staff in planning, implementing, and evaluating a unit-based in-service education offering. A 10-step checklist serves as a practical tool that can guide the presenter in developing a unit-based program.

References

Alspach, J.G. (1995). *The educational process in nursing staff development.* St. Louis, MO: Mosby.
American Nurses Association. (1998). *Standards of clinical nursing practice* (2nd ed.). Washington, DC: Author.
American Nurses Association. (2000). *Scope and standards of practice for nursing staff development.* Washington, DC: Author.
DeYoung, S. (1990). *Teaching nursing.* Redwood City, CA: Addison-Wesley Nursing.
Incalcattera, E. (1999). Is it nursing continuing education or is it in-service? *New Jersey Nurse, 29*(6), 11.
Lockhart, J.S., & Bryce, J. (1996). A comprehensive plan to meet the unit-based education needs of nurses from several specialty units. *Journal of Nursing Staff Development, 12*(3), 135–138.
Lockhart, J.S., & Resick, L.K. (1997). Teaching cultural competence: The value of experiential learning and community resources. *Nurse Educator 22*(3), 27–31.
Mager, R.F. (1984). *Preparing instructional objectives* (2nd ed.). Belmont, CA: David S. Lake Publishers.

Oermann, M.H., & Gaberson, K.B. (1998). *Evaluation and testing in nursing education.* New York: Springer Publishing.

Reilly, D.E., & Oermann, M.H. (1990). *Behavioral objectives: Evaluation in nursing* (3rd ed.). New York: National League for Nursing.

Shirts, R.G. (1977). *BaFa BaFa: A cross-cultural simulation.* Delmar, CA: Simile II.

UNIT 4

Helping Staff Develop as Professionals

CH

Getting Involved in
and Community C

As mentioned earlier in Chapter 2, professional development is a lifelong, continuous process expected of professional nurses (American Nurses Association [ANA], 2000). Although nurses need to assume primary responsibility for developing themselves professionally, others, such as staff development educators and employers, also have a responsibility to assist nurses in this process (ANA). Staff development educators can achieve this goal by serving as models in the multiple roles they assume (e.g., educator, facilitator, change agent, consultant, researcher, leader) (ANA) and through mentoring other nurses. Educators also are responsible for their own professional development through involvement in professional nursing organizations and the community (ANA). Unit-based educators need to mirror the behaviors of staff development educators and help clinical nurses develop themselves as professionals.

Nurses can participate in a variety of professional and community-based activities. Although many professional activities reflect more structured efforts with nurses who hold similar interests, other methods of professional development include more informal, self-directed activities (DiMauro, 2000). This chapter will discuss the benefits of being involved in the profession and community and provide examples of opportunities for nurses.

Benefits of Involvement

As a unit-based educator, you probably have heard comments such as these from some nurses who were questioned about their professional involvement: "Why should I become involved in professional organizations or community activities? Isn't my performance as a professional nurse at work enough? I don't have time to do anything else besides go to work every day and take care of my personal responsibilities at home. I do have a life besides nursing!"

Responses such as these may be a common occurrence at your workplace, especially in light of the multiple changes that have occurred in nursing and health care over the past decades (see Chapter 1). As a unit-based educator, you need to respond in an effective way to such statements. You also need to clarify your own questions regarding the expectations of nurses related to the professional development process.

Being an active, professional nurse offers a variety of advantages to you as the participant, to the recipients of your efforts, to the nursing profession, and to the

ons with which you affiliate. Armed with this information, you need to
ine their priorities at this time in your professional career.

Professional Rewards

Nurses can benefit professionally by participating in activities at their own
workplace, within the nursing profession, and in the community. Although some
of these professional rewards meet job-related expectations or specific personal
needs, others relate to your overall development as a professional nurse. Each of
these will be discussed separately.

Job-Related Rewards

First, some rewards gained by professional development are directly job-related.
In fact, work-related improvements were identified as significant benefits of membership in professional organizations by nurses who held these memberships as
compared with nurses who did not (Deleskey, 2003). Whether you are an experienced nurse or a new graduate who has just passed the licensure examination,
evidence of your participation in various nursing and community organizations
can give you an advantage over other applicants when seeking employment or
promotion opportunities. This is true whether you are seeking your first nursing
position, moving to a new clinical unit, or changing jobs to work at another
healthcare agency.

If you are in the process of finding a job, evidence of your participation in various professional organizations sends a positive message to prospective employers. It reflects that even though you have not found a nursing position to date, you
still have taken the responsibility to become involved in professionally related
activities with which you have some control. This behavior tells prospective employers that you have assumed a leadership role with regard to your professional
development. You, as a prospective employee, have the potential to support team-
building efforts and to promote a positive professional attitude. It also reflects
your concern about the consumers who reside in the community. Employers may
make the assumption that, if hired, you will continue this professional behavior to
the benefit of patient care and to the successful operation of their healthcare organization.

Being active in professional and community associations may be an expectation for promotion within some institutions that emphasize clinical advancement
programs. This activity within these organizations is viewed as an example of
professional behavior. These behaviors require active involvement, the use of leadership skills, and a sense of personal responsibility. Possessing these behaviors
may set you apart from others who have not yet assumed that level of professional
development in their nursing careers.

Remember to use your participation in professional organizations and activities in the community as a strategy to maintain or secure your present nursing
position. A great deal of the success in using this tactic depends upon the value
that your organization and manager places on these behaviors. As a result, you
may need to help your employer understand the importance of professional involvement as well as the benefits it offers. Your explanation is vital in this era of
organizational downsizing or right-sizing, especially at a time when it is important for nurses to be perceived as valuable and indispensable leaders of healthcare
organizations.

Meeting Specific Needs

Belonging to a professional organization can help you meet specific needs that relate to your development as a professional nurse. For example, many professional nursing organizations offer benefits that reflect their mission, goals, and purposes. As a result, various opportunities are made available to their active members, such as being eligible to apply for funding. These often include research and literature review grants and scholarships for pursuing education, either formally through a school of nursing or informally through continuing education programs. Many organizations offer opportunities for certification to nurses who meet specific clinical requirements. Other organizations offer members travel grants so they can attend their national conference or financial awards that pay for the cost of certification examinations.

Some professional organizations recognize demonstration of professional behaviors. Some groups offer awards to members who demonstrate outstanding overall leadership in nursing or who display exceptional performance in specific areas, such as clinical practice, teaching, research, or community service. Other nursing associations have writing contests or offer competitive awards to local chapters. Finally, some organizations recognize their members who provide outstanding service to their mission and goals.

Professional Development

Professional rewards can influence your professional development. Involvement in professional and community organizations can help you develop a professional career plan. Your involvement also can help you attain your professional goals. Benefits can occur through activities such as working on an assigned project, interacting with other members, or organizing committee work. All of these activities provide you with an opportunity to learn and practice leadership skills and mentor others in these skills. More information on career planning and goal setting will be discussed in Chapter 15.

Participating in professional organizations enables nurses to network with experienced nurses who possess admirable leadership qualities and demonstrate professional management skills. Clinical nurses, through their active involvement, have an opportunity to develop their own leadership skills. Figure 8-1 provides a partial list of leadership skills that can be developed through involvement in professional organizations.

Although many professional behaviors can be observed in members of nursing organizations, it is unrealistic to assume that the behaviors of all members are positive. However, it is important for you to not only recognize these differences but also to learn from them. Negative behaviors usually serve a member's personal interests or goals, but they often pose barriers to meeting organizational

• Communication skills (oral and written)	• Goal setting
• Organization skills	• Strategic planning
• Time management skills	• Organizing work or projects
• Leading groups or teams	• Allocating resources effectively
• Being a group or team member	• Budget planning
• Managing conflict	• Conference or program planning
• Using negotiation skills	• Developing creativity
• Running a productive meeting	• Motivating others
• Defining a mission	

Figure 8-1.
Skills Valued by Professional Nursing and Community Organizations

goals. Try to use the "less-than-admirable qualities" you may observe in some nurses as examples of what not to do.

Members of professional nursing organizations also can serve as a professional support system for nurses, forming a link or network among individual members within and outside the organization. Networking with colleagues has the potential to positively impact your professional career and personal goals (Cardillo, 1998) and help you cope with changes that result from the many healthcare trends discussed in Chapter 1. For example, networking can help you acquire a mentor who can assist you in developing expertise identified in your professional career plan. This mechanism can help members form interest groups composed of nurses who share a common interest, such as clinical teaching, health promotion, or research.

Finally, being active in a professional organization or community agency provides you with current information related to its focus. For example, members of organizations usually receive a newsletter that shares information about other members, events, and opportunities at local, regional, national, or international levels. Membership often includes being placed on the mailing list of various related associations that inform members about upcoming workshops, new products, or special services. Some organizations provide members with access to valuable information on their Web site. The Internet also provides nurses with an opportunity to network with other professionals through access to e-mail lists, news groups, and membership databases (Washer, 2002). This information helps professional nurses keep abreast of new knowledge within a specialty and share ideas with other professionals with similar interests.

Recognition for Your Organization

Being an active and productive member in professional and community associations can bring public recognition to your employer, school of nursing, and organizations to which you belong. Your success sends a positive message to the public about you and your affiliations. This, in turn, adds to the reputation of your workplace or school within the community.

Serving as an officer of a national nursing organization is a professional accomplishment that can bring prestige to your school of nursing. In fact, the success of both you and other alumni has the potential to add to the national status of your school, as well as to its marketability for future applicants. Be sure to remind your employer of the benefits to be gained by your active role in organizations.

Positive Image and Identity

As mentioned earlier in this chapter, being active in both professional and community organizations is an integral part of the professional nursing role (ANA, 2000). Visibility of nurses within the community creates a positive image and identity for the profession. It reflects support by nurses for each other and demonstrates nurses' concern for the health and welfare of the community. This positive image also can contribute to the future of nursing by encouraging the recruitment of individuals into the nursing profession.

Dedicated members within a professional nursing organization can collectively influence others, especially making changes that are in the best interest of the organization, the nursing profession, and the quality of patient care (Deleskey, 2003). For example, members of a professional nursing organization can lobby legislators who influence laws or regulations that govern the nursing profession.

Nurses also can form alliances with other organizations or groups and function as a powerful team to influence decisions that affect nursing.

Consumer Benefits

Consumers can benefit both directly and indirectly from nurses' involvement in professional and community organizations. The knowledge and skills gained by nurses through their involvement in professional nursing organizations can impact the quality of nursing care that consumers receive. For example, results of unit-based research projects supported by a nursing organization can be used in patient protocols on the unit. Journal publications and presentations at nursing conferences enable other nurses to change their nursing practice. Finally, consumers can reap the benefits of healthcare resources gained through the lobbying efforts of professional nursing organizations. All of these factors can potentially impact both the quality of care that consumers receive and the outcomes of this care.

Other nurses and assistive personnel (AP) can benefit from nurses' involvement with professional and community organizations and model the professional skills and leadership behaviors exhibited by these nurses. They can enhance their clinical performance through mentor relationships and attendance at educational offerings sponsored by nurses within these professional organizations.

Personal Advantages

Playing an active role in community and professional organizations has its personal rewards for nurses. For instance, working on specific task forces with set goals can provide you with a sense of belonging to that group. Being an active member of a group can help you learn skills and overcome personal challenges. Participating in these activities can help you realize that your professional and personal qualities are valued, adding to your self-esteem. You may obtain personal satisfaction in knowing that you made a difference in the lives of others, your organization, and the nursing profession. You can apply the leadership skills you developed to your work setting and personal situation. Finally, you can mentor other nurses.

Ways to Share Your Professional Expertise

Although nurses can function in community groups as lay people, it is important that they offer their special talents and expertise as professionals. Nurses have a variety of opportunities to demonstrate their in-depth knowledge and skills that are valued and needed by both community and professional organizations.

Speaker at Educational Programs

One way to share your professional expertise with your local community is to volunteer as a presenter for an educational program. For example, if your expertise is cardiovascular nursing, contact your church representatives and explore their learning needs. Offer to sponsor a program on cardiopulmonary resuscitation (CPR) or one that deals with the risk factors for heart attacks. Share your talents with your own organization, its outreach agencies, or schools of nursing. Consider presenting a unit-based in-service education program; coordinating a learning activity such as

Grand Rounds on your clinical unit; or volunteering to sponsor a booth on smoking cessation at your hospital's annual health fair. Be sure to include other healthcare workers as learners, such as AP, physical and occupational therapists, physicians, nutritionists, and social workers. Volunteer to teach educational programs for your professional nursing organization, and explore local, regional, and national opportunities. Help develop a CE program for nurses through the local chapter of your nursing organization. Be sure to consider a variety of potential learners in your community who could benefit from your expertise as a professional nurse. Chapter 14 will focus on details of developing CE programs and marketing yourself and colleagues in the community.

Consultant

Think about offering your professional nursing expertise with others as a consultant. Start this process by taking an inventory of your professional talents. Identify those things with which you are particularly good. Maybe you possess clinical expertise and expert knowledge in a specialty such as oncology nursing. Perhaps you have advanced skills in trauma nursing or nursing leadership, or maybe you were instrumental in designing a highly successful ambulatory care unit in your organization.

Once you have identified your strengths, brainstorm about individuals or groups who need your services. Ask your colleagues for help with this step. Many law firms use experienced nurses as expert witnesses in legal cases that involve questions related to nurses who provide patient care. Many local chapters of community organizations such as the American Cancer Society (ACS) sponsor professional education programs that use the expertise of an experienced oncology nurse. Consider helping with projects in the community through your local division of the American Heart Association (AHA) or at a child abuse program in your local community.

Finally, investigate ways to market your expertise to individuals you have targeted, then develop a plan to implement your services. If being an expert nurse witness interests you, investigate ways to communicate your interest with law firms in your community. Contact professional organizations, such as the American Association of Legal Nurse Consultants, for guidance regarding this role. If you are interested in assisting community organizations, then contact your local chapters and explore the opportunities. Consider appearing on a local television program or radio station to discuss timely topics related to health care. Offer to write a column on a health topic for a local newspaper or community publication. Some nurses choose to start their own for-profit businesses and market their services in this manner.

Mentor

Have you been fortunate to have a mentor or role model, a person who helps you with decisions regarding your professional development? Even if you have never experienced such a relationship, think about becoming a mentor for an inexperienced nurse.

You can begin this goal of becoming a mentor in a variety ways. Start by volunteering to serve as a preceptor for a nursing student or a new nurse on your unit, or try joining the membership committee of your local professional nursing organization. Sometimes mentor-mentee relationships develop informally through working with others on projects within professional organizations, community agencies, or affiliations.

Community Volunteer Activities

Consider volunteering your services to organizations within your community, such as AHA, the American Red Cross, or ACS. Offer to speak about various health needs and concerns at locations such as schools, prisons, or community clinics.

Approach this goal using a well-developed plan. Start by making a list of community agencies that relate to your career goals, to the clinical specialty with which you have some interest or expertise, or to your professional strengths. Perhaps you pride yourself in being an effective teacher, a compassionate listener, or a productive group leader. Start by first focusing on these strengths.

You can find a list of community agencies in the Human Service Agency section of your telephone book, through your public library, or on the Internet. For example, if you are interested in pediatrics, select several community organizations that reflect this interest. Be sure to investigate available opportunities for professional nurses within each organization. Even if an organization does not have a defined role for nurses, explore the possibility of developing a unique position. Next, select the organization that best matches your goals. Examples of some professional activities appropriate for a professional nurse include the following: organizing a community support group, teaching CPR or childbirth classes, providing instruction in parenting, and coordinating public and professional education programs.

Getting Started: Possible Sources for Involvement

What is the best way to start getting involved in professional nursing and community organizations? In reality, there are many options from which to choose and no single correct way to start the process. In fact, sometimes an individual's involvement begins purely by accident. For example, a colleague asks you to attend a program sponsored by the local chapter of a professional nursing organization. You belong to this organization but have not been active. At this meeting, you are asked to serve on a committee. Before you know it, the group elects you to chair the committee. The satisfaction you gain from your involvement influences you, and you decide to run for an elected office the following year. Later, you serve on a task force for the organization at its national level. Keep in mind that all of these events occurred without planning them from the start.

But what if you choose to be active in an organization from the start? Simply join the organization as a member, then indicate that you would like to explore volunteer opportunities with them. Attend the organization's meetings and educational programs to gain a better understanding of the organization and to meet other members.

When planning your involvement in a professional nursing organization, you need to consider several factors. First, try to match your choice of organizations with the goals you identified in your career plan. More discussion on developing a career plan is presented in Chapter 15.

Second, choose the pace with which you want to become involved within an organization. Start by deciding where you want to be within that organization using a specific time frame. For example, is your goal to chair a committee by next year? Do you want to master the role of a committee member first before you decide to run for office two or three years down the road?

Next, select your desired level of involvement within the organization. Do you want to be active as a general member, a committee member, chair of a committee, or an elected officer? Decide if you are interested in being active at the local, regional, or national levels of the organization. Consult other nurses who hold positions to which you aspire. Ask for their perspective on which position to seek and how to prepare for that role. In the meantime, observe their leadership skills and take detailed notes. Incorporate their advice into your career plan.

Finally, think about your overall involvement in professional nursing organizations. Because it is highly likely that there may be more than one organization that matches your professional interests, decide which ones to join and at what level you plan on participating in each. Although it is common practice to belong to several different nursing organizations at the same time, you will need to carefully plan how to divide your time among them without feeling overwhelmed with commitments you cannot keep. Regardless of your decision, be sure that the quality of your performance does not suffer by the quantity of your involvement. Think about being just a "card-carrying member" in some organizations for a while, as you rotate your participation among them.

Professional Nursing Organizations

Nurses can choose to belong to a variety of professional nursing organizations. Figure 8-2 is a partial list from the more than 200 professional nursing organizations currently available. ANA regularly updates this information on its Web site and provides you with a link to each organization's home page. Although most of these organizations are national or international associations, many have regional or local chapters in which nurses can become actively involved.

How does one go about choosing an organization with which to belong? To help nurses understand more about this topic, Piemonte and Redman (1997) organized professional organizations into three primary categories based on their focus: broad purpose professional organizations, specialty practice associations, and special interest associations. Regardless of its category, select an organization whose purpose matches your particular career interests.

Broad Purpose Professional Organizations

The first category of professional nursing organizations, broad purpose professional organizations, advances the nursing profession within a broad context that concerns most nurses regardless of their clinical specialty (Piemonte & Redman, 1997). Organizations like ANA and National League for Nursing are examples of broad purpose organizations. If your career interests include these concerns, then consider membership in these nursing organizations.

Specialty Practice Associations

Specialty practice associations focus on specific clinical areas that exist in nursing practice (Piemonte & Redman, 1997). These may include specialties such as on-

- Academy of Medical-Surgical Nurses
- Air and Surface Transport Nurses
- American Academy of Ambulatory Care Nursing
- American Assembly for Men in Nursing
- American Association for Continuity of Care
- American Association of Critical-Care Nurses
- American Association of Legal Nurse Consultants
- American Association of Neuroscience Nurses
- American Association of Nurse Anesthetists
- American Association of Nurse Attorneys
- American Association of Occupational Health Nurses
- American Association of Spinal Cord Injury Nurses
- American College of Nurse Practitioners
- American Heart Association Council on Cardiovascular Nursing
- American Holistic Nurses Association
- American Medical Informatics Association
- American Nephrology Nurses Association
- American Psychiatric Nurses Association
- American Public Health Association
- American Radiological Nurses Association
- American Society for Parenteral and Enteral Nutrition
- American Society of Ophthalmic Registered Nurses
- American Society of PeriAnesthesia Nurses
- American Society of Plastic and Reconstructive Surgical Nurses
- American Thoracic Society
- Association for Child and Adolescent Psychiatric Nurses
- Association of Black Nursing Faculty in Higher Education
- Association of Community Health Nursing Educators
- Association of Nurses in AIDS Care
- Association of Occupational Health Professionals
- Association of Pediatric Oncology Nurses
- Association of Perioperative Registered Nurses
- Association of Rehabilitation Nurses
- Association of State and Territorial Directors of Nursing
- Association of Women's Health, Obstetric and Neonatal Nurses (formerly NAACOG)
- Chi Eta Phi Sorority
- Consolidated Association of Nurses in Substance Abuse International
- Council on Graduate Education for Administration in Nursing
- Dermatology Nurses Association
- Developmental Disabilities Nurses Association
- Drug and Alcohol Nursing Association
- Emergency Nurses Association
- Hospice Nurses Association
- International Nurses Society on Addictions (formerly National Nurses Society on Addictions)
- International Society of Nurses in Genetics
- International Society of Psychiatric Mental Health Nurses (ACAPN, SERPN, ISPCLN)
- Intravenous Nurses Society
- National Association of Clinical Nurse Specialists
- National Association of Directors of Nursing Administration in Long Term Care
- National Association of Hispanic Nurses
- National Association of Neonatal Nurses
- National Association of Nurse Massage Therapists
- National Association of Nurse Practitioners in Reproductive Health
- National Association of Orthopaedic Nurses
- National Association of Pediatric Nurse Associates and Practitioners
- National Association of School Nurses
- National Association of State School Nurse Consultants
- National Black Nurses Association
- National Gerontological Nursing Association
- National League for Nursing
- National Nurses Society on Addictions (or International Nurses Society on Addictions)
- National Nursing Staff Development Organization
- National Organization of Nurse Practitioner Faculties
- National Student Nurses Association
- North American Nursing Diagnosis Association
- Nurses Organization of Veteran's Affairs
- Oncology Nursing Society
- Philippine Nurses Association of America
- Respiratory Nursing Society
- Sigma Theta Tau International
- Society for Vascular Nursing
- Society of Gastroenterology Nurses and Associates
- Society of Otorhinolaryngology and Head-Neck Nurses
- Society of Pediatric Nurses
- Society of Urologic Nurses and Associates
- Wound, Ostomy and Continence Nurses Society

Figure 8-2.
American Nurses Association Affiliated Organizations

Note. From "ANA Affiliated Organizations," by the American Nurses Association (2003, June 11). Retrieved June 19, 2003, from http://nursingworld.org/affil/index.htm Copyright 2003 by the American Nurses Association. Reprinted with permission.

cology nursing, medical-surgical nursing, or ear, nose, throat, and head-neck cancer nursing. Organizations such as the Oncology Nursing Society, the Academy of Medical-Surgical Nurses, and the Society of Otorhinolaryngology and Head-Neck Nurses are examples of these specialty practice associations. Join these specialty organizations if you are interested in ensuring standards of care and the needs of nurses within a specialty (Piemonte & Redman). Many of these organizations provide certification, education, research, and publication opportunities related to their area of focus. Other organizations in this category, such as the Nursing Staff Development Organization, focus on nursing education and the role of the staff development educator in healthcare organizations.

Special Interest Associations

Third, special interest associations focus their efforts on interests common to select groups of nurses (Piemonte & Redman, 1997). Examples of these organizations include Sigma Theta Tau International and the Transcultural Nursing Society. Join these organizations if their interests align with yours.

Nursing Alumni Associations

Finally, nursing alumni associations can be conceptualized as a fourth type of professional nursing organization. Although similar to special interest associations, nursing alumni associations limit the majority of their membership to graduates from a respective school of nursing. Although specific goals vary among alumni associations, they often foster the needs of its members, current students, and the school. Nursing alumni associations provide excellent opportunities to develop mentor relationships between alumni and students, and they offer alumni an opportunity to shape the future direction of their alma mater and its future graduates.

Employer Affiliations in the Community

Investigate potential opportunities for involvement with community organizations that are affiliated with your workplace. These places may include community wellness clinics, nurse-managed centers, homecare settings, urgent centers, or daycare centers for seniors and children.

Neighborhood and Religious Organizations

The community in which you reside may need the expertise of a professional nurse. Various neighborhood citizen associations, religious groups, such as churches or synagogues, homeless shelters, and school districts are examples of organizations that can benefit from your knowledge and skills as a nurse. For example, join a parish nurse group if your goal is to work within a faith community doing health screenings, health education, and referrals. If you are unsure what opportunities exist in your area, conduct a community assessment with the help of your local librarian.

Maximizing Your Involvement

Regardless of your choice of professional involvement, be sure to communicate your participation in professional and community organizations with others.

Sharing this information serves two purposes. First, it creates an awareness that may encourage similar behaviors in other nurses. Second, communicating your involvement results in recognition for you, your colleagues, your workplace, and your school.

Be sure to communicate your involvement using both verbal and written methods. Record your involvement appropriately in your professional files through documents such as your portfolio (Chapter 11) and resume (Chapter 12). Write about your experiences in your local community or nursing newspaper, school newsletter, or employer's newsletter. Share the details of your involvement in a manuscript for publication (Chapter 9), or present it as a poster at a nursing conference (Chapter 10). Share your efforts with your colleagues in a unit-based in-service program (Chapters 6 and 7) or informal roundtable presentation. Finally, communicate your accomplishments in an interview with the public relations representative at your workplace.

Summary

This chapter explains reasons why nurses need to be involved in both professional and community organizations. Specific opportunities and directions to promote this activity are described.

References

American Nurses Association. (2000). *Scope and standards of practice for nursing professional development.* Washington, DC: Author.

Cardillo, D. (1998). How to network successfully: Build a team to help you reach your professional and personal goals. *Nursing: Career Directory,* p. 7.

Deleskey, K. (2003). Factors affecting nurses' decisions to join and maintain membership in professional associations. *Journal of Perianesthesia Nursing, 18*(1), 8–17.

DiMauro, N.M. (2000). Continuous professional development. *Journal of Continuing Education in Nursing, 31*(2), 59–62.

Piemonte, R.V., & Redman, B.K. (1997). Professional associations. In K.K. Chitty (Ed.), *Professional nursing: Concepts and challenges* (2nd ed., pp. 88–104). Philadelphia: W.B. Saunders.

Washer, P. (2002). Professional issues. Professional networking using computer-mediated communication. *British Journal of Nursing, 11,* 1215–1218.

CHAPTER 9

Helping Clinical Nurses Share Their Expertise Through Publishing

Sharing clinical expertise with others through publishing is one way that nurses can develop themselves as professionals. Nurses often assume they are not capable of being good writers or publishing an article in their favorite nursing journal. Some nurses think that it is always that "other" nurse with special talents who publishes. Perhaps, after reading an article related to your clinical area, you thought to yourself, "I could have written that!" Maybe you said, "We did that over two years ago at our agency!" You may have remarked to your colleagues, "We had a more effective approach to that clinical problem than the one published in that article."

As a unit-based educator, you may be involved in mentoring nurses on your clinical unit who are interested in preparing an article for publication, or perhaps you are interested in submitting a manuscript yourself. Regardless of your goal, it is important for you to understand the publishing process so that you can offer helpful suggestions. It is also beneficial if you have experienced this process first-hand before you help other nurses.

Most nurses think of journal articles, book chapters, or textbooks when they hear the phrase "writing for publication." However, there are a variety of other ways that nurses can participate in the publishing process. In fact, there are many ways that most nurses already have become involved in publishing. For example, think about the ways you use your written skills at work. Your contributions to your agency's standards of care, patient teaching materials, as well as policies and procedures are a beginning form of professional writing. Think about courses or educational programs you have conducted or talks and poster presentations you have developed. Include the articles you have published in your organization's newsletter or local community newspaper. In some way, you already have had some beginning experience using your professional writing skills.

Why Publish?

Why should clinical nurses, like you, publish? You will be glad to know that this is a common question that nurses often ask themselves. Your educational background and clinical expertise provide you with valuable first-hand knowledge and insight into what is important for your patients and colleagues. Most likely you have been involved in research projects or clinical protocols and have witnessed the impact of these projects on patients and their families. These experiences prepare you to be able to contribute valuable information to the nursing literature. In addition to your clinical expertise, other reasons to publish involve the needs of your patients, nursing profession, employer, and yourself.

Positive Effects on Patient Outcomes

One reason why clinical nurses should publish involves its indirect benefits on nursing care and patient outcomes. Whether you are a student just learning about patient care or an experienced nurse who needs to develop expertise in caring for patients who require special nursing skills and knowledge, print resources, such as articles, can help you meet your needs.

Think about questions you ask yourself in the clinical setting. How should I teach the patient to care for his new appliance? What is the best way to handle that new procedure? What is considered safe clinical practice? You as an expert practitioner in your clinical specialty have the responsibility to answer these questions for other nurses.

Think about the print resources you have read as a nursing student while learning to care for patients. In addition to your nursing text, you probably searched the published literature for journal articles that gave you current information about meeting the needs of your patients and their families. Remember how helpful those articles were to you and how they enabled you to develop your current clinical competencies? Recall how you relied upon information presented in these articles to understand how to care for your patients. Realize the impact that these references have had on your current skills. Now that you possess expertise in your clinical specialty, you need to help other nurses develop this knowledge and these skills. As an experienced nurse, you are in a prime position to help nurses who are just learning about patient care.

Experienced nurses also may rely on the nursing literature to help themselves maintain their clinical competencies or to develop new competencies. As mentioned in Chapter 1, the downsizing and restructuring efforts that have occurred in healthcare organizations resulted in the closing of clinical units and departments. These changes required many nurses to relocate to clinical units unfamiliar to them and to care for patients with health-related needs that were new to them. Nurses who have the clinical expertise in this area can publish articles that describe the nursing care these patients require. This information can assist these relocated nurses as they develop their knowledge and skills in this specialty.

It is important for you to publish articles that may be helpful to assistive personnel (AP) who provide direct care to patients. AP need your expertise as an RN to help guide them through many of the complex patient situations they encounter. AP rely on your leadership skills as they attempt to implement patient care that is delegated to them. They also need print resources that will help them understand how to function as a team member in this restructured healthcare environment. You as the RN are the most appropriate healthcare professional to guide them.

Patients as consumers can benefit directly from your clinical expertise through accessing health-related literature published by nurses. The public can benefit from your expertise by reading articles on topics such as explanations about medications and procedures, the illness experience, and health promotion practices. Lay caregivers, such as spouses and a patient's significant other, need your help as they assume greater responsibility at home for their loved ones. Print resources, developed especially for them, can support their expectations as caregivers.

Finally, consider publishing an article that focuses on controversies in patient care practices or about current healthcare trends. Offer other nurses and consumers an opportunity to view multiple perspectives of an issue so that they can make informed decisions regarding their health care.

Positive Impact on the Nursing Profession

Publishing also contributes significantly to both the present and future status of the nursing profession. It would not have been easy for you to learn about nursing without having access to nursing literature that was both current and applicable to nursing. How would your nursing instructors have gained information about what or how to teach? Nurses often take it for granted that someone else creates the knowledge base so that nurses can learn about patient care.

Publishing can strengthen the history of the nursing profession. Without the printed word, only oral accounts would be available to preserve nursing's knowledge base, practice, and traditions. There would be no documentation describing the evolution of the nursing profession and no research findings to support nursing practice. Nurses would not realize the best way to provide nursing care and teach patients and families. Publishing is an excellent way to document these landmarks and issues.

Benefits to Your Employer and School

The organization in which you are employed benefits by your publishing in the nursing literature. By including your clinical agency or workplace among the bylines, readers will realize where you work. This information is free publicity for your employer and offers a great deal of prestige for your organization. Readers interested in the topic assume that your organization(s) is the place to work or be a patient. Your employer may be viewed as a trendsetter that offers the latest advances to its patients and employees. Because both you and your institution get recognized in an article, your success in publishing is also your employer's success.

Publishing also benefits the school of nursing from which you graduated. Evidence of various scholarship activities, such as publishing, is one of several outcomes tracked by schools of nursing through their alumni surveys. Evidence of graduates' performance are valued by organizations that accredit schools of nursing, such as the National League for Nursing Accrediting Commission (NLNAC, 2003) and the Commission on Collegiate Nursing Education (CCNE, 2003).

Personal and Professional Rewards

Publishing provides personal as well as professional rewards for you as the author (Oermann, 2002). It is rewarding to view your work and name among the pages of an established nursing journal, or perhaps one of your colleagues, while browsing through the latest specialty journal, sees your article and compliments you. What about nursing students on your unit using your article to prepare their plan of care? Or the nurse, living across the country, who just read your article and contacts you to ask for your help with a clinical situation? What about a concerned family member who e-mails you requesting guidance for his or her loved one who needs the surgical procedure you described in your article?

Although these outcomes can obviously boost your self-esteem, publishing also can positively impact your professional nursing career (Tonges, 2000). Once your work is published, people who read it assume that you are an expert on that topic. As a result, other publishers who want you to write for them may contact you. A professional nursing organization may invite you to speak on this topic at its local chapter meeting or conference. A law firm may contact you to serve as an expert witness in a legal case or may ask you to provide your professional opinion on litigation involving a nurse who cared for a patient in a clinical scenario or topic similar to the one you published in your nursing article.

Consulting and job offers can result by others viewing your publications. You may be asked to give advice on a new research or clinical tool you developed or to share your expertise on developing a research project.

Publishing can be a means of validating your clinical expertise for promotion purposes at work. If publishing is among the criteria for clinical nurse advancement at your healthcare organization, then that means your employer values publishing. Publishing, therefore, can provide professional benefits to both you and your colleagues.

The process of preparing a manuscript, in itself, also has its rewards. Although you may choose a topic with which you are already familiar, your additional research on it can expand your knowledge base on that subject and strengthen your competency in that area (Oermann, 2002). In fact, your writing efforts can lead to the development of a book or even a new journal targeted toward your area of expertise.

Publishing with other colleagues can result in lasting friendships and a professional network. Now, rather than being simply a consumer of nursing literature, you are also a contributor to a particular area of nursing knowledge. This in itself helps you develop as a professional nurse.

Finally, consider other rewards associated with publishing. Some nurses view writing as a creative outlet and enjoy it (Zilm, 2002). Most publishing companies provide you with a free copy of the journal in which your article appeared. Although most companies do not pay their authors for their work, the personal benefits you gain by seeing your name and article in print can be rewarding (McConnell, 1999).

Ways to Overcome Barriers on a Unit-Based Level

If your official role on your clinical unit or department includes encouraging your colleagues to publish, there are a variety of ways to get started with the process. You may be interested in writing yourself. Before you begin, think about some common reasons most nurses give for not publishing. Then, develop a plan that includes strategies to overcome these barriers.

Maximize your approach by developing small writing work groups on your unit. One way is to identify either existing formal work groups or informal groups on your unit, and encourage them to publish using their clinical projects as examples. Journal clubs are one informal way that nurses can get involved in the publishing process. Journal clubs are groups of nurses who meet on a regular basis, such as once a month, to discuss published articles of interest to them (Polit & Beck, 2004).

Introduce this activity as part of your professional nursing organization's local chapter activities. Because nurses who participate in these organizations most likely will have interests similar to yours, this strategy can help nurses develop ideas and gain support.

For example, suppose a group of RNs just returned from presenting a clinical project on critical pathways at a national nursing conference. Develop a plan that will take advantage of the current excitement of this group. Suggest that they turn their presentation into a manuscript. If you have an opportunity to talk with them before they present, ask them to audiotape their presentation. Once they transcribe the tape, they will have a draft of their manuscript. Because their abstract was accepted for a national presentation, there probably is an audience that would like to have it in print form. Even if they did not get a chance to tape their presentation, suggest they tape it as they repeat their presentation at a unit-based conference for the nurses or at a local chapter of a professional nursing organization.

Consider capturing the essence of a poster presentation as a manuscript. The work that you already put into organizing your poster will help you develop an outline to structure your draft.

Encourage members of formal work groups on your clinical unit to publish. Approach members of the patient education committee to transform their recent success with patient-focused critical pathways into a journal article, or encourage members of the staffing work group to document the novel approach they devised to meet the staffing needs of several specialty units. Survivors of an organization's merger can help their colleagues, who have not yet experienced a restructuring, benefit from their insight. Nurses who have first hand experience with new events, such as restructuring, can provide leadership for others to follow their successes and to avoid their pitfalls. Sharing (in writing) the challenges that you faced and strategies you used to manage them is vital.

Henninger and Nolan (1998) described the success of two group education programs designed to promote publication in hospital-based nurses. Both programs included sessions on instruction, guidance, and encouragement and resulted in positive outcomes. The authors attributed the success of these strategies to the positive value that was placed on publishing within the organization and having a clear idea for a manuscript at the start of the program. This group approach was considered more cost-effective and used fewer resources when compared with traditional one-on-one instruction on publishing.

Lack of Time

Many nurses cite lack of time as a reason why they do not publish (Oermann, 2002). They claim that their job, family, and personal life consume most of their day. These nurses feel that someone else can publish because it is too much work for them. Do these comments sound familiar? It is very easy to talk yourself out of devoting the time it takes to write.

Assuming that you and others are interested in professional writing and want to make it a priority in your nursing careers, think of creative ways to incorporate writing into your existing schedule, either at home or at work. This task is essential if publishing is among your professional goals.

If you plan to write alone, first determine during what part of the day you feel most creative and in the mood to write (Oermann, 1999a). Maybe it is the early morning hours before work or one afternoon during the weekend. Lunchtime at work also can provide some productive time for writing. For some individuals, writing flows best in the evening or late at night. Regardless of the time you choose to write, set aside some time that is best for you.

Next, determine how much time you can dedicate to publishing. Whether it is one hour or two, any block of time allotted to your writing project will help you progress in the right direction. For example, a couple of hours of writing on the weekend can accumulate significantly over time. Try to record something down on paper, even on the days when you feel less creative. You will be surprised how much progress you can make with small, continuous additions to your project. Establish a time schedule with a mentor or former teacher in which small portions of a manuscript are due on a specific date. This approach may help you get past some of those small hurdles or delays in writing that you may encounter.

Another way to capture the time to publish is to coauthor a manuscript with a colleague. Although this approach may take a little more coordination with schedules than when writing by yourself, working with a partner also has its benefits. Besides contributing to only part of the total manuscript, writing with a partner may encourage you to meet deadlines. You do not want to disappoint your colleague or become embarrassed by your lack of productivity on the project.

If you prefer to author a manuscript by yourself, try bouncing your publishing ideas off other colleagues or friends. They can serve as a preliminary editor of your work and provide you with encouragement.

Fear of Failure

Some nurses may delay or totally avoid writing for publication because they fear they will fail (McConnell, 1999; Oermann, 1999b). For some individuals, this fear may be the possibility of having their manuscript rejected by a journal editor. Other nurses may resist receiving constructive criticism or feedback about their work from manuscript reviewers. Some writers may perceive preparing a manuscript as an overwhelming task. As a result of these feelings, prospective authors may either procrastinate writing or avoid the project entirely.

There are several ways that you can overcome these feelings. First, realize the strengths you already possess related to publishing, such as the oral and written communication skills you use every day at work (Stepanski, 2002). Second, think about the worst scenario that can happen. For example, an editor may reject your manuscript, a possible outcome that will be discussed later in this chapter. Even the most experienced and successful nurse authors have had their share of rejection letters and have survived to talk about it, along with their publication credits.

There are a variety of reasons why your article might be rejected, other than your writing style. The editor should provide you with specific reasons why your manuscript was rejected so that you can strengthen it for the next submission. For instance, perhaps your topic was not appropriate for the readers of the journal, or maybe the idea was already published two years earlier by that journal or by another journal.

Keep in mind that only the journal editor and you will know that your manuscript was rejected and the reasons why it was rejected. Because your name is removed from your manuscript as it is reviewed (blind review), none of the peer reviewers knows the identity of the author. It is your prerogative to tell others about your rejection letter or to keep this information private. It is important to remember that you have control over the situation.

Remember that writing for publication takes practice and faith in yourself. You needed hours of practice, repetition, and help from experts in perfecting your clinical skills over the years to become the competent practitioner that you are today. This same process of practice and guidance applies to developing your professional writing skills. Before you were a novice nurse, and now you are a novice author. Allow yourself some time, lots of practice, and encouragement from others. Just tell your story, believe what is in your heart, and share it. Give yourself credit for trying and heading in the right direction.

Try sharing your ideas with other colleagues before submitting your manuscript. Ask for their honest opinion about things such as the importance of the topic, the way you organized the manuscript, and your writing style and grammar. Ask them if additional tables or figures would help clarify the content. This will provide you with some input before you receive the reviewers' comments. This strategy also may provide you with the self-confidence you need to complete the project.

Some authors deal with their fear of failure by teaming up with an experienced author, especially for their first manuscript. This approach can give you that extra assurance that will help you to move forward. Consider using networks that already exist in your personal and professional life. For instance, approach a clinical nurse specialist who has a successful publishing record to write an article together. Because faculty in university-based schools of nursing usually are experienced in the publication process and are expected to publish, ask a former nursing instructor to join you in coauthoring a manuscript based on a class project you recently completed.

Finally, consider coauthoring a manuscript with a colleague that you met at a national conference sponsored by your professional nursing organization. Try communicating with your colleague using a variety of methods, such as e-mail, postal mail, fax, and telephone. Jacob and Cherry (2000) shared their success in using electronic communication while coauthoring a text. This approach increased their productivity and reduced their costs when compared with traditional methods. It also required them to strengthen their planning and communication skills. Brandi, Lockhart, and O'Hare (2003) claimed similar benefits by using e-mail in developing a keypal project between American and Japanese nursing students. The authors were successful in preparing a published manuscript describing this student project, relying on e-mail and fax.

Limited Resources

Some nurses are worried that they may not have access to resources needed for producing a manuscript. Earlier, this chapter described ways to obtain additional human resources for your project, as well as finding time to fit writing into your schedule.

Preparing a manuscript has some costs associated with the process. Main costs may include conducting a literature search, duplicating references, preparing a computer-generated final product with computer disk, and mailing manuscript copies to the editor. In some cases, you also may need to produce camera-ready figures, illustrations, or photographs that will enhance your manuscript.

Although the costs associated with these steps of the publishing process may vary depending on your project, they often can be minimized if you do them yourself, share them with coauthors, or combine them with other projects in which you are involved. For example, the literature review that you completed for you recent project in graduate school can serve as a good beginning for a manuscript. Even the background research that you conducted to prepare your presentation for the local professional organization can provide the basis for a paper.

If typing is not your strongest skill, you can create a manuscript draft and contract with a typist who can prepare your final product on a computer. This holds true with any pictures or computer-generated tables you may need to develop to accompany your manuscript.

Some journals have recently implemented a Web-based management system in place of the traditional paper approach to submitting a manuscript. These systems require potential authors to submit their manuscript materials online through a specific Web site. This approach not only facilitates the submission process for authors but also allows them to track the progress of their manuscript as it proceeds through the peer-review process. This online management system also enables peer-reviewers to access manuscripts they are assigned to review and to submit their comments and recommendations online.

Difficulty Generating Ideas

Finding a specific topic or idea about which to write poses a barrier for some nurses, especially when you are under pressure to do so. A good way to avoid this obstacle is to create a file folder labeled "writing ideas." As you think of topics, just write them down on a piece of paper and store them in this folder. You will be surprised how they come in handy later. As time passes, you may opt to organize your ideas into a publishing binder that contains several file folders, each labeled with a different topic. You also may want to store your general references on publishing here, as well as some sample articles from various journals. It is also a good place to keep your writing style manual or similar references you use in preparing a manuscript so they can be easily retrieved.

Record ideas for articles as soon as you think of them. Sometimes ideas come to you in the strangest situations, such as when you are driving your car, waiting for a doctor's appointment, or listening to a speaker at a nursing conference. Audiotape your ideas as they come to you, if you prefer this approach. Remember, the more details that you record about your proposed article, the easier you will be able to recall them. Later, this chapter will present creative ways you can use to capture the ideas that are publishable.

Unfamiliar With the Publishing Process

"I don't know how to publish!" If this is your claim, then approach this problem in a similar fashion as you have in the past with other skills you have tried to master. Seek out sources of instruction that can help you with various aspects of the publishing process. If writing is not your strength, then enroll in a creative writing class for adults at your community college. Ask you local bookstore or librarian to locate available "how-to" books on publishing that can help you get started.

Consider enrolling in a writing for publication course sponsored by a school of nursing. Lockhart (2000) described the successful implementation of such a course that was conducted through a partnership between a hospital and school of nursing. The course resulted in several publications by graduate nursing students and clinical nurses who enrolled in the course. The project enabled both organizations to attain additional goals related to recruitment and professional development.

If you are not sure about what to do once you have sharpened your writing skills, attend sessions sponsored by nursing organizations that deal with publishing. Invite a nurse who is an expert in publishing to speak either to a group of interested colleagues at work or to nurses at the next meeting of your local nursing organization. Investigate the library for written sources on publishing, including select chapters on publishing in texts. Try searching the Internet for resources on writing for publication. The "how-to" of writing for publication will be discussed later in this chapter.

Few Incentives to Publish

Because publishing can be considered a change in behavior for some nurses, try relying on the approach you usually use when implementing a new policy or piece of equipment to staff on your unit. For example, start by identifying the positive things that nurses might value regarding publishing. Identify the negative features they perceive. Positive features may include a group's desire to publish or the benefits that publishing can have on advancing up the career ladder. On the other hand, negative features might include reasons that were already discussed in this chapter, such as a lack of time or fear of failure. Develop a plan for nurses on your clinical unit that emphasizes the benefits of publishing and minimizes the negative factors. Continue to provide the nurses with ongoing support throughout the process.

Include various strategies in your plan that will help you meet your goal. One way is to appeal to your colleagues' sense of reason by promoting all of the positive aspects related to having an article published. Or perhaps you may want to try a different approach, and remind your colleagues that publishing is a criterion for promotion. Third, try showcasing a group that has been successful in publishing. Once a few nurses on your unit start publishing, others may feel out of place by not publishing. Over time and with the right support systems in place, other nurses may be encouraged to participate.

Understanding the Publication Process: The 10-Step Approach

Once you overcome some of the emotional and logistic barriers to publishing, you will need to focus on the practical aspects of writing for publication. If you have never published before, it is likely that do not know how to begin. The following section reviews the publishing process, using a clinical journal article as an example.

Figure 9-1 displays the process involved using the 10-step approach to preparing a manuscript for publication in a journal (Lockhart, 2000). There may be instances in which you may begin at a step anywhere along the process or situations in which you will need to repeat previous steps. Because each writing experience may differ, it is important not to be discouraged along the way.

Figure 9-1.
The 10-Step
Approach to
Publishing

Note. From "Writing
for Health Care Publi-
cations: A Partnership
Between Service and
Education," by J.S.
Lockhart, 2000, *Nurse
Educator, 25*(4), p.
197. Copyright 2000
by Lippincott Williams
and Wilkins. Re-
printed with permis-
sion.

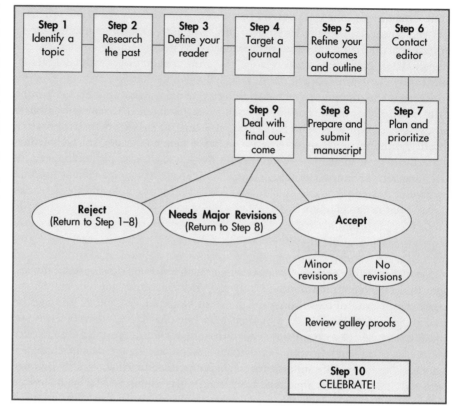

Step 1: Identify a Topic or Idea

Start the publishing process with a general topic or idea in which you have an interest. If available, start by reviewing the notes you recorded in your file folder, as described earlier in this chapter. If you have not developed an idea for a manuscript, then you will need to know where to search for publishable topics. Remember that it is essential to clearly identify a topic of interest and fully develop it before discarding the idea altogether.

You can use a variety of strategies to identify an idea that you can develop into a manuscript. First, consider writing on a topic on which you have previously searched the literature and were unsuccessful in finding anything, or perhaps you found a few articles on the topic, but these articles did not meet your needs.

A second way to define an idea for a manuscript is to reflect on your clinical experience with patients and families. Try recalling a particular incident that stands out in your mind, such as when a patient avoided a postoperative complication because of your astute nursing assessment skills. Consider a situation in which your creative adaptation of nasogastric tube taping relieved your patient's discomfort. Think about the teaching tool you developed for patients so they could easily remember to take their medications on schedule at home.

A third method you can use to identify publishable ideas is to reflect on your clinical strengths. For example, do nurses from other clinical units call you for advice to learn how to care for the patient who has a tracheotomy? Do your colleagues contact you for help when they need to prepare a poster presentation? Do you have a unique role (e.g., a case manager, unit-based educator) on your clinical unit? Consider sharing information about your role, which can benefit other interested nurses. By recording your experiences like these in print, you can guide other nurses in their professional development efforts.

School papers or projects can serve as a fourth method to identify a publishable topic. For example, consider adapting the debate that you presented on the advantages and disadvantages of obtaining a nursing specialty certification into a manuscript. Other nurses considering certification can benefit from your research on this topic. Think about sharing how you managed juggling multiple roles while finishing your nursing degree. Review some of your school papers, and determine the value of their topic for a manuscript. Although your actual school paper usually cannot be submitted as a manuscript, it can provide a good draft after some revisions are made.

Another source of manuscript ideas includes your involvement in community projects or professional organizations. For example, think about sharing how you developed an electronic newsletter for your local nursing organization. Write about the volunteer activity you experienced immunizing children in an underserved region of the country or the vision-screening program that you developed for school-age children in your community.

Although most of these strategies focus on your role as a nurse, think about providing other nurses with insight about your personal experience as a patient or family caregiver. For example, consider writing about your experience as caregiver for an elderly parent following a debilitating illness or when you needed to make a decision regarding life support for a loved one. Also think about sharing your personal experiences as a patient. For instance, describe how you coped with a diagnosis of cancer and what the nursing staff did that helped you or did not help you. Many of these experiences have the potential to benefit others that may face similar situations.

Include writing about topics that reflect strategies that your organization has used to deal with current healthcare trends and issues. For example, think about describing the innovative ways that nurses on your clinical unit have dealt with the nursing shortage. Write about the novel patient education approach you recently implemented to help nurses deal with patients' shortened lengths of stay following surgery. Discuss the critical pathways that you formed or the creative staffing approach that you developed. Talk about the strategies you used to cope with the stress associated with recent restructuring and downsizing at your workplace. These strategies have the potential to help other nurses who may be experiencing these changes.

Finally, ask your colleagues to help you generate publishable ideas. For example, they may comment on the admirable way you handled a conflict with a physician or the effective manner in which you worked with APs on your clinical unit. Perhaps they acknowledge the effective way you preceptored a senior nursing student last semester.

Step 2: Research the Past

After identifying a publishable idea, confirm and clarify your idea by searching the current nursing literature. This search can be accomplished using both formal and informal approaches. One informal approach is to thumb through recent issues of nursing journals. Start by reviewing recent issues of journals that you often refer to as resources or journals to which you subscribe. Examine the topics in their tables of contents, as well as the perspectives used by the authors. This approach may help you identify what topics have been already published or those that have not been addressed.

Next, conduct a systematic literature review on your topic in the recent nursing literature. Unless you need articles that are considered classic works, limit your search to articles published within the past four to five years (Buchsel, 2001). Even if you did not find an article on your topic in the journals you reviewed by hand, it may have been published in journals with which you may not be as familiar. The best way to systematically review the literature is to conduct a computerized literature search on your topic using healthcare databases, such as the Cumulative Index to Nursing and Allied Health Literature (CINAHL®) or MEDLINE. Ask for the librarian's assistance so that you can be sure you have completed a comprehensive review of your topic.

This first literature search is aimed at helping you clarify your topic in the nursing literature. You will need to review the literature again as you prepare the details of your manuscript to develop your reference list (Sigler, 1999).

Do not be alarmed if you discover that your idea has already been published. Then, consider being creative by developing a manuscript using a different perspective on the same topic or targeting a different audience.

For example, suppose your literature review revealed that someone has already published an article about the nursing care of patients following a total laryngectomy. Think of other creative options that involve this topic, such as focusing on the care of laryngectomy patients at home or describing effective teaching methods you have used to promote self-care. If you are experienced in perioperative nursing, write about this phase of patient recovery. If your interest lies in the office setting, describe the assessment skills you used with patients prior to their admission for surgery. Finally, back up a step further and focus on health promotion practices that individuals can use to prevent laryngeal cancer.

Researching the nursing literature also helps you create an updated reference list to use in developing your manuscript. The search can help you determine which journals you can target for publishing your manuscript.

Step 3: Define Your Readers

After developing a publishable idea and searching the literature, clarify your target audience. This step will help you establish a focus for your manuscript and will assist you later as you develop objectives for your manuscript. Knowing your readers also can help you in selecting potential journals that may publish your work.

If you decide that your target audience is clinical nurses, then determine their practice area. Consider if they work on a medical-surgical unit or in a specialty area. If these nurses are generalists, try to clarify if they work in specific settings, such as ambulatory care, acute care, home care, or long-term care. If they are specialists, clarify the way in which their practice areas are defined, such as critical care, emergency, or oncology nursing.

If nurse educators are your target audience, use the same process to determine the specific needs of your readers. Determine if these educators function in roles such as patient educators or faculty in schools of nursing. You may want to target staff development educators or community-focused educators employed in wellness centers.

Try a similar approach with readers such as nurse managers or nurse research-ers. The more specific you are, the easier it will be to develop your manuscript and identify potential publishers. Remember to consider consumers, families, and other healthcare workers such as AP, student nurses, physical therapists, occupa-tional therapists, and physicians as possible target audiences for your manuscript.

Step 4: Target Specific Journals

Once you have completed the first three steps of the publishing process, develop a strategic plan to use in targeting potential journals in which to publish your manu-script. You can use a variety of approaches to identify these journals. You may start by selecting journals with which you are familiar, as mentioned earlier.

You also can access a listing of nursing journals and a description of their characteristics through the Internet or in print sources (e.g., a list of print and elec-tronic publications through PubList.com). This site provides detailed information about numerous journals with links to each publisher's Internet home page (PubList.com, 1998–2001). The CINAHL Database is another helpful site for in-formation about journals (CINAHL, 2003). ONLINE™ Nursing Editors provides readers with a list of more than 200 nursing journal and book editors. This site provides you with contact information for each editor and a direct link to the journal's author guidelines (Oermann, 1999b).

If you are interested in learning more about publications outside the United States, a review of publishing opportunities by McConnell (2000) is a resource you may find helpful in refining your publishing plan. This article provides you with details about journals, such as their circulation, acceptance rate, and issues published annually. It also tells you whether a journal is refereed, a topic that will be discussed later in this chapter.

Although these articles provide you with an overview of publishing opportuni-ties, obtain detailed information from the journal's author guidelines. They will tell you about the purpose of the journal, its targeted readers, and the type of ar-ticles the journal publishes (Carroll-Johnson, 2001).

Key information about journals can be very helpful to you as a prospective author. For example, you may decide to submit your manuscript to a specific journal because, if published, it will be exposed to a large readership. You may wish to choose a journal that publishes several issues each year or a large numbers of pages per issue, with the assumption that this may increase your odds of having your manuscript published in a timely manner.

These resources on journals also provide you with helpful information about the way you will need to prepare your manuscript (e.g., required format, number of copies you will need to submit, need for a query letter). Details on the purpose and development of a query letter will be provided later in this chapter.

This information also informs you about what happens to your manuscript once it is received. An important feature to know about the review process is whether the journal is refereed. Being a refereed journal means that your manuscript is reviewed by peers—other nurses across the country who have expertise in both your topic and in publishing (Polit & Beck, 2004). These content experts share their comments with the editor of the journal, who incorporates them into the fi-nal decision regarding publication of your manuscript. Obviously, having your manuscript withstand the scrutiny of expert nurses in your field adds prestige and value to an article.

You may want to review each journal's acceptance and rejection rates, as well as the average time it takes for your manuscript to be reviewed and published once it has been accepted. This information can help you estimate your chances of getting published in a specific journal. As a result, you may want to consider the odds of having your manuscript accepted when you choose a journal. Knowing that it can take as long as one year from the time of your manuscript's acceptance to see it in print may help you put the process in its proper perspective.

After reviewing the list of prospective journals, identify two to three journals you think would be appropriate sources for your manuscript to be published, and list them in order of preference. Considering more than one journal initially will save you time later, in the event your manuscript is not accepted. This approach also may lessen the tension you may experience in thinking that you have only one opportunity to publish.

Other factors, such as your idea, approach, and target audience, can influence your choice of journals to target. For example, suppose you want to prepare a manuscript dealing with the care of patients diagnosed with laryngeal cancer. You have no specific audience in mind.

Because you possess expertise in caring for these patients, support your journal selection with rationale based on your experience in clinical practice. You are frequently consulted by nurses who work on medical-surgical units asking for your advice in caring for laryngectomees recently being admitted to their unit for cardiac problems following surgery. In networking with your colleagues at a nursing conference, you discover that they also have experienced similar requests at their organizations. You conduct a literature search, and find that very little has been recently published on this topic.

After speaking with the medical-surgical nurses, you discover that most of them rely on two primary journals to keep them current. A brief trip to your local nursing library reveals two other general journals. A crosscheck with your literature search confirms that nothing on this topic has been published in these journals. This information will help you in designing your publishing plan.

While you are at the library, record key information, such as author guidelines, from the most recent issue of each journal. These guidelines often are located near either the front or back of most journals. If you cannot find this page, record the editor's name, address, telephone number, and e-mail address. Use this information to contact the editor to obtain a copy of the guidelines. Many journals post their author guidelines and sample articles on their home page accessible via the Internet.

Remember to duplicate sample articles from each journal, selecting examples that most closely resemble the one you have in mind. These are useful to refer to as you develop your final manuscript.

Finally, confirm the purpose of your manuscript and target audience with those of each journal you selected. Journals usually publish this information either near the front of the journal, in the author guidelines, or on the Internet.

Step 5: Refine Your Focus With Outcomes and Outlines

After identifying the journal that is your first choice, use the journal information to develop objectives for your manuscript. Although you already have a general idea and purpose for your manuscript, generating objectives is essential to refine your focus. This step is frequently a difficult one for authors. One approach is to ask yourself, "After nurses read my article, they will know what? Be able to do what?" Limit your manuscript to two or three key objectives or outcomes.

After identifying your objectives, develop an outline for your manuscript using resources you obtained from the literature review and the sample articles you duplicated. The more specific your outline is, the easier it will be to prepare your manuscript. Expect to spend sufficient time on this planning step.

After you have realized the overall content and tone of your manuscript, start thinking of a creative title for it. The style of the title should be consistent with those of other articles in the same journal, short in length, and yet unique enough to capture the reader's interest. Remember that the working title may change as you develop your manuscript or be changed by the journal editor after your manuscript is accepted and edited.

Step 6: Contact Prospective Editors

This next step of the publishing process involves contacting the editor of the journal you selected to determine his or her interest in your manuscript. It is acceptable to send queries to more than one journal at the same time (Carroll-Johnson, 2001).

Some editors prefer written contact from prospective authors, called a query letter, whereas others prefer to be contacted by telephone or e-mail. You can find this information in the author guidelines. Some editors prefer no prior communication and request that you submit your manuscript directly. You also can inquire about their interest by discussing your manuscript in person with journal editors often available during conferences sponsored by professional nursing organizations. Regardless of the approach, you will need to do some work in advance.

Essential elements you will need to share with the editor are illustrated in Figures 9-2 and 9-3. Figure 9-2 is a sample of a query letter, and Figure 9-3 is a sample of an e-mail query. It is suggested that you address the e-mail directly to the editor and include your name and manuscript title in the subject heading (Johnson, 2003).

If you are unfamiliar with formal letter writing, be sure to use your library's writing reference texts for composing the basic structure of a letter. In Figure 9-2, the query letter consists of three primary sections: an opening, body, and closing. Each of these components will be discussed in greater detail.

Opening

In the opening section of the query letter, be precise with the spelling and format of the editor's name, credentials, and title of the editor exactly as it appears in most current issue of the journal, in the journal's author guidelines, or on the journal's Web site. When in doubt, contact the journal directly to obtain this information.

Body

The body is the most crucial part of the query letter in which you logically convince the editor that your manuscript is exactly what the journal needs. In presenting your case, be sure to answer the following questions:

What? Provide the title of the proposed manuscript as well as a brief overview of its contents. An attached outline of your manuscript will help clarify your point.

Figure 9-2.
Sample Query
Letter

June 16, 2004

Jane Smith, PhD, RN
Editor, *Journal of Nursing*
375 Bayside Road
Philadelphia, PA 15202

Dear Dr. Smith:

As an experienced Clinical Staff Nurse in the Head and Neck Oncology Unit at Nursing University Medical Center, I recently assumed the additional responsibility for meeting the in-service education needs of nurses who work on several patient units in our facility. As a result, I developed a strategy that not only facilitates the implementation of unit-based in-service programs on these units but also fosters the professional growth of the staff nurses.

Following an annual written assessment of education needs for these units, I devised a six-month plan to fulfill these requests. Because nurses chose unit-based conferences as their preferred learning method, I developed and implemented a unit-based in-service program. This one-hour program focuses on the process involved in presenting an in-service offering, assessment of learner needs, development of a lesson plan, implementation, and evaluation. A 10-Step Checklist was created to help nurses track the details. Since I have implemented this program in July, several staff nurses have developed lesson plans and have presented excellent programs.

I hope that you will find this manuscript that describes this strategy appropriate for readers of *Journal of Nursing*. Nurses who assume similar responsibilities in staff education will find this information extremely valuable as they seek innovative strategies to meet the multiple requests for in-service education and professional staff development. I would be able to have this manuscript available to you for review within the next four to six weeks.

Your consideration of my request will be greatly appreciated. Please feel free to contact me at my e-mail address (lockhartj@dsd.com) or via telephone at work at (413) 376-8640 during the day anytime between 8:30 am and 5 pm.

Sincerely,

Joan Such Lockhart

Joan Such Lockhart, BSN, RN, CORLN
1344 Treeline Drive
Pittsburgh, PA 16439

Why not? Convince the editor of the importance of your topic. Stress how innovative it is and how it may affect nursing practice and patient outcomes.

Why you? Describe your expertise, especially why you are qualified to write this article. Be sure to include your formal and informal education, clinical experiences, and certifications.

Why now? Emphasize the timeliness of your topic. Explain how it fits into what is currently happening in health care or its anticipated focus in the near future.

Why them? Explain how your idea matches the focus of the journal and will appeal to its targeted readers. It is a good idea to mention the journal's name in the letter.

When? Inform the editor when you foresee your manuscript being ready and submitted. Depending on your topic, it is a good idea to keep your timeline realistic yet marketable.

Closing

Finish the letter with a formal closing. Be sure to sign your name directly above the typed version. Include your credentials (e.g., RN, BSN) and certifications, if appropriate.

General Guidelines for Query Letters

Because a query letter often is your first contact with an editor, both its content and appearance need to make a good first impression. Be sure it is neatly typed and spaced on the page, preferably computer-generated, and printed on quality paper. Use these same guidelines in preparing the envelope. Be sure to sign your name to the letter.

Unlike manuscripts, it is appropriate to send query letters to more than one journal editor at the same time. If you do this, be sure to customize the content of each letter to match its respective journal. This is also a good time to request author guidelines from the editor, if needed.

From: Joan Lockhart (lockhartj@dsd.com)
To: Dr. Eileen Carter
Subject: Manuscript Query: Being Alert After Routine Procedures (Joan Lockhart)
Date: Mon, 17 June 2004 16:45:17

Dear Dr. Carter:

As an experienced medical-surgical staff nurse at City Hospital, I recently encountered a clinical emergency that would be appropriate for your Emergency! feature column.

An elderly man diagnosed with cholangiocarcinoma returned to his room following a percutaneous transhepatic cholangiogram (PTC). This radiological procedure, used to visualize the biliary structures, is frequently performed as both a diagnostic test and a therapeutic intervention.

Unfortunately, the patient developed one of the common risks associated with a PTC, bleeding at the injection site. His preexisting liver failure and associated deficiency of clotting factors only complicated the situation. The nurse's assessment of early changes in the patient's mental and hemodynamic status and prompt treatment saved his life.

I hope that you will find this manuscript appealing to your readers, because nurses play a pivotal role in detecting early complications in patients following routine invasive procedures. I would be able to have this manuscript available to you for review within the next month.

Your consideration of my request will be greatly appreciated. Please feel free to contact me at my e-mail address or by telephone at (413) 376-8640 during the day at work anytime between 8:30 am and 5 pm.

Sincerely,

Joan Such Lockhart, BSN, RN
Clinical Staff Nurse II, Community Hospital
Pittsburgh, PA 26667
E-Mail: lockhartj@dsd.com

Figure 9-3.
Sample E-Mail Query

Remember, a promising response from an editor to your query letter only means that your idea may be a publishable one for the journal. It is not an automatic guarantee that your manuscript will be accepted once it is received. Your manuscript will undergo a review process as described earlier in this chapter. Timely submission of your manuscript after receiving a positive response from an editor has the potential to make a difference in the final outcome of your manuscript. For example, if you wait too long to submit your manuscript, it may be received by a new editor that may have different goals in mind for the journal than the previous editor, and your proposed idea may not be one of them.

Step 7: Plan and Prioritize

Based on the response to your query letters, prioritize your journal selection again. Then start preparing your manuscript or finalizing changes.

Step 8: Prepare and Submit Your Manuscript

Some authors prepare their manuscripts prior to sending query letters, whereas others wait for the editor's response before finalizing their manuscript. Over time, you will develop your own preference and style. If it is your first attempt at publishing, you may want to have something prepared in writing ahead of time. Developing a manuscript in advance permits you to make minor changes in a timely fashion and submit it. Its drawback is that you may need to make major changes if you need to target a different journal than the one you used to prepare it.

Regardless of your choice, prepare your manuscript using the outline you developed, the sample article, and the author guidelines for that journal. Keep the objectives you initially developed in mind. Before you complete your manuscript, visualize what your finished product will look like in publication. Attempt to draft a preliminary layout of your article, considering the use of supplements such as figures, tables, graphics, or photographs.

Unlike query letters, submit your manuscript to only one journal at a time until you are notified that your manuscript was rejected (Carroll-Johnson, 2001). This point is crucial, because lack of compliance may be considered a violation of copyright laws.

As the author, you are responsible for ensuring that the information in your manuscript is accurate (Wong, 1999). Pay extreme attention to items such as references, data, and other citations. Double-check your final manuscript for errors, and ask a colleague to provide a second review to check for its accuracy.

When preparing your manuscript, be alert to issues related to plagiarism, fabrication, and falsification. Plagiarism basically means that you submitted someone else's work as your own (American Psychological Association [APA], 2001). Avoid plagiarism by carefully citing sources in your text according to guidelines cited in publication manuals. Fabrication is "making up data or facts" included in your manuscript, and falsification means "changing or misrepresenting data or facts" (Flanagin, 1993, p. 359).

Creating a Title

Think of a title for your manuscript that is creative yet captures the essence of your project. The title should reflect the general meaning of your manuscript. Others may use key words of your title when they conduct computer searches on the topic.

One way to arrive at a title is to write down several key words that are essential elements of your manuscript. Then, try to logically arrange them. Refer to sample articles, especially those published within your targeted journal, for ideas. Start with a title draft, and then refine it after you have completed your manuscript.

Deciding Authorship

If you are preparing a manuscript with the help of others, you will need to deal with several issues concerning authorship. First, before you prepare your manuscript, decide who will be authors, and explain the expectations of an author. To be considered an author, the individual should have made a significant contribution to the manuscript (International Committee of Medical Journal Editors [ICMJE], 2001). According to ICMJE, authorship means meeting three criteria. First, the individual made a significant contribution to the conception or design, data collection, data analysis, or interpretation described in the manuscript. Second, the individual should have played a part in drafting or revising the manuscript for substantial content. Third, the individual must have reviewed the final draft of the manuscript before it was submitted to the journal and provided approval. If individuals who helped with the manuscript do not meet all these criteria for authorship, recognize them in the article in an acknowledgment paragraph.

Next, determine the order in which the authors will be listed. The first author is the person who assumes most of the work related to the manuscript process, such as the preparation, submission, and follow-up (Oermann, 2002). The first author is usually the contact person, the individual with whom the editor corresponds throughout the publishing process. Try to determine the order of the remaining authors using a cooperative approach. Arrive at an understanding about authorship prior to submitting your manuscript to avoid misunderstandings (Oermann, 2002).

Once your manuscript is accepted for publication, the editor may ask each author to complete a brief biographical form that includes questions about your clinical expertise and educational background. You may be asked to sign a document declaring any conflict of interest and to transfer copyright to the journal. Return these forms promptly to avoid delay in processing your manuscript.

Guidelines for Preparing the Manuscript

Follow the author guidelines for your target journal very carefully while preparing your manuscript. Most journals specify a maximum page length for a manuscript, as well as minimum font and margin sizes. Arrange the parts of your manuscript as specified. Most often this consists of a title page, abstract (limited to a specified numbers of words), narrative text, reference list, and appendices (tables, charts, figures, and photographs). Duplicate your manuscript as indicated, making sure that all copies are complete and legible. The editor will send these copies to the reviewers. Include a copy of your work on disk, if requested. Label the disk with your name, manuscript title, file name, and software used. If the journal prefers online submissions, follow the specific guidelines provided by the editor.

Prepare your manuscript appropriately using the manual of style, such as APA's or the American Medical Association's, suggested by each journal. If you are unfamiliar with these formats, ask your local librarian for help. Use articles published in that journal as a guide. Be alert to things such as person or style used by the journal. Make sure your references are current and relevant to your topic.

Double-check that references cited in the body of your manuscript are listed in your reference list.

After drafting your manuscript, let it sit a day or longer. Then reread it aloud. This helps you focus on the rhythm of your writing and helps you recognize deficits. Ask a friend, one who is not a nurse, to review the manuscript for you and provide an objective critique.

Including Visuals

Explore if the articles published in your target journal include visual items, such as tables, figures, or photographs. If these items are included, plan on enhancing your manuscript with these visuals. Include bullets, boxed material, or bold print to highlight important points, if appropriate. Limit yourself to the graphics used by each journal. For example, some journals do not use photographs in their publications, or some journals may only use black-and-white photographs. Remember to reflect back upon that mental image of your article when you first started this process.

If you plan on using photographs in your manuscript, be sure to obtain written permission to print these. Even if these photographs are of your students, colleagues, or family, you need to obtain their written permission. Most institutions have prepared permission forms available for such situations. Check with the editor to see if he or she has other preferences regarding the use of color, slides, and negatives.

If you plan on using a photograph or other visual from a printed source, you will need to obtain permission to reproduce it, called copyright permission. It is a good idea to photocopy a sample of the visual and the exact source in which it was published, including page numbers, to attach with your letter. Because obtaining permission may take several weeks, be sure to allow yourself sufficient time. You also will need to cite the source and reprint information next to the visual, once published. Some journals have an artist on staff. If this is the case, they may redraw a picture that you submit. Explore this option with the editor.

Cover Letter

Be sure to submit a cover letter with your manuscript. This letter should be addressed to the editor of the journal, similar to your query letter. It should explain your past correspondence with the editor. Although some journals acknowledge the receipt of manuscripts in writing, be sure to obtain validation that they received it in the mail.

Keep a File

Be sure to keep copies of all the materials you used and submitted during the preparation of your manuscript, including the return receipt or letter acknowledging receipt of your manuscript. Because this process may take more than one year, these come in handy if questions arise or if clarification is needed. For example, you may be asked to respond to a letter written to the editor in reference to your article; also, materials such as references may be useful when you prepare your next article. These letters may be helpful to use as examples as you mentor other nurses who want to publish.

Step 9: Deal With the Outcome

Waiting for a final response from the editor can be an exciting yet stressful time. Most journals acknowledge the receipt of your manuscript by a letter, postcard, or e-mail. As mentioned earlier, the final decision regarding your manuscript will vary depending on the journal. In most situations, you can expect three possible outcomes regarding your manuscript: (a) acceptance, with or without minor revisions; (b) major revisions needed and resubmit for second review; or (c) rejection.

Acceptance

Congratulations! Your manuscript was accepted. Consider yourself very fortunate if you have no revisions to make. It is common to be asked to make minor revisions as suggested by the editor and manuscript reviewers. Read these suggestions very carefully as you incorporate them into your draft, and resubmit your manuscript in a timely fashion. Be sure to contact the editor if you have any questions about the comments or if you disagree with some suggestions.

The editor probably will ask you to complete some documents at this time. You will need to sign an author's agreement form that describes your role in the publishing process, such as copyright and ownership issues (Sigler, 2001). This means that the journal will be the legal owner of your work and that you have not submitted or published it in any other journal. Be sure to ask the editor to clarify any questions you may have before signing these forms.

The editor may ask you to revise your manuscript slightly and submit a hard copy of it, along with a computer disk version. You also may be asked if you are interested in purchasing reprints of your article once it is published. Most journals provide each author with a complimentary copy of the journal in which the article appears.

You will be given a tentative date of publication at this time, which may be as long as two years from the date your manuscript was accepted (Carroll-Johnson, 2001). Although this date may change, it will give you an estimate of when to expect a computer-generated page layout of your manuscript, called the galleys, to review (Carroll-Johnson). You may be expected to review this galley in a very short turnaround time, so be prepared to make this task a priority. Check this galley for accuracy against your original manuscript. Do not be surprised if the galley looks very different from the manuscript you submitted. Make a copy of the galley pages, and keep them in your file folder.

Revision

You may be asked to revise and resubmit your manuscript. Some journals ask authors to make major revisions in their manuscript, rewrite it, and resubmit it for a second review. Although this response is not an acceptance, neither is it a rejection. It may be best to consider this response as a second chance. Depending on the comments, go back to the steps described previously and repeat what is needed. Follow the same author guidelines as you did when you first submitted your manuscript.

When developing your revised manuscript, carefully review the comments made by the editor and reviewers, and respond to each comment (Cupples, 2001). You can address each of these comments in a cover letter attached to your revised manuscript. Another approach is to highlight your revisions using a table with three columns labeled with these headings: "reviewer's comments, author's response, and manuscript changes (revised manuscript page, paragraph, line)" (Cupples, p. 3). Contact the editor if you are unclear about a particular comment or if, in your expert opinion, a comment does not warrant a change. Be open to suggestions when discussing these issues.

Rejection

No one likes rejection. It is important to remember that the editor rejected your manuscript, not you. After you have had some time to react, look closely at the comments and try to understand them from the reviewers' perspective. Remember that learning to write for publication is similar to perfecting clinical skills in that they both take practice and time. Be sure to ask the editor for specific suggestions on how to improve your manuscript and for ideas on where to submit your manuscript in the future.

Many things may have occurred as the result of your manuscript being rejected. Perhaps you reacted emotionally with anger or despair, or maybe you concluded that you were a failure and vowed to never write again as long as you live. It is all right to feel that way. Just set your manuscript aside for a few days until your negative emotions clear. Then take a closer look at your manuscript and try to be objective.

Learn something positive from the rejection of your manuscript while keeping the situation within the proper perspective. How important is this one experience in the total scheme of things? You did not lose anything, but rather you experienced a delay in meeting your goal. Start incorporating those changes into your manuscript, and begin the process over again, targeting the journal that was your second choice. Be sure to reflect upon the tips for successful writing listed in Figure 9-4.

Figure 9-4.
10 Tips for Becoming a Successful Author

Tip #1: Think positive.
Repeat to yourself, "I know I can do it!" Try to visualize yourself as an author. Imagine what your article will look like once it is published.

Tip #2: Be creative.
Think of a creative way to meet the objectives of your manuscript. How would you, as the learner, be best able to understand the content?

Tip #3: Do your homework.
Conduct a self-assessment on yourself as an author. List your strengths and weaknesses. Develop a plan to strengthen areas that are not strong. Take a noncredit writing course, or attend a presentation on writing for publication. Seek out an experienced mentor or a self-help book.

Tip #4: Use proper English.
Time to review your old English notes. Proper grammar and sentence structure are a must.

Tip #5: Follow the rules.
The journal set specific guidelines to follow for a reason. Do not jeopardize your chances for successful publication by not complying with details. If this is not your strength, then ask a friend who is strong in this area for help.

Tip #6: Follow your plan.
Follow the strategic approach described above. Do not get discouraged if you need to use all your targeted journals. Learning to write is a process that often takes time.

Tip #7: Think like an editor or reviewer.
Imagine you are a reviewer who just received your manuscript. What impression does it make?

(Continued on next page)

Tip #8: Practice. Practice. Practice.
Attempt to gain all the writing experience you can. Volunteer to write for your nursing organization's newsletter. Write a letter to the editor in your local newspaper or nursing journal.

Tip #9: Celebrate successes.
Celebrate your article with your peers, and encourage them to publish.

Tip #10: Don't give up!
Be persistent and keep trying.

Figure 9-4.
10 Tips for Becoming a Successful Author
(Continued)

Step 10: Celebrate!

Congratulate yourself on your success. Remind yourself of the reasons why nurses need to publish that were mentioned earlier in this chapter. Share your success and your article with your colleagues in your organization's newsletter. Keep a copy of your manuscript in your professional portfolio, which will be discussed in Chapter 11. Send a copy of your article to your supervisor for your work file and a copy to your faculty advisor at school. Submit your article for display during the National Nurses Week celebration at your organization.

It is a good idea to keep your original journal in a file folder with the information you collected in preparing the manuscript. This will allow you to retrieve it for future articles or in the event a reader poses a question for you. Now, it is time to get started on your next manuscript and help other nurses get involved in publishing. You already are an experienced writer.

Summary

This chapter presented an overview of the publication process, using a 10-Step Approach. Both the benefits and barriers to publishing were discussed, along with creative strategies to overcome the barriers. Details highlighted practical points that can be used by unit-based educators in preparing a manuscript for publication in a nursing journal.

References

American Psychological Association. (2001). *Publication manual of the American Psychological Association* (5th ed.). Washington, DC: Author.

Brandi, C.L., Lockhart, J.S., & O'Hare, D. (2003). Overcoming barriers to implementing an international keypal exchange program between Japanese and American nursing students. *Nurse Educator, 28*(4), 156–160.

Buchsel, P.C. (2001). Researching and referencing. *Clinical Journal of Oncology Nursing, 5,* 7–11.

Carroll-Johnson, R.M. (2001). Submitting a manuscript for review. *Clinical Journal of Oncology Nursing, 5,* 13–16.

Commission on Collegiate Nursing Education. (2003). *Standards for accreditation of baccalaureate and graduate nursing programs.* Retrieved June 26, 2003, from http://www.aacn.nche.edu/accreditation

Cumulative Index for Nursing and Allied Health Literature. (2003). *CINAHL® database.* Retrieved June 22, 2003, from http://www.cinahl.com/prodsvcs/cinahldbbody.htm

Cupples, S.A. (2001). Responding to reviewer's comments. *Nurse Author and Editor, 11*(1), 1–4.

Flanagin, A. (1993). Fraudulent publication. *IMAGE: The Journal of Nursing Scholarship, 25,* 359.

Henninger, D.E., & Nolan, M.T. (1998). A comparative evaluation of two educational strategies to promote publishing by nurses. *Journal of Continuing Education in Nursing, 29*(2), 79–84.

International Committee of Medical Journal Editors. (2001). *Uniform requirements for manuscripts submitted to biomedical journals.* Retrieved June 22, 2003, from http://www.icmje.org

Jacob, S.R., & Cherry, B. (2000). Publishing a nursing textbook: Collaborating through "seamless technology." *Computers in Nursing, 18*(5), 230–236.

Johnson, S.H. (2003). E-mail queries to editors. *Nurse Author and Editor, 13,* 6.

Lockhart, J.S. (2000). Writing for health care publications: A partnership between service and education. *Nurse Educator, 25*(4), 195–199.

McConnell, E.A. (1999). From idea to print: Writing for a professional journal. *Health Care Supervisor, 17*(3), 72–85.

McConnell, E.A. (2000). Nursing publications outside the United States. *Journal of Nursing Scholarship, 32*(1), 87–90.

National League for Nursing Accrediting Commission. (2003). *2003 accreditation manual.* Retrieved June 27, 2003, from http://www.nlnac.org/Manual%20&%20IG/2003_manual_TOC.htm

Oermann, M.H. (1999a). Extensive writing projects: Tips for completing them on time. *Nurse Author and Editor, 9*(1), 8–10.

Oermann, M.H. (1999b). Writing for publication as an advanced practice nurse. *Nursing Connections, 12*(3), 5–13.

Oermann, M.H. (2002). *Writing for publication in nursing.* Philadelphia: Lippincott.

Polit, D.F., & Beck, C.T. (2004). *Nursing research: Principles and methods* (7th ed.). Philadelphia: Lippincott Williams & Wilkins.

PubList.com. (1998–2001). *The Internet directory of publications.* Retrieved June 22, 2003, from http://www.publist.com

Sigler, B.A. (1999). Writing for publication. Part III–References. *ORL–Head and Neck Nursing, 17*(3), 27.

Sigler, B.A. (2001). Signing on the dotted line. *Clinical Journal of Oncology Nursing, 5,* 17–18.

Stepanski, L.M. (2002). Becoming a nurse-writer: Advice on writing for professional publications. *Journal of Infusion Nursing, 25*(2), 134–140.

Tonges, M.C. (2000). Publishing as a career tool: Don't forget to write. *Seminars for Nurse Managers, 8*(4), 212–214.

Wong, D.L. (1999). Publishing "cutting-edge" information. *Nurse Author and Editor, 9,* 8–9.

Zilm, G. (2002). The write time. *Canadian Journal of Nursing Leadership, 15*(2), 25–30.

CHAPTER 10

Sharing Your Expertise Through Oral Presentations and Posters

Imagine that you have been asked to present a paper at a national conference for a professional nursing organization, or maybe you are interested in preparing a poster for a local clinical nursing workshop. Most of your colleagues have given presentations such as these, and you feel left out. Perhaps there are other reasons why you want to present, such as requirements for advancement within your workplace or for your own personal satisfaction. Where do you start? On what topic could you possibly present?

If you are like most nurses, you have mixed emotions when you are asked to prepare a formal presentation for other nurses or healthcare professionals. Part of you is thrilled that you were asked to share your nursing expertise, but another part of you is scared to death, wondering why you ever agreed to do it or even volunteered in the first place.

Do not be alarmed, because you already have what it takes to create an excellent project. As a nurse, you have encountered many complex, stressful experiences, especially in the clinical setting. You came through most of them with increased skills and confidence in dealing with other similar clinical situations.

The approach you need to take to be effective at presentations is very similar to that of learning new clinical skills in nursing practice. You need to carefully assess the situation, develop a strategic plan, complete your homework, and practice, practice, practice. Try to rely on the leadership and interpersonal skills that you learned in nursing school for this experience, and remember to always visualize a positive outcome, because you *can* do it.

As mentioned in Chapter 2, staff development educators are expected to serve as role models for staff nurses in professional development activities, such as presentations at professional nursing organizations (American Nurses Association, 2000). Educators also are expected to share their expertise and mentor others in continuing their professional development. As a unit-based educator, it is important that you demonstrate these professional behaviors not only in your own role but in helping staff nurses on your clinical unit to do the same.

Types of Presentations

Presentations can be viewed as being either formal or informal. A formal presentation usually involves speaking in front of an audience, either at a podium or in a more relaxed environment. This oral or paper presentation, as it is sometimes called, is accompanied by some type of audiovisual, such as a Microsoft®

PowerPoint® presentation, slides, or overhead transparencies. At some conferences, several speakers may present on related topics during a special session called a symposium.

Informal presentations can include options such as roundtable sessions, panel discussions, and poster presentations. During a roundtable discussion, presenters informally share their projects with others in a discussion format. Panel presentations consist of a group of experts who contribute their expertise related to a particular topic. Each panel member may briefly present and respond to questions posed by the audience. If you are scheduled for a poster session, you must prepare a visual representation of your project using a poster format. You stand next to your poster during your scheduled session and discuss questions with the viewers. Some conferences ask poster presenters to provide a brief oral summary of their poster for the participants during a formal part of the conference.

Both formal and informal presentations are effective and efficient methods of sharing clinical projects with peers. Although both types of presentations involve some preparation, each option relies on different skills by the presenter. Depending on the conference, you may be either asked or told which option to present. If it is your first time presenting, choose the option with which you feel the most secure and have resources to complete. Figures 10-1 and 10-2 list the advantages and disadvantages of both oral paper and poster presentations.

Figure 10-1.
Advantages and
Disadvantages of
Oral Presentations

Advantages
- Viewed as more prestigious than posters, by some sources
- Content is portable and conducive to travel.
- Presenter has more time to convey message than poster presenter.
- Audiovisuals (images or slides) can be used in other projects.
- Creativity can be used to influence content.

Disadvantages
- Audiovisual production may be costly.
- Oral presentation may be overwhelming or anxiety producing.
- Requires good oral presentation skills
- Requires the presenter to convey information to learners

Choosing a Topic to Present

You can investigate several sources to arrive at a topic to present. These include such sources as clinical practice, research, teaching, or educational projects. Topics derived from either professional issues or life experiences can serve as rich sources for presentations. A poster, for example, can be an effective way to update peers about policies and procedures in the workplace. Many of these ideas are similar to those generated as topics for publication purposes previously discussed in Chapter 9.

Before you choose a topic, be sure to match your idea with the objectives of the conference or its overall theme. Discover who the learners (audience) will be and what their expectations may be regarding your topic.

If you have a specific topic in mind, this process may only involve rethinking the perspective from which you present it. For example, a presentation that describes the steps involved in performing a neurologic assessment is quite appropriate for a clinical nursing conference attended by RNs who provide direct care for patients at risk for neurological impairments. The focus of your presentation, in this case, is on the content of the assessment. However, if the conference is geared toward nurse educators, you may want to describe the creative teaching strategy you developed that was effective in helping nurses learn how

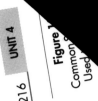

Advantages	Disadvantages
• Most of the preparation work is completed prior to the conference.	• May be viewed as less prestigio... some sources, but gaining popu...
• Permits individual interaction between viewer and presenter	• May be time-consuming to prep... yourself
• Permits informal sharing and networking with viewers	• Often costly to have commercially... pared
• May be less intimidating than an oral presentation	• Requires artistic talent or resource...
• Primary focus is on questions posed by the viewer.	• May pose barriers related to portal...
• Mutual learning on shared interests may occur between viewer and presenter.	• Limited time and space to convey m... sage
• Learning may occur without the presence of a presenter.	• Requires assembly, dismantling, and storage space
	• Difficult to reuse pieces in future projects

to conduct a neurologic assessment. The perspective of the topic, in this case, is on the teaching strategy used, rather than the content.

Anticipate Resources in Advance

Before you start to develop your presentation, carefully determine the resources you will need to carry out the project. Be sure to match your specific needs with those resources available to you at your workplace.

Resources can consist of people who are experts, money, or special services. All of these sources can expand your expertise with a project and maximize your success with your presentation. The resources available to you also will determine how you ultimately structure and present your topic.

Media and Artistic Talent

Check if your workplace has a media center or instructional designer who can help you create audiovisuals, such as a PowerPoint presentation, slides, or overheads for a formal presentation or photographs and other illustrations for a poster. Start by making an appointment to meet with someone in the center to discuss your project plans before you begin your presentation. Ask questions that may be pertinent to your project. Appropriate questions may include the following: In what format (e.g., handwritten, typed, computer file, photographic, text picture) do you prefer audiovisual sources? What is the turnaround time from submission to actual development of audiovisuals? What is the anticipated cost of the media center's involvement on a project such as yours? Also, check with your supervisor or advisor to see if your employer or school can share any of this cost.

Supplies

Next, think about other supplies or services you may need for your presentation. This may include such items as typing for your project, duplication of handouts, or actual construction of your poster. Figure 10-3 lists common supplies needed to construct your own poster. Enter the cost of these items in your projected figures for your presentation.

• Material for backboard and content areas (e.g., foam board, poster board)	• Pencil and soft eraser
• Material to connect sections of backboard (e.g., adhesive-backed loop and hook tape)	• Ruler
	• Masking tape (to mark outline for mock display)
• Adhesive (rubber cement, spray adhesive, or double-sided tape)	• Adhesive letters (if needed)
• Razor-like art knife for cutting foam board (art supply cutting knife)	• Computer word-processing or graphic software
	• Additional decorative edging
• Wooden surface upon which to cut board	• Photographs or images for poster display
• Scissors	• Plastic bag to carry poster
• Material upon which to print text (paper)	• Paper towels and protective cover to be used during gluing

Cost

After you have researched your need for resources and other supplies, develop a tentative budget for your project. Include anticipated costs such as typing, conducting literature searches, creating slides and overheads, duplicating handouts, and making poster materials. The specifics of these projects will be discussed in more detail later in this chapter. Do not forget the other costs associated with the conference. Some organizations either offer a reduced fee or waive this fee for speakers.

Once you see the figures on paper, you may need to make decisions that may keep your project within a cost range reasonable for your budget. For example, if your total costs exceed your budget allotment, you may choose to make your poster yourself, rather than paying a media center to do this. Perhaps you decide to use a PowerPoint presentation or overhead transparencies to accompany your oral presentation, rather than using more expensive slides.

Timeline

Be sure to create a timeline to keep you on schedule as you develop your presentation. Start from the time your topic was accepted to the actual day of presentation. Indicate the major steps in this process so that you do not rush to prepare at the last minute. Figure 10-4 illustrates the essential steps when developing your timeline for presentations.

Although individuals require different timelines, give yourself several weeks to prepare, organize, and carefully think through your project. Allow time for unexpected events, such as family and work crises, mistakes, retyping, or obtaining supplies.

Developing the Content

The next step is to plan the actual content for your presentation. Use an approach similar to the detailed outline described in Chapter 7, in which you learned how to develop content for an in-service program, and in Chapter 9, where you learned how to prepare a manuscript. If you plan on presenting a research project, consider relying on the major headings used for most research proposals, such as purpose, specific aims, review of literature, and methodology. Details on research projects will be discussed in Chapter 13.

If you are presenting at a conference, ask the person who is coordinating the education sessions, or your contact person, if there are any specifications for your presentation. Perhaps your topic came about as the result of a needs assessment conducted by the conference planning committee. If this is the case, the contact person may have some additional information that may help you develop your project. If there is no background information about your topic, think your project through logically as though you were a member of the audience.

Identify a Topic

From these discussions, decide upon a topic for your presentation. You may need to research it as described previously in Chapter 9.

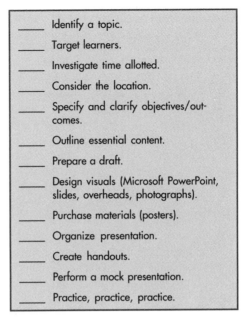

_____ Identify a topic.

_____ Target learners.

_____ Investigate time allotted.

_____ Consider the location.

_____ Specify and clarify objectives/outcomes.

_____ Outline essential content.

_____ Prepare a draft.

_____ Design visuals (Microsoft PowerPoint, slides, overheads, photographs).

_____ Purchase materials (posters).

_____ Organize presentation.

_____ Create handouts.

_____ Perform a mock presentation.

_____ Practice, practice, practice.

Figure 10-4.
Essential Steps Included in a Timeline for a Presentation

Identify and Target Learners

Who will be the learners or audience? It is vital that you know this as you prepare your presentation. You need to tailor both the content and level of your presentation according to the learner's existing knowledge level. If your learners possess a beginning level of understanding of your topic, then establish a baseline. If your audience consists of learners with a more advanced knowledge level of your topic, then customize your presentation at a higher, more complex level. Perhaps you may find a need to quickly review the basics before you start your presentation at a more involved phase. Regardless, you want to be in synchrony with your learners to maintain their interest. Attempt to create a balance between their being bored and becoming overwhelmed.

Investigate Time Allotted

Find out how much time is allotted for your presentation. If you have 20 minutes, be sure to subtract some time for introductions, questions, and other procedures. It is often to one's advantage to end a presentation a little earlier than scheduled, rather than to extend the program or to take some of the next speaker's time. Practice staying within your allotted time frame. It is also helpful to investigate what presentation learners will most likely attend before and after yours. If they have experienced several formal lectures before they arrive at your presentation, you may prefer to change yours to a discussion format with more audience participation.

If you are presenting a poster, most likely you will be given specific directions that explain times when conference participants will view your poster. You will be told when to set it up and dismantle it. Be sure to schedule your time so that you will be available to stand next to your poster and answer questions that the viewers may have at that time. As mentioned earlier, some conference formats have a scheduled time during the conference when each poster presenter provides a brief summary of their project to all conference participants.

Consider the Location

Find out as much as you can about the general conference location planned for your presentation. As soon as you have the opportunity, visit your assigned space. Doing this well in advance of your presentation will afford you some time to make last minute changes in your approach, if necessary.

If you are scheduled for an oral presentation, visit the room in which you will present. It is a good idea to do this when no one is in the room, such as during breaks or when the conference has finished for the day. Walk up to the podium and attempt to simulate your presentation. Try out your PowerPoint presentation and practice using the remote control. If you are using slides, place them in the projector, and practice advancing them with the controls.

Try to use the laser pointer if it will help with your presentation. Be sure to dim the lights appropriately. Evaluate how your slides project on the screen. Check if you will be able to see your slides during your presentation. Determine if you have sufficient lighting at the podium to see your notes. Practice using the microphone.

Next, look at the seating arrangements, and plan where you will sit prior to your presentation. It is often helpful to sit close to the front so that you will not take too much time getting to the stage prior to your talk. Examine how the audience seating is designed and its conduciveness to hearing your presentation. If possible, listen to several speakers present their topics in the same room before you present. Carefully observe what works for them.

If you are giving a poster presentation, possibly visit the location ahead of time where the posters are scheduled to be exhibited at the conference. Later in this chapter, specific features to observe will be discussed.

Specify and Clarify Objectives

Think about the overall purpose of your presentation, and try to state it succinctly to yourself. An example might be, "The purpose of this presentation is to describe the development of a unit-based education program for RNs assigned to a specialty unit." Keep the knowledge level of your learners in mind as you do this.

Then, outline specific objectives or outcomes that you hope learners will be able to demonstrate following your presentation. This will help you focus the direction of your content. Remember that objectives must be learner-centered. They should be neither too simple nor extremely difficult. Develop these objectives using a process similar to the one described for in-service programs in Chapter 7. The number of objectives you develop is influenced by a variety of factors, including the length of your presentation. For example, two to four main objectives may be appropriate for a presentation 20–40 minutes long. If you are preparing a poster, design it so that viewers will be able to capture the essence of your poster within the few minutes they have available to them.

Outline Essential Content

This next step begins with you systematically researching information related to your topic. Perform this as described in Chapter 7, when creating an in-service offering, or in Chapter 9, when developing a manuscript. As before, do not forget to explore either the assistance of your local librarian or the Internet. Be sure to talk with various experts in the field, and supplement your content with materials prepared by community agencies, if appropriate.

Once you have the materials carefully organized, draft a detailed outline of your presentation. Be sure to follow the direction established by your objectives, because the content should help the learner meet these objectives. If your presentation is a description of a research project, use the main headings of your proposal to guide you, as mentioned previously in this chapter.

Prepare a Draft

Finally, prepare a draft of your presentation that is based on your outline. The amount of detail needed for your draft will depend on whether you plan to read your presentation verbatim or closely follow the primary points. Although some presenters prefer preparing a script ahead of time, others record only general thoughts and use their slides as cues. If it is your first presentation, it may be best for you to have your talk written verbatim on paper. You can rely on it if the other option fails. Although the decision is yours, be sure to practice your approach before you decide on the method.

One of the most convenient ways to prepare your script is to type it using computer word-processing software. With a computer, you can change the print font to a larger size and double-space the text to facilitate reading it in dim lighting. The use of upper and lower case letters is more readable than using all capital letters. Attempt to use the least amount of paper during your talk; this minimizes the chance that shuffling papers will distract participants. If you record your speech on small note cards, be sure to write sufficient information.

If you are developing your presentation using PowerPoint software, you can use its various features to develop your script, including its handout option that records keynotes next to your slide images. Regardless of what option you choose, be sure you select a strategy with which you feel comfortable.

Plan for Visuals

Once you are fairly satisfied with the overall outline and draft of your presentation, plan for some type of visual that enhances it. You need to use an audiovisual that is appropriate for your presentation and matches both your resources and your budget. Conference planners will ask you in advance what equipment you will need for your presentation.

One approach is to divide your presentation into major sections of content (e.g., outline sections A, B, C) and identify at least one image or slide (or overhead transparency) for each section. You can use slides that contain words or illustrations that reflect each section of your presentation. Creating a grid or storyboard that contains categories based on your purpose may help you visualize the overall picture.

Do not forget to start with an image that depicts your workplace, school, or the agency that is sponsoring you to attend the conference. Talk with your public affairs representatives and ask them for assistance with this. Pay close attention to authorship issues discussed earlier in Chapter 9, giving appropriate acknowledgment.

Develop Audiovisuals

Now that you have decided on the content of visuals that match your presentation, finalize the type of audiovisual you will use. Most presenters use PowerPoint software, whereas others rely on color slides or overhead transparencies. Using overheads is an option for presentations that are more informal, interactive, and involve discussion. Some speakers also incorporate a short piece of videotape into their presentation. Regardless of your selection, be sure to adhere to copyright standards. Check with your contact person to determine what audiovisual equipment is available for your presentation.

Images and Slides

If you decide to use PowerPoint for your presentation or color slides, it is vital that you work closely with an expert in the department or laboratory that will help you prepare and/or develop them. As mentioned earlier in this chapter, you need to do this well in advance of the date of your actual presentation. This software program is fairly easy to master, but seek the help of an expert the first time you create a presentation.

There are several ways that you or others can create slides. One way is with the help of computer software programs, such as PowerPoint. This program assists you in designing slides that contain text or graphics, such as charts or pictures, and has color options that can be chosen or predetermined by the computer. If you decide to use this method, ask your media center how to save the files on a computer disk. These files then will need to be transferred to film for processing if you choose to create slides.

You can use the images you created and save your presentation as a PowerPoint file. Realize that the use of images in addition to text may increase the size of your computer file, requiring it to be saved on a compact disc rather than on a floppy disk. You will need to use an LCD projector to project your presentation on a screen.

LCD projectors currently are replacing the use of slide and overhead projectors at professional conferences (Everson, 2003). This machine connects directly to a laptop computer and projects PowerPoint presentations onto a screen so participants can view the images. LCD projectors vary in their available features, such as size, weight, brightness, resolution, and cost, and are compatible with most laptop platforms (Everson). However, not all conferences may have access to LCDs for their speakers. Check with your conference contact person in advance to determine if this equipment is available and if there is an added charge to use it at the conference. Investigate if a laptop computer is provided for speaker or if you will need to bring your own.

Some centers have the ability to copy pictures or graphics from books or journals using a scanner and transform them into slides. If you are talented in this area, use color slide film in your camera to photograph the images you need. Be sure to factor in some extra time for retakes. If you need to capture a very close shot outside the focal range of your camera, you may need to rely on expert help. Regardless of your resources, prepare to hold the interest of your audience with slides that contain both text and graphic images.

Do not forget to address issues such as font size, the color of text and the background, and the numbers of words per line. If you use computer graphics software to prepare your slides, these issues usually are handled within the program itself. Ideal color combinations of text, background, and style often are predetermined for the user.

Once your slides are developed, arrange them in order based on their appearance in the presentation. A slide-viewing screen that is especially designed for this purpose makes this step easier. This screen consists of a semi-opaque plastic sheet placed in front of a box with a light source behind it. It looks similar to an X-ray viewer box placed horizontally on a table. If you do not have a viewer to use, then hold each slide up to a bright light, against a white background, or view them within a commercial plastic sleeve that holds many slides.

Next, flip (turn and reverse) your slides so that they are in the proper upright left-to-right position during projection. Once your slides are in the proper sequence, use a permanent felt-tipped marker to label each slide with a number in the upper right-hand corner. Either place the slides in a slide tray with the safety lid attached, or keep your slides in the plastic sleeve. Be sure to label the tray with your name and topic. You can purchase plastic slide sleeves in photography shops or paper supply stores. You may choose to use the sleeve if you are traveling a distance. Although most conferences supply empty slide trays, be sure to confirm this. Regardless, keep your slides with you as you travel; avoid checking them with your baggage if at all possible.

Overhead Transparencies

You may choose to enhance your presentation using overhead transparencies. Most transparencies are clear 8.5 x 11-inch pieces of plastic on which an image can be imprinted using a variety of methods. Some transparency film is available in color. The benefit of using transparencies rather than slides is that transparencies are cheaper and can be more versatile, especially if your presentation involves informal group discussion. Unlike slides, using overheads does not require dimming of lights to visualize them. However, overhead transparencies are not as effective as slides to convey photographic images.

As with slides, various computer word-processing and graphic software programs can be used to create professional-looking overheads. These programs often control factors such as font size and number of characters per line or page. These programs can incorporate graphics into your presentation, as well. This image can be printed directly onto a transparency film especially made for your printer. Depending on the capability of your printer, you can make overheads in either black and white or color.

Transparencies also can be created using other means. Regardless of the approach you choose, be sure to purchase transparencies made especially for the method you select. Overheads can be made from an image placed in most copy machines. Make sure the film you purchase can be used in your specific copier. If you want your overhead to be in color, you must duplicate a color image onto a transparency using a copier that has this capability; otherwise, your image will be in black and white. Overheads also can be created using a machine that uses heat to create a black and white image. They also can be made by hand using either permanent or temporary felt-tipped markers made especially for this purpose. These may not look as professional as typed versions. Be careful not to touch the print on overheads made with temporary markers because of possible smearing.

As with slides, organize your overheads ahead of time. Be sure to number them in some fashion that is not obvious to the audience. You can secure each overhead in a cardboard frame especially made for overheads. Another convenient method used to organize overhead transparencies is to place them in commercially made plastic sleeves that are secured within a three-ring binder. The overhead can be viewed through the sleeve by simply removing it from the binder.

If you plan on using overheads to enhance your presentation, decide whether you or someone else will place them on the overhead projector during the talk. If the environment requires that you stand at a podium that is a distance from the overhead projector, you may need someone's assistance with this activity. Again, be sure to plan this ahead of time so your presentation proceeds as planned.

Videotape

If you plan on using videotape with your presentation, start by obtaining written permission from the proper authorities. As with slides and transparencies, practice using the video with your presentation. Be alert to details such as accurate timing of the video and proper match in size between the videotape and the video player. Using the seating arrangement in the room, make sure the audience can both see and hear the video adequately. If an audiovisual expert is not available at the conference, arrange for someone with experience in using this equipment to control the viewing and to troubleshoot, as needed.

Handouts

It is helpful to supplement key points of your presentation for the audience with printed handouts. This allows the learner to spend time listening to your presentation, rather than focusing on note taking. A few good handouts also can be a method to add additional content to your topic, especially if you have limited time to present.

Handouts are useful to supplement a poster presentation, as well. If your poster is research-based, a printed abstract of your project, reference list, or details on data analysis can help to enhance the content. Do not forget to add your name and a way that conference participants can contact you at a later date. Sharing your mailing address, telephone number, or e-mail address is a common way to develop a network with others across the country who may be interested in your topic.

If you plan on using handouts, investigate if the computer software program used to prepare your slides or overheads also has the ability to generate a smaller version of your presentation that can be used as handouts, as in the case with PowerPoint. Talk with your contact person from the conference planning committee to decide whose responsibility it is to duplicate handouts. If it is your responsibility to provide handouts, ask conference planners for the number of participants anticipated to attend your presentation. Be sure to prepare a few more in case unexpected participants arrive.

Using Posters to Share Clinical Expertise

Poster presentations can be a very creative and effective way to communicate your clinical and research expertise with others. In fact, poster presentations have gained increased recognition for their value, compared with oral presentations, by the nursing profession over recent years (Moore, Augspurger, King, & Proffitt, 2001).

Poster presentations often allow you a way to share your ideas with colleagues in a more relaxed, informal environment than exists with oral presentations (Taggart & Arslanian, 2000). This setting allows you, as a presenter, to interact on a one-on-one basis with conference participants and offers you the opportunity to develop professional networks.

Spend some time consulting with other nurses who recently have prepared posters. Nurses who have experienced this process can be helpful sources of information and support and can provide insight (Moore et al., 2001). Include nurses from your own organization, such as staff development educators and clinical nurse specialists, as well as faculty from affiliating schools of nursing.

Depending on your available budget, you can either choose to create a poster — *future* yourself or use the assistance of a professional media service at either your workplace or in your community. Regardless of your choice, it is important that you focus on the message your poster conveys.

Design a Mock Layout

Before you start creating your poster, you will need to design a mock layout to map the essential content. First, decide on the main content areas and headings that you want to include on your poster. These major categories can be easily — *got from AACN* adapted from the outline you developed previously. Do not forget the title of the poster, along with the names of authors and places of employment, if appropriate. Be sure to acknowledge any sources of funding for your project, such as grant monies.

Next, discover what the display specifications are for your poster. Most often, this information will be supplied to you by the conference planning committee. It will tell you whether you should design your poster to be free standing using a table or easel or attached directly to a large bulletin or display board provided at the conference. The committee also should provide you with details such as the outside dimensions of the bulletin board or table upon which you will place your poster.

Once you know the maximum outside dimensions for your poster, develop a mock version of your poster. This step will enable you to plan the content of your poster and to adjust its content to be aesthetically pleasing. One helpful way is to create an outline of your poster with masking tape marking the outside dimensions. Use a flat surface such as a large tabletop or the floor. Once you have typed a draft of each content area, trim the paper to size. Then, organize these pieces within the marked outline. Be sure to leave plenty of space for non-text content such as photographs or other graphics to add interest and balance your poster. Adjust the size of each content area as needed.

Consider the Aesthetics of Your Poster

Be aware of both the content and physical appearance of your poster presentation. Your poster must create a good "first impression" before participants may choose to read it.

Simple, Yet Creative

Remember to keep your poster simple and professional. It should look appealing yet contain essential content. One way to accomplish this is to replace the details of tables and other data using color visuals, such as pie charts, bar graphs, or photographs. Because viewers have little time to spend at each poster, add graphics such as arrows or lines to provide direction and guide them through the essential points of your poster.

Use of Color

Color can be used either in the text or background, but be sure it is readable and appealing. Test the colors both at a distance and in the lighting anticipated at the poster session. Incorporate the use of color and color combinations when deciding on the poster background and frames for each content area. Use colors or color combinations that complement each other. If appropriate, use color combinations that reflect your workplace, school, conference theme, or project topic. Prepare a draft of the color scheme before you finalize your plans.

Factors to Consider With Text

If possible, rely on computer software, such as word-processing or graphics programs, to create the text for your poster. Be certain to allow space around the edges for a sufficient border surrounding the text. Choose a print style that is attractive yet simple and readable. Fancy styles, such as italics or gothic, may interfere with your poster's legibility. Avoid using punctuation in your poster, unless necessary. Make sure your print is large enough to enable viewers to read your poster at a reasonable distance. Print the text for your poster using a quality printer, such as a laser. Enlarge images if needed using a quality copier.

If you do not have access to a computer to generate text, neatly type the text or use commercially prepared adhesive letters. Use larger letters for headings and smaller ones for the text. Carefully arrange these letters and erase any pencil marks you made during the preparation phase.

Use of Photographs and Graphics

Enlarged photographs can be used to enhance the appearance of a poster presentation, especially to illustrate the poster's overall theme or concepts. An enlarged photographic image can be made either through the help of a photography service or a color copier. Photographs should be enlarged so viewers may see them at a reasonable distance. Photocopy enlargement often is less expensive than enlarging through film development and requires a shorter time for processing. As with manuscripts, be sure to obtain permission to use photographs from the proper authorities.

Balance Text and Graphics

Create a poster that is pleasing to the viewer's eye. One way is to offer a balance between text and graphics. Once you have developed your draft, stand a distance from your poster and judge its overall appearance for this feature.

Choosing Materials

Think about your poster in two sections: the backboard and the content areas. A backboard can be constructed using a variety of available materials. Its overall size usually is dictated by specifications made by the conference planners and/or available resources. Backboards can consist of freestanding commercial felt-covered boards, foam board, poster board, or corrugated cardboard. The latter three materials can be purchased from an art or office supply store. In fact, some stores sell freestanding poster displays that contain three connected cardboard panels that are coated with a white or black finish. They require no additional preparation.

As mentioned earlier, large bulletin boards often are provided as backboards at some conferences. These boards can be left natural (white or cork) or covered with colored paper or cloth, if desired.

Although commercial backboards usually are freestanding, other materials such as foam board can be connected to become a freestanding poster. Adhesive-backed hook and loop strips, one side is split and attached to the back of two connecting boards and the other side is left whole and intact, serve as a convenient way to connect the sections. Try connecting two or three pieces of board along the seam using masking tape. This process will create a flexible poster that can stand alone. If hook and loop strips are used, one side (with the protector on the adhesive side remaining) can be removed to permit easy dismantling and storage of the poster sections.

The smaller content sections of the poster can be made, depending on the backboard, using similar materials such as foam board, poster board, or paper. These sections can be created with rubber cement or spray adhesive and adhered to the backboard with small pieces of adhesive hook and loop tape. This permits easy removal and storage of the content areas. If you plan on using the display or bulletin board as a backboard, affix content sections of your poster with attractive thumbtacks. Staples may be used in some cases. Long metal pushpins often are required to penetrate the depth created by several layers of either poster board or foam board.

In addition to constructing your own poster, some organizations and imaging companies have the ability to duplicate a PowerPoint presentation as one large document or as slides fused to individual pieces of foam board. Although these commercially prepared posters are attractive and appear professional, they also are more costly than posters made by hand.

Ways to Enhance Your Poster

In addition to computer word-processing and graphics software, there are several ways to enhance your poster with the use of special features. Consider the use of an enlarged poster title or institution logo resting separately or suspended by thick wire above the main body of your poster. Borders, either made from professional edging tape or double pieces of colored paper purchased at an art supply store, can add zest to simple text. Cover the bulletin board with colored paper or material such as felt. Be sure to include a holder for your business card, abstract, and handouts.

Attempt to use creative yet professional approaches for your poster presentation. Remember that you need to get your message across to viewers in a very brief time. If appropriate, consider a novel approach, such as a poster shaped like a hand, for reporting a clinical project on hand washing or infection control. You could also try a poster shaped like a head when conveying information about an educational program on cranial nerve assessment.

One display method used by some presenters is a large one-piece photograph of a poster. Although this approach is frequently more expensive than the methods described previously, it serves as an attractive and portable way of presenting a poster. You will need to investigate more about this method at your media center.

Consider Poster Assembly and Portability

In designing your poster, plan for certain features such as the ease of its assembly, portability to the conference site, and storage. This is especially true if you need to carry your poster a distance when traveling. You want to design a poster that requires minimal time to assemble and dismantle.

Depending on your needs, you may decide to check a large poster as baggage using a commercial cardboard box, or carry it as dismantled pieces in a garment bag or suitcase. If your poster is flexible, it can be rolled and carried in a protective cardboard cylinder.

Capture the Final Product

Now that your poster is finished, take a picture of it. You can use this photograph to supplement your portfolio, discussed later in Chapter 13, or to help you develop future posters. Figures 10-5 and 10-6 illustrate some examples of posters.

Use this opportunity to evaluate the content and overall appearance of your poster. Look at the photograph objectively to determine if it contains the quali-

Figure 10-5.
Health Beliefs of Nicaraguan Women of Childbearing Age

Note. Photo courtesy of Leah Vota Cunningham, Duquesne University School of Nursing

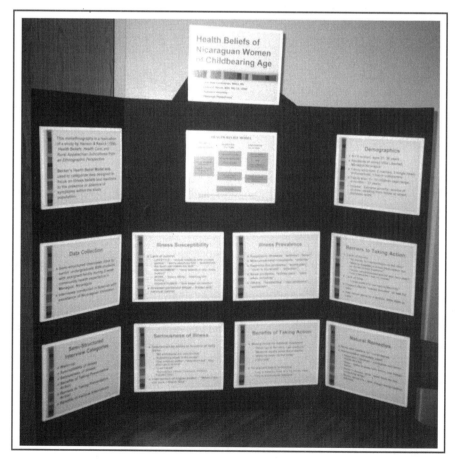

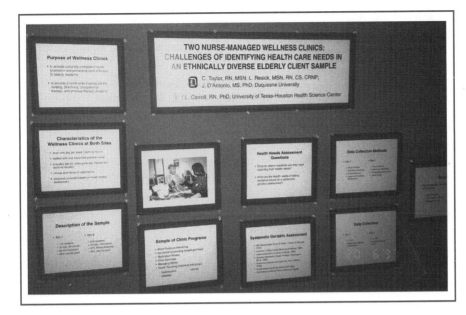

Figure 10-6.
Two Nurse-Managed Wellness Clinics: Challenges of Identifying Healthcare Needs in an Ethnically Diverse Elderly Client Sample

Note. Photo courtesy of Leni K. Resick, Duquesne University School of Nursing

ties mentioned previously. Judge if the overall message of your project is conveyed.

Finally, when you arrive at the conference, compare the quality of your poster with others. Take notes about features of other posters you particularly enjoyed. If permitted by the authors, photograph posters that were especially well done. Review these images when it is time to develop your next poster presentation.

Overcoming Presentation Jitters

Most presenters have experienced their share of the "jitters" prior to their presenting. In fact, even the most experienced presenters report some degree of anxiety associated with this activity.

Although you cannot control all aspects of the situation when presenting, there are certainly several methods within your control that you can use to help decrease your anxiety. These methods start by anticipating the worst that can happen, and then preparing for it. Just as in writing for publication, presentations involve a great deal of homework and practice.

Know Your Topic

Knowing your topic thoroughly can reduce some anxiety associated with a presentation. This involves not only memorizing your presentation but also truly understanding the topic. You should be able to describe your project to someone without notes. Prior research that you conducted on your topic will help you accomplish this.

Refine Your Presentation Skills

Once you understand your topic, try to refine your presentation skills through practice. Discover what approach is most comfortable to use. Although some presenters read verbatim from their notes, others let their slides and a few notes guide their presentation.

One helpful way to gradually perfect your presentation skills is to practice them at various local meetings or conferences. These settings may pose a lesser threat to you and help you perform better in the future at larger national conferences.

Take the opportunity to closely observe experienced presenters as they share their work in front of others. Watch how they organize their content and how they present themselves. Decide what was impressive and what could be improved. You may decide to attempt to model some of these successful behaviors in your own presentations.

If you have the opportunity to listen to some of the speakers before it is your turn to present, be alert to content that is related to your topic. Then, during your presentation, try to address these issues and incorporate them into your talk, if appropriate. This adds to the overall continuity of the program.

Know Your Equipment

Be certain that you are comfortable with the equipment you plan to use for your presentation. As mentioned earlier in this chapter, practice with the equipment both at home and at the conference. Many large conferences have speaker-ready rooms where presenters can review their audiovisuals prior to their presentations.

Dress the Part

It is important that you create a good impression as a presenter. Start by dressing appropriately for the conference and your presentation. Most often, a conservative business-like outfit is suitable. Dress in an outfit that is comfortable yet professional. Feeling good about yourself often creates a positive visual image of yourself in your mind. This can boost your confidence and help you perform well. Have faith in yourself.

Do not forget that your presentation needs to be just as professional as your physical appearance. Place your speech or notes in a nice plain folder. Because no one will see your notes, you can mark them as needed. However, it is not impressive for the audience to see you carrying various unorganized pieces of paper to the podium.

Perform a Mock Presentation

Conduct several mock presentations well in advance of your scheduled talk. Try capturing your practice sessions on audiotape or videotape, unless this increases your anxiety. As you review your mock session, try to be objective. Watch for distracting gestures such as hand or head movements when you speak. Be alert to errors with pronunciation and especially the use of extraneous words such as "uh" or "OK?" Be sure that you are speaking at a proper speed. Most often, nervous speakers talk too fast. Focus on reducing these problems in future taping. Imagine yourself as an admired speaker, then act the part. Be sure to smile and make eye contact.

Anticipate the Worst

Even with the most experienced presenters, an unexpected situation can arise. One way to lessen your anxiety is to anticipate and prepare for the worst that can happen. The following are situations that may occur when giving both formal and informal presentations. After each problem situation, a solution based on preparing ahead of time is provided.

Situation #1
You become short of breath and nervous during your presentation.

Solution
Remember that there is a difference between your feeling nervous and others being aware that you are nervous. Most often, you may feel more nervous than others perceive you to be. If you find yourself a little breathless during your presentation, stop for a few seconds. Take several deep breaths, then start again. The time period may seem like forever, but in reality it is only a brief moment.

If your presentation is a more informal one, this is a good time to pose a few questions to the audience and to talk with others. Do not assume the audience is focused on you. Most likely, their attention is focused on your audiovisuals or handouts.

Regardless, slow down, make eye contact, and smile. Some presenters relax if they mingle with the participants before their presentation. Do not forget that the lights will be low. Try wearing a turtleneck or scarf if this makes you feel more at ease while presenting.

Situation #2
Your mind goes blank during your presentation. You lose your place within your talk.

Solution
No problem. You have prepared some backup notes clearly marked with the headings of your content. Take a few seconds to regroup your thoughts.

Situation #3
Your talk does not match the audiovisual on the screen. Your slides will not advance.

Solution
Perhaps you got a little ahead of yourself with your slides. Excuse yourself to the audience and advance or reverse to the appropriate slide. Because you have marked your script with the appropriate slide number or image that accompanies it, you can easily relocate your place. If your slides do not advance, ask for assistance. While this is happening, proceed with your presentation to keep you and the next speaker on schedule. Once your slide projector is working, briefly run through the main ones, if appropriate and time permits.

Situation #4

You are running behind schedule or have less time than previously thought to present.

Solution

Quickly regroup your thoughts. You may need to advance ahead to the essential portions of your presentation. Maybe you can use the question and answer time of the program to finish. Then you can agree to meet with participants, who may have questions, during the break or lunch. Practice and careful timing of your presentation could minimize the risk of this happening to you. Again, it may be useful to prepare a shorter version of your talk in the event that you have less time than anticipated.

Situation #5

You do not know the answers to questions posed by the audience. Some participants become rude and challenge your patience.

Solution

Remember that no one expected you to know the answers to all questions. Your prior research on your topic should enable you to know most of them. Do not hesitate to say that you do not know the answer to a question. Ask the audience for assistance. You may choose to investigate the question later, and get back to the participant via telephone. You should be courteous and professional to participants, even the most annoying ones. Do not be intimidated. Remember that you are the one making the presentation.

Situation #6

You lose your presentation.

Solution

No problem, because you have kept duplicate copies of your talk in your carry-on luggage and in your check-on baggage. Prevent this from happening by keeping your slides and presentation with you at all times prior to the conference. Do not check your only copy. It is also a good idea to have an extra copy of your presentation at home so it can be faxed to you in the event of an emergency.

Evaluate the Results

Now that it is over, be objective and personally evaluate the strengths and not-so-strong areas of your presentation. If you audiotaped it, you can use the tape to critique your efforts. Give yourself credit for your strong points, and decide to work harder on the areas that were not as strong.

Learn to Accept Constructive Criticism

Most conferences request participants to evaluate each presentation. They often supply presenters with a summary of these scores. If not, ask the conference planners for them.

Look at the general consensus of the audience. Presenters have the habit of focusing on the one negative comment in a collection of 30 good evaluations. You cannot please everyone. Remember that some individuals have not learned how to offer criticism in a polite and constructive manner.

Measure Learner Outcomes

Reflect back to the primary purpose of your presentation. Determine whether the learners actually gained information. Reflect on your predetermined outcomes or objectives.

Publish Your Presentation

While the topic is still fresh in your mind, think about making the most of your efforts. Attempt to transform your project into a manuscript for publication. As discussed in Chapter 12, begin this process by audiotaping your presentation and transcribing it. You already have the beginnings of a manuscript. Perhaps you can purchase an audiotape copy of your presentation, if your conference provided this service to members.

Share Your Presentation With Colleagues at Work

Before you disassemble your presentation, be sure to share it with your coworkers. Think about presenting it at a unit-based inservice program as described in Chapter 7. Figures 10-5 and 10-6 are examples of poster presentations created by nurses.

Summary

This chapter described the steps involved in preparing both formal and informal presentations. Specific suggestions were provided for oral and poster presentations, including all aspects from developing the idea or topic to evaluating the final product.

References

American Nurses Association. (2000). *Scope and standards of practice for nursing professional development.* Washington, DC: Author.

Everson, F.P. (2003). Buying an LCD projector for emergency nursing continuing education: One ENA state council's experience. *Journal of Emergency Nursing, 29*(2), 168–170.

Moore, L.W., Augspurger, P., King, M.O., & Proffitt, C. (2001). Insights on the poster preparation and presentation process. *Applied Nursing Research, 14*(2), 100–104.

Taggart, H.M., & Arslanian, C. (2000). Creating an effective poster presentation. *Orthopaedic Nursing, 19*(3), 47–52.

CHAPTER 11

Recording Your Professional Achievements in a Portfolio

As a professional nurse, you realize the important role that meticulous documentation plays in validating and tracking key elements of patient care. On a more personal note, documentation of your professional accomplishments serves a similar purpose with respect to your career goals. Whether you are a recent graduate or an experienced nurse, maintaining a systematic and accurate record of your professional life is an essential activity that serves a variety of purposes.

After you have collected and organized your professional accomplishments, place them together in a professional document referred to as a portfolio (American Nurses Association [ANA], 2000). A portfolio not only provides a way for you as a staff development educator to record your professional development but also serves as a method for you to record your "career planning, demonstration of learning, and maintenance of continuing professional competence" (ANA, p. 25).

As a unit-based educator, you will need to not only maintain your own portfolio but also to mentor other staff nurses on your unit in this process (Brooks & Madda, 1999). Attempt to complete this task by using creative strategies that will accomplish the purpose of a professional portfolio and meet the organizational needs, as well. For example, one medical center provided their nurses with a portfolio binder in recognition of National Nurses Week (Brooks, Barrett, & Zimmermann, 1998) and used completed portfolios as documentation of standards during a Joint Commission on Accreditation of Healthcare Organizations accreditation visit.

Validating the Need to Document

Why should you spend time collecting and organizing data that reflect your professional achievements? There are a variety of reasons, some of which are global in nature and others that are more specific and personal. However, only you can determine what is essential for you to do at this point in your career.

Progress Toward Career Goals

Assembling, organizing, and documenting your professional accomplishments are good ways to help you keep focused and evaluate progress toward your career goals (Oermann, 2002). It is a way to take charge and responsibility for your own learning. Although developing a professional career plan will be discussed in more detail later in Chapter 15, the following example may help to clarify this purpose.

Suppose you are interested in pursuing a career as an oncology nurse in home care and have developed a plan to accomplish this outcome. During the current year, you have targeted several specific steps or strategies that will help you move toward the goal of becoming a homecare oncology nurse. As you collect and organize your professional records, you have an opportunity to reflect upon the status and nature of your accomplishments to date. This gives you a chance to either alter your selection of activities or stay on track with what you have accomplished. Your choice to engage in new opportunities can be evaluated based on their match with the focus of your career plan.

Promotions and Job Opportunities

Although you still need to develop a resume when you are applying for a job, many potential employers value a professional portfolio when you are interviewed (Brooks et al., 1998). This document enables prospective employers to review your professional achievements and examples of your work that support them.

Keeping a record of your professional activities can help you prepare for an upcoming performance appraisal and/or merit raise. Use the criteria listed on your position or job description as a guide to document essential outcomes.

Maintaining a professional record can give you the edge on promotions within your organization as well as opportunities outside your workplace. Use documented criteria for promotion, such as those identified in your organization's clinical advancement or career ladder guidelines, to direct you.

Coping During Organizational Downsizing

Collecting written evidence of professional work such as projects or other types of activities has been suggested as one way to help nurses cope with organizational changes, such as downsizing in the workplace or career transitions (Brooks & Madda, 1999). This proactive strategy of developing a work portfolio can be used to confirm your level of nursing knowledge and clinical skills and help you prepare for an unexpected layoff or career move. This approach forces you to organize your professional past while you are actively employed, rather than while you are experiencing the emotional distress of being jobless. This strategy also may provide you with a sense of control over your future, especially during a time of uncertainty or great change in healthcare organizations.

Recognition and Validation of Expertise and Competency

It is helpful to have an organized record of your professional accomplishments when applying for awards such as scholarships, grants, or other types of professional recognition. Similarly, validation of items such as clinical practice hours, continuing education (CE) programs attended, and contact hours earned often can help you when verifying specialty nursing certification requirements. This need will be discussed further in Chapter 14. Perhaps you need evidence of teaching cardiopulmonary resuscitation (CPR) classes to maintain your volunteer position as a CPR instructor.

An organized collection of documents that reflect your clinical competency in a particular area can be used when pursuing formal educational preparation in nursing. Some schools–because they focus on assessing learning outcomes–

accept portfolios as verification of one's past professional achievements, accomplishments, and other personal learning experiences. Following careful evaluation of this portfolio, faculty determine the learner's individual strengths and weaknesses and use this information to develop an individualized plan that builds upon existing competencies. In some instances, a school also may grant advanced standing credits or some type of recognition for these prior learning experiences.

Preparation of Professional Documents

Organizing and filing your professional achievements provide a mechanism to develop and update your resume and other professional documents, such as a portfolio. Because most of the data and vital documents you need to record fall into one of several major content categories used in both resumes and portfolios, this makes the process of both creating and updating them much easier. Details on how to prepare a resume will be provided in Chapter 12. This current chapter will focus on how you can develop an effective professional portfolio.

Documents to Collect, Organize, and Record

What data and documents are important to record and file? There are a variety of essential materials upon which you may want to focus your efforts. Most of the materials can be categorized into one of several content headings. As you review your professional materials, sort them accordingly. Be sure to place valuable original documents such as official school transcripts, diplomas, licenses, and certifications in a safe place. Use copies of these documents, if acceptable, for the purposes of your portfolio.

Educational Experiences

First, organize documents that deal with your formal educational preparation. Include materials such as copies of your school transcripts, diplomas, and the results of required admission tests. Be sure to keep a copy of the school catalogue that contains the curriculum with which you were involved. This includes the program of studies and course descriptions with objectives. You also may want to keep some key correspondence that describes your progress, such as admission, advanced standing, program completion, evaluations, and financial agreements. Samples of outstanding papers or projects you completed during school can be useful in documenting your creativity and writing skills.

Professional Work Experiences

Similar to how you organized your education experiences, collect and organize evidence related to your clinical performance. Start by focusing on your present job, and then reflect back to previous ones. Keep a copy of your position or job description along with samples of any evaluations received from your supervisors and peers. Hopefully they were all positive. However, retain the not-so-good ones as well in order to document your progress in certain areas. File copies of any other correspondence, such as thank-you letters received from patients and their families, peers, and supervisors. Include the letter of appreciation you received from the faculty member regarding the nursing student you just preceptored in your clinical unit.

In addition to these obvious documents, be sure to keep a daily record of your clinical successes, specifically those things that set you apart from your colleagues. Perhaps it was the individualized plan of care you developed for your patient, or the standard you created for patients following a total laryngectomy. Explain how you introduced a new piece of equipment or procedure on the unit, such as the IV controller or discharge form. How about the new scheduling system that you devised last year? Describe other changes that you have implemented with the staff in your department.

Share information about the unit-based in-service program you presented on chemotherapy safety precautions for your coworkers. Try to recall a specific clinical situation or critical incident in which your nursing skills and behaviors positively influenced the outcome. Whether it is participation in committees or unit-based projects, be sure to salvage some documentation of the project along with any evaluation comments or feedback received. Do not forget to document your success on the annual clinical competency test.

Licensure, Certifications, and Certificates

Maintain a copy of your nursing license along with any certifications or certificates you have obtained. You also may choose to keep any correspondence related to these items, such as test scores or certification results.

Awards, Honors, and Special Recognition

Copy documents that reflect awards or honors you have received, such as membership in Sigma Theta Tau International Honor Society for Nursing, outstanding work accomplished, or being on the dean's list at school. Include recognition of outstanding professional or community work you received, as well.

Professional Memberships

Document membership in professional nursing organizations such as ANA or the Oncology Nursing Society. Keep copies of membership cards and correspondence that describe your involvement on committees or as an elected official. Be sure to note any evaluative comments you receive about the nature of your work in these organizations.

Publications

As mentioned in Chapter 9, keep the original and copies or reprints of any publications with which you were involved. Include both formal and informal publications. Formal publications include documents such as journal articles, editorials, topical journal issues, and chapters or books. Be sure to mention experience as a manuscript or book reviewer. Clinical publications of a more informal nature consist of items such as patient teaching guides, clinical or critical pathways, policies and procedures, discharge guides, staff education materials, newsletters, and charting samples, such as patient assessment forms or discharge instructions. Be aware of confidentiality standards when recording these documents.

Research Participation

Keep a copy of your participation in research activities. Documentation of your participation in research can range from a letter written by the principal investigator or researcher thanking you for helping with data collection or the literature review, to actual publication of the results in a journal. Perhaps you organized and led a unit-based journal club conference in which staff nurses read and discussed clinical research articles. Do not forget to file a copy of any research grant(s) submitted or accompanying correspondence. Be sure to maintain a copy of the abstract that describes the completed research project.

Consulting

Include any experience you may have as a consultant. For example, document your efforts when you served as an expert witness for a legal firm. Perhaps you shared your clinical expertise with the nursing staff of an affiliated homecare agency on the postoperative care of patients with head and neck cancer.

Presentations

Include a copy of any professional presentations you have completed. Also include photographs of posters you developed both within your organization and outside at professional organizations. Try to keep the original conference flier that lists you as a participant. Be sure to include any evaluations or copies of correspondence that address the quality of your efforts.

Community Volunteer Activities

Just as with presentations, be sure to document any volunteer activities in which you participated. Especially include those that relate to your expertise as a professional nurse. Enclose any feedback received about the outcomes of your involvement.

Attendance at Continuing Education Programs

Keep an ongoing record of the CE programs that you have attended, along with evidence of contact hours earned or certificates of completion granted. Be sure to include any independent learning or home study modules you may have completed at work or through nursing journals. Keep records as to the date of the conference, title, speaker name, location (city and state), organization that sponsored the program, length of program, and any contact hours earned. Figure 11-1 illustrates one example of recording and organizing your attendance at conferences.

Date	Title	Speaker(s)	Location	Sponsor	Length	Contact Hours

Figure 11-1. Example of a Method for Documenting Attendance at Professional Conferences

Letters of Recommendation

Save any letters of recommendation you received during your professional career; also include documents such as thank-you notes that reflect your professional performance.

Other Helpful Materials

It is a good idea to obtain a small professional photograph of yourself along with several copies. A black and white or color wallet-sized photo will do. Ask the media center at your workplace or the copy center in your community for details. Photographs come in handy when you are asked for one in a hurry, such as for the newsletter at your workplace or for a local professional organization to which you belong. Sometimes editors request a photograph to accompany manuscripts for publication.

Consider including copies of your recent health records, such as immunizations or tuberculosis skin test results (Brooks et al., 1998), and liability insurance, if appropriate.

Keep your old calendars or appointment books until you have had a chance to transcribe their content. Recording professional events and personal accounts on your calendar provides a helpful means of making sense and organizing your yearly professional activities.

Developing a Painless Record-Keeping System

What is the best way to start collecting and organizing these professional documents? Keeping track of all these details can be a nightmare unless you develop an organized record-keeping system. Create a system that is sophisticated enough to accomplish the outcome, yet easy to use. This way, you are more likely to use it and make it work for you.

Identify a Time Frame for Your Records

Begin this process by choosing a 12-month time span that matches your needs. For some nurses, this may be a calendar year that starts in January and ends in December. For others, it may comprise a fiscal year, one that begins July 1st and goes to June 30th of the following year. Or maybe you choose to organize your record-keeping system in accordance with your date of hire or annual performance appraisal. Whatever timeline you choose, match it with your needs.

Develop a System to Collect and Organize Data

Once you have established a suitable time frame, develop a system that you can use to collect and organize your professional data. Use your personal calendar or appointment book to record important events and other occurrences such as clinical successes. This helps to create an overall picture for the year.

Now that you know what to record, how do you start the system? One simple approach involves the assembly of several file folders in an expandable accordion-like file pocket. Use colored file folders for easy identification. Label each folder with the headings shown in Figure 11-2. Then go through your documents and place each in the appropriate folder based on the topic. Develop a three-ring notebook with dividers labeled according to your categories of documents.

A similar approach can be attempted using computer software programs. Create the headings using a traditional word-processing program or a spreadsheet, and then record the data. Save both a hard copy and the disk for your files. Combine the two approaches using the folders or binders for storage and the computer for recording and organizing data. Regardless of the approach you use, it needs to be manageable for you.

- Educational experiences
- Professional work experiences
- Licensure, certifications, and certificates
- Awards, honors, and special recognition
- Professional membership
- Publications
- Consulting
- Presentations
- Community
- Letters of recommendation

Figure 11-2. Suggested Headings for Record Folders

Incorporate Data Into a Meaningful Project

Now that you have your data organized and sorted, take advantage of this ideal opportunity to transform all the pieces into a professional document. As mentioned earlier, try transforming the data into a useful resume or portfolio. Retrieve each folder as needed to create these documents. If possible, start your system with new folders (or empty the old ones) for each 12-month time frame.

Creating a Professional Portfolio

Faculty in schools of nursing traditionally have used portfolios to assess competence in nursing students (Gallagher, 2001; McMullan et al., 2003). Portfolios also have been used by faculty to document the scholarship of teaching (Reece, Pearce, Melillo, & Beaudry, 2001). However, some healthcare organizations promote the use of portfolios with staff nurses (Brooks & Madda, 1999), and some employers require their nurses to submit a professional portfolio when applying for promotion or clinical advancement. A portfolio has been suggested as a mechanism to communicate one's professional capabilities to prospective employers (Brooks et al., 1998).

Understanding the Process

If you need to develop a professional portfolio, ask the individual requesting it for specific guidelines as to its development. It is important for you to know such things as the specific focus or purpose of the portfolio, the content required, and the outcomes to be measured. If you plan on developing a portfolio for your own satisfaction, use the content areas listed above as a guide.

Putting It All Together

Be creative when developing your portfolio, and tailor it to meet your specific needs. Unless otherwise specified, you can develop a portfolio using a variety of practical approaches. For example, create a portfolio incorporating a file folder with two or more pockets. Try making one with a three-ring binder to organize data. Some experts suggest organizing your portfolio according to a chronological or alphabetical order or by topic titles (Brooks et al., 1998). Whatever method you use to compile it, be sure that your portfolio is more than just a collection of documents.

It is essential that you apply both the portfolio development process as well as the portfolio itself to your best advantage. The portfolio development process can be viewed as an exercise along with the portfolio as a tool or worksheet as you plan and evaluate your career development. By using both the process and the outcome or product, you can assess your professional accomplishments and reflect upon your strengths and weaknesses. These data enable you to develop a plan based on your career goals that includes specific interventions or strategies to help you meet these goals. Finally, you can evaluate your success in meeting your goals.

Remember, include personal reflections of experiences that illustrate your professional knowledge, skills, and attitudes in nursing. Include introspective evidence that reflects the qualities that make you a unique, competent, and exceptional professional nurse.

Summary

This chapter describes the importance of recording your professional achievements, especially for the purpose of resume and portfolio development. Practical tips are provided to help make the record-keeping procedure a systematic and organized process.

References

American Nurses Association. (2000). *Scope and standards of practice for nursing professional development.* Washington, DC: Author.

Brooks, B., Barrett, S., Zimmermann, P.G. (1998). Beyond your resume: A nurse's professional "portfolio." *Journal of Emergency Nursing, 24,* 555–557.

Brooks, B.A., & Madda, M. (1999). How to organize a professional portfolio for staff and career development. *Journal for Nurses in Staff Development, 15*(1), 5–10.

Gallagher, P. (2001). An evaluation of a standards based portfolio. *Nurse Education Today, 21*(3), 197–200.

McMullan, M., Endacott, R., Gray, M.A., Jasper, M., Miller, C.M., Scholes, J., et al. (2003). Portfolios and assessment of competence: A review of the literature. *Journal of Advanced Nursing, 41,* 283–294.

Oermann, M.H. (2002). Developing a professional portfolio in nursing. *Orthopaedic Nursing, 21*(2), 73–78.

Reece, S.M., Pearce, C.W., Melillo, K.D., & Beaudry, M. (2001). The faculty portfolio: Documenting the scholarship of teaching. *Journal of Professional Nursing, 17*(4), 180–186.

CHAPTER 12

Preparing Your Resume and Cover Letter

You are faced with a dilemma. You need to prepare a resume for a new position that is available in a local community center but are not quite sure where to begin. You also are not sure what information should be included in a resume.

To answer your question, you search your dictionary that describes a resume to be a "summary; a brief account of one's education and professional experience submitted with a job application" (Webster's Third, 1976, p. 1937). Although nurses frequently associate preparing a resume with the job-searching process, nurses develop a resume for a variety of other professional reasons.

A resume should be more than just a summary of your past experiences. In fact, some individuals perceive a resume as being a visual representation of one's professional image or self-image. Your resume needs to tell those who read it who you are as a professional nurse. It should reveal your identity and be framed within your experiences, accomplishments, and progress in self-development activities. An effective resume can send a message that tells others how motivated you are as a professional and how you differ or stand apart from other nurses.

You may have heard the term "curriculum vitae" or "CV" and are not sure how it differs from a resume. Which of these documents do you need to develop: a resume or a CV? The dictionary defines a CV as "a brief account of one's life; a brief statement including biographical data" (Webster's Third, 1976, p. 557). Although some sources use the terms "resume" and "CV" interchangeably, in reality, a CV is a more lengthy and detailed account of an individual's professional life, not just a description of educational and professional experience (O'Connor, 1999). A CV usually is required of nursing faculty who work in schools of nursing within university or college settings.

Markey and Campbell (1996) described the difference between a resume and a CV using an analogy. They likened a resume to an "advertisement" and a CV to an "owner's manual of information" (p. 192). This example of comparing resumes and CVs can help you decide which document to develop, based on its intended purpose.

Regardless of your choice to create a resume or a CV, the process described in this chapter can be helpful in designing either one. Be sure to adhere to specific guidelines, if provided, by individuals to whom you plan on submitting your resume or CV. For example, if a newspaper ad for a nurse educator position requests applicants should submit a one-page resume, then adhere to that request.

Reasons for Preparing a Resume

There are several reasons why nurses need to prepare a resume. Most nurses will agree that it is an expected practice to submit a resume when you are applying for a new position or when you are changing work settings. However, developing a resume for other professional events can help you create a good first impression that may help you with many of your professional career goals. A professional resume can set you apart from other nurses competing for the same opportunity. Finally, having your resume prepared and current is a strategy to help nurses deal with unanticipated changes in the work setting (DeMello & Pagragan, 1998).

Even though a formal resume is not required in all professional situations nurses encounter, they often are asked to provide content that is similar to that contained in a resume on various applications. For example, application forms needed for admission into a school of nursing request information such as prior education and work experience. If your resume is up-to-date and readily available, using it as a reference will save you a great deal of time and aggravation.

Developing your resume is very similar to conducting a professional self-assessment. In fact, the process of developing a resume can help you realize your strengths or accomplishments, as well as your weaknesses or areas that need developed. Because a resume traditionally contains several categories related to your professional development, it can be used as a focal point upon which to guide your career plan. Chapter 15 will provide additional information on developing a professional career plan.

Perhaps while you were drafting your resume, you discovered that you have nothing to enter under categories such as "Professional Organizations," "Continuing Education Programs Attended," "Community Involvement," or "Publications." Rather than fretting about not having these activities, view this finding within its proper perspective. By preparing your resume, you discovered potential areas in which you may focus your career goals. Use this experience as a learning opportunity. Plan to explore the professional activities that are missing in your resume, such as writing an article, and incorporate them into your career plan. Include publishing an article in a nursing journal among one of your short-term goals.

As a unit-based educator, developing your resume first can help you as you mentor other staff nurses in creating their own resumes. You will already be familiar with the process and the content that needs to be included. Consider using creative teaching strategies when helping staff nurses on your clinical unit develop their resumes. For example, Freed and Kettler (1999) described modeling a resume after one they developed based on the accomplishments of Florence Nightingale. This helped nursing students not only to learn how to develop a meaningful resume but also to appreciate the accomplishments of this historical nursing leader.

Job Application

As mentioned earlier, resumes are commonly used when applying for a job, whether it is your first nursing position or a change in jobs. A resume provides your prospective employer with a summary of your professional experience that is needed for the advertised position and can influence whether or not you obtain an interview for that job (Brooks, Barrett, & Zimmermann, 1998). For example, a professional-looking resume that accurately reflects your educational background, clinical expertise, and teaching or preceptor experience can result in a follow-up interview when applying for a part-time clinical teaching position at your local school of nursing.

A resume often is used to supplement the information asked on an agency's job application. A well-prepared, professional, and attractive resume can set you apart from others who are applying for the same position. As mentioned in Chapter 11, your resume should be part of your professional portfolio.

Promotion or Clinical Advancement

In addition to securing new positions, resumes also can be viewed as an important career management tool (Clarke, 2000). Depending on your workplace, resumes may be required or preferred as part of the promotion process, especially in clinical advancement programs. Resumes are an effective means of summarizing your overall accomplishments and demonstrating your progress within your career plan.

Admission to School

A resume is appropriate to include, along with your application, when applying for admission to a school of nursing. Your resume sends a message to members of the admissions committee that you recognize key activities that comprise professional nursing practice. A resume also can reflect the consistency of your contributions in areas such as clinical practice, nursing scholarship, and community service.

Scholarships, Awards, and Recognition

Include your resume when applying for opportunities such as scholarships and awards, grants, or other forms of recognition. The next time you ask your former employer or teacher for a letter of recommendation, attach an updated resume with your request. Your resume can help these individuals organize the content of their letter so that it accurately reflects your accomplishments.

Conference Speaker

A resume or a biographical sketch, a document that resembles a resume, is requested of nurses who present papers or posters at professional nursing programs that award contact hours for attendance. Sponsors of these continuing education (CE) programs submit this information to a specific organization, such as their state nurses association, that approves the program and allows the sponsor to award nurses who attend the program with contact hours. Contact hours are a standardized unit that measures the amount of time that is spent during an educational offering (American Nurses Association [ANA], 1994). This term will be explained in detail in Chapter 14.

Once you are confirmed as a speaker, the conference planning committee may send you several forms to complete prior to the conference. Even if a formal resume is not required, information available from your resume can make this process a very simple one. Resumes also are used by conference planners to introduce you to the participants immediately prior to your presentation.

Manuscript Reviewer

If you are interested in serving as a manuscript reviewer for a nursing journal, a resume can provide an editor with an overall impression of your professional qualifications. Once you have become a manuscript reviewer for a journal, be sure to add this accomplishment to your resume.

Consultant

Maybe you possess expertise in a particular area of nursing, such as establishing an early discharge program for new mothers or providing nursing care for patients diagnosed with head and neck cancer. Perhaps you have the expertise to serve as a legal nurse consultant on cases where professional judgment of nursing care is required. Regardless of the type of consulting you provide, a resume can inform others of your qualifications.

What to Include in a Resume

Although there are minor variations, most resumes contain common categories or content areas. Begin your resume by collecting your data. Spend time organizing, prioritizing, and polishing this information into the appropriate format, discussed later in this chapter. Start this process by recording the headings or categories illustrated in Figure 12-1 on a sheet of paper. Use a word-processing program on your computer if this is your preferred way to accomplish this task. Be sure to leave sufficient space after each category so that you can fill in your specific information.

Figure 12-1.
Main Categories Frequently Used in a Resume

- Identification information
- Career objective (optional)
- Education
- Professional work experience
- Licensure, certifications, and certificates
- Awards, honors, and special recognition
- Professional activities
  - Membership in professional organizations
  - Publications
  - Research
  - Consultant
  - Presentations
- Community volunteer activities
- Attendance at CE programs (past five years)
- References

Although computer word-processing software can be extremely useful for this step, a handwritten approach can be just as effective for now. You can reorganize these handwritten sections by cutting and pasting them before your final transcription, or use small adhesive note pads that can be easily moved on a page. Do not worry about being neat right now, because this is your personal worksheet. Only you need to understand it at this point in the process.

Next, read the following sections in this chapter, along with their detailed descriptions. Using them as a guide, record this information as examples from your personal files. As you complete this step, try to be accurate and record detailed information. Pay less attention to style, format, or order of content at this point.

Depending on your experience, you may need to search several sources in obtaining this information. These sources may include items such as your personal calendar, certificates received from attending CE programs, school files, conference records, presentations, and performance evaluations. Ask the nurse educator in the staff development or nursing education department at your workplace for more details about the programs you have attended, if needed. You also may need to review your professional file at work to fill in some gaps. A brainstorming session with your peers can be a productive means of completing missing data such as conference dates or college courses. If you have nothing to add under a heading on your resume, then omit the category for now.

Identification Information

This section of a resume contains simply what it says, identification information, and provides the heading for your resume. Record your full name followed by your credentials; your highest degree in nursing appears before the RN listing. Be sure to include any certifications you may have, such as RNC, OCN®, or CORLN. Follow this information with your mailing address, telephone number, and e-mail address. Avoid using your work e-mail address if you are applying for a position at another healthcare organization.

Because this information may be used by the receiver to contact you, it is important that it is both accurate and current. Omit personal or confidential information on your resume, such as your social security number, age, marital status, or names of family members.

Career Objective

Include a career objective next on your resume, especially if you are applying for a job. This objective informs prospective employers of your career goals. It also helps them determine a match between your goal and their needs. If your resume is intended for a reason other than job placement or promotion, you may want to omit this category.

An example of a career objective might be, "To obtain a beginning staff nurse position in cardiovascular nursing." Perhaps you are an experienced RN interested in obtaining a nursing management position. If so, your objective may look like this: "To obtain a first level management position within a progressive university-affiliated medical center." Tailor your career goal to the agency to which you are applying. Keep it realistic, concise (one to two sentences), and within the limits of your qualifications.

Education

Use this category to describe your educational background that is relevant to the overall purpose of your resume. Include the name of the educational institutions you have attended, such as your school of nursing and college or university. If you attended a college and earned several credits there but did not complete a degree at that site, you may choose to include it and indicate this status. If you are currently completing a degree, include your anticipated date of graduation. Be sure to add the location of the schools, the years attended, your major and/or minor area of study, and degree(s) awarded. Some nurses choose to supply their grade point average at each school attended. In most instances, it is not necessary to list your high school education.

For example, you might list a diploma in nursing, an associate degree in nursing, bachelor's degree in nursing, or a master of science degree in nursing. Check your school transcript or official diploma if you are uncertain of the wording of your degree. Most likely, your major is in nursing, although you may possess a minor in another discipline such as psychology or a language. If nursing is your second degree, be sure to list your previous degree.

This information informs readers of your formal preparation in nursing and other fields. It also makes them aware of any advanced nursing preparation you have received.

Professional Work Experience

This section affords you the opportunity to describe your previous professional employment (paid) experiences. As mentioned before, include content that is essential to the purpose of your resume. Start by listing your present and past job titles or positions, dates of employment, agencies, and their respective locations. Provide a succinct review of your major responsibilities. Include activities such as serving as a clinical preceptor for nursing students or new employees on your unit. If you are applying for your first position as an RN, include your experience working as a nursing assistant or participating in student internships at your healthcare agency.

List each major responsibility as a separate, brief statement. Begin each statement with an action verb like the ones listed in Figure 12-2. Unless you want to emphasize a particular point, provide more details about your most current position and fewer details about your previous positions. You may choose to include your membership on various committees at work in this section.

If possible, try to organize your past positions so that they demonstrate progression or make some sort of sense. For example, if you have had several nursing positions within one organization, develop a creative way to illustrate how these positions were connected. Avoid making them appear simply as a listing of jobs. If you are applying for your first job as an RN, list those jobs that represent your positive qualities, such as your ability to organize and lead groups, your independence and competence when completing assignments, and your effective communication skills.

Licensure, Certifications, and Certificates

List any current licensure that you hold. Include the state in which you received licensure and the expiration date. In this category, include any specialty certifications you have attained such as an OCN® or CORLN, the sponsoring agency providing the certification, and the dates during which your certification is effective. Be sure to include special certificates you may have obtained in such areas as cardiopulmonary resuscitation (CPR) or advanced cardiac life support. Specify if you are qualified as an instructor or instructor-trainer in these areas. As mentioned earlier, list the sponsoring agency and effective dates.

Although proof of licensure as a professional nurse is a requirement when obtaining an RN position, certifications tell the receiver that you voluntarily excelled above and beyond in a nursing specialty. You assumed a leadership role by choosing to prepare for and take the certification examination. These activities can set you apart from other RNs who possess similar professional work experience.

Awards, Honors, and Special Recognition

List any awards, honors, or special recognition you have received, especially those that have resulted from a review of your accomplishments by your peers.

The following is a list of action words that you may want to use in your resume. These words are action-oriented and represent skill areas you may have that would be beneficial to the prospective employer.

accelerated	conducted	eliminated	initiated	negotiated	recommended
accomplished	conserve	enlarged	inspected	observed	recruited
achieved	consolidated	entertained	installed	obtained	reduced
activated	constructed	established	instituted	operated	reinforced
adapted	consulted	estimated	instructed	organized	reorganized
administered	controlled	evaluated	interpreted	originated	repaired
analyzed	coordinated	examined	intervened	participated	researched
appraised	corresponded	exhibited	interviewed	performed	responsible for
arranged	counseled	expanded	invented	persuaded	reviewed
assembled	created	expedited	investigated	pioneered	revised
assisted	delegated	explained	judged	planned	rewrote
bargained	delivered	explored	launched	predicted	scheduled
budgeted	demonstrated	facilitated	lectured	prescribed	simplified
built	developed	formulated	located	presented	solved
calculated	diagnosed	fostered	logged	presided	strengthened
charted	directed	founded	maintained	processed	supervised
classified	discovered	generated	managed	produced	taught
coached	dispensed	governed	mastered	proficient at	tested
collected	displayed	handled	measured	programmed	trained
compiled	distributed	implemented	mediated	promoted	translated
completed	dramatized	improved	moderated	proposed	updated
composed	earned	increased	monitored	received	wrote
conceived	edited	indexed	motivated		

Figure 12-2.
Examples of Action Words

Note. From *The Career Services Center 1997 Career Guide*, Duquesne University (p. 7), by Duquesne University Career Services Center, 1997, Atlanta, GA: Career Publishing Network. Copyright 1997 by the Career Publishing Network. Reprinted with permission.

Include the name of the award, the sponsoring agency, and the date. Examples include attaining membership into Sigma Theta Tau International, attaining the dean's list at your school, receiving a professional nursing organization's literary award, or other service awards.

This information tells the receiver that you not only have experience in particular areas within the profession of nursing but also were recognized by your colleagues or community members for your accomplishments.

Professional Activities

This section of a resume contains an assortment of professional experiences in nursing. These activities can either be grouped together or listed separately. This decision needs to be made by you based on what experiences you have had in these areas. If you have very few activities to list under these subheadings, then you may choose to organize them together under the heading of "Professional Activities." On the other hand, if you have many experiences, list them separately under each subheading. Exclude any subheadings for which you have no experience. Avoid the practice of listing headings or subheadings followed by the explanation "none."

Membership in Professional Organizations

List any professional organizations to which you belong as a paid or nonpaid member. These may include international, national, state, local, or private organizations (e.g., Oncology Nursing Society, ANA, Sigma Theta Tau International

Honor Society of Nursing). Include memberships you hold within these organizations at local chapter and state levels. Try clustering smaller state and chapter groups under the larger parent organization to provide a sense of order to your listing.

Be sure to include the official name of the professional organizations (and initials), dates of membership, and your specific role within the organization. This role may be that of member, committee chair, or other office held, such as treasurer or president.

This section tells the receiver that you are an involved professional who is concerned about what is happening within nursing and your specialty. Holding an office or committee chair position demonstrates your ability to lead or direct others related to a particular project. It also speaks of your communication skills. Because your peers voted for you to lead them, holding an elected office reflects that your skills are valued.

Publications

List any publications that you have authored or coauthored, if available. Unless specified, use any publication style to document the details of your publication(s). If you are listing an article, be sure to include the author(s) full names and first initials, year of publication, the title of the article, journal name, number, volume, and inclusive pages. If you are citing a book, include the book title, the city and state of the publisher, and the publishing company. When noting a chapter, indicate the author(s) and title of the specific chapter you are citing. Use a consistent format or publication manual style when citing your entries. You can obtain copies of these manuals through your library reference section. The sample resume shown in Figure 12-3 illustrates publications formatted according to the American Psychological Association (APA, 2001), a style that is frequently used to cite references in nursing journals.

Listing your publications informs the receiver of your diversification as a professional nurse. The reasons for publishing were discussed in Chapter 9.

Research

This section provides you an opportunity to share any research activities with which you have been involved. Research experience often varies among nurses and frequently depends upon the type of job you have, the research opportunities available at work or school, and the guidance available to conduct research. Research participation can be viewed as either formal or informal. Formal activities in research often involve assuming the role of an investigator or researcher. Informal participation may include helping a unit-based research team with various activities that are needed to carry out the research process. These may consist of conducting the review of literature, assisting with data collection on the clinical unit, or helping with data entry.

If appropriate, describe the extent of your involvement in any research project, along with the following information: list of investigators (specify who was the principal investigator or leader of the project), title of the study, agency that funded the study and the amount in dollars awarded (if applicable), and year(s) during which the research was conducted. If the research is still in progress, clarify this point. If you are not listed as a formal investigator, then provide information that

Figure 12-3.
Sample Resume

EMILLIE M. BROOKS, BSN, RN, OCN®
126 Oaktree Drive
Pittsburgh, PA 35871
(617) 333-8979 (Work) (617) 987-4957 (Home)
E-mail: brooksem@cmm.org

OBJECTIVE: Obtain a staff nurse position in oncology home care.

PROFESSIONAL WORK EXPERIENCE
University Medical Center, Pittsburgh, PA 15213
Clinical Nurse II, Medical Oncology Unit (1999 to present)
• Provided direct care to medical patients with cancer
• Supervised staff nurses and ancillary healthcare workers
• Functioned as charge nurse as needed
• Chaired the Patient Education Committee
• Coordinated a unit-based education program
• Served as a preceptor for staff nurses during cross-training

EDUCATION
BSN, Nursing, 1999, Duquesne University School of Nursing, Pittsburgh, PA

LICENSURE AND CERTIFICATIONS
PA RN License (1999 to present)
OCN®, Oncology Nursing Certification Corporation (2001 to present)
Basic Cardiac Life Support, American Heart Association (1999 to present)

AWARDS AND HONORS
Sigma Theta Tau International Honor Society of Nursing, 1999
Graduated summa cum laude, Duquesne University, 1999

MEMBERSHIP IN PROFESSIONAL ORGANIZATIONS
Oncology Nursing Society (1999 to present)
Sigma Theta Tau International Honor Society of Nursing, Epsilon Phi Chapter (1999 to present)

PUBLICATIONS
Brooks, E.M. (2003). Teaching the medical oncology patient. *Nursing Journal, 1*(4), 123–125.

COMMUNITY ACTIVITIES
Volunteer for Eastside Shelter, Pittsburgh, PA, 1998 to present

CONTINUING EDUCATION PROGRAMS ATTENDED
Cancer Nursing Course, Oncology Programs Inc., March 3–7, 2004
Case Management, L. Jones, Townsend Conferences, June 5, 2003
Pain Management, J. Goodman, University Hospital, January 5, 2002

REFERENCES
Available upon request

describes your specific role in the project, as mentioned earlier. If you worked on this project as a research assistant or student while in school, be sure to indicate this, as well.

This section on research tells the receiver about your involvement and initiative in nursing scholarship and related clinical problem-solving activities. It also illustrates many of the reasons for participating in research described in Chapter 13.

Consultant

Describe your involvement in consulting activities, such as serving as an expert witness for a law firm. Be sure to provide details, including your general area of consultation, such as labor and delivery or trauma nursing, along with the dates you were involved in this activity. To maintain confidentiality, avoid disclosing the names of the parties involved in the case. Use the same guidelines for other opportunities you may have had as a consultant.

This section tells the receiver that your nursing expertise is recognized and valued by others. It also provides opportunities for jobs related to your specialty area.

Presentations

List any paper or poster presentations you have had at local, regional, national, and/or international levels. Be sure to include the title of your presentation, the conference and organization for which it was presented, the date(s), and the location (city and state).

The presence of presentations on your resume informs the receiver of your ability to disseminate professional information. It also reflects that you assumed a leadership role in communicating with groups such as the professional nursing and lay communities.

Community Volunteer Activities

Use this section to identify any community activities in which you volunteer your expertise and time. Perhaps you serve lunch at a local homeless shelter and provide its members with monthly educational programs on health promotion topics. Maybe you taught CPR to a neighborhood community group. Be sure to list the dates involved, the name of the volunteer organization or group, its location, and a general statement about the specific service(s) you provided.

This listing of community activities tells others that you share your nursing expertise voluntarily with the community. It demonstrates that you recognize the need to participate in community service as a healthcare professional.

Attendance at Continuing Education Programs

List any professional CE programs you have attended. Try to limit this list to the past three to five years. Start with the most current program you have attended, and go back in time. Include the following with each entry: date(s) attended, title of the presentation, speaker, sponsoring organization, and location (city and state). Be sure to keep track of the contact hours you received. If your list is a particularly long one, prepare this section as an appendix or attachment to your resume.

Regular attendance at clinically relevant professional conferences tells the receiver that you take personal responsibility to keep abreast of changes in your discipline.

References

If appropriate, supply the names, addresses, and telephone numbers of individuals who are willing to serve as professional references for you. Choose two or three individuals whose expertise matches the goal of your resume. References should include people who know you on a personal level as well as colleagues who can speak on the quality of your professional work. In some instances, you may be asked to choose names of individuals as references who possess particular backgrounds or specifications, such as a former clinical instructor or supervisor.

Be sure to obtain permission from these individuals before you list their names as references. It is unprofessional to assume that they will grant permission without your asking them. You might want to call and ask them to serve as a reference for you. Follow the call with a note or letter that explains the details of your request. A sample cover letter is described later in this chapter that explains the details of your request. Supply a copy of your resume for their review. Because some agencies ask for references written on an official application form rather than in a letter form, be sure to investigate this point prior to making arrangements.

Organizing the Content of Your Resume

Once you have recorded the main content of your resume, then organize the data you compiled under each heading. Decide what content areas you plan on including, combining, or eliminating. Decide on the order in which the headings will be presented in your resume. Although most resume guides suggest a similar sequence of headings, you can design your resume to emphasize certain areas for the receiver. Although you want to avoid "padding" or adding false information to your resume, you have the freedom to fashion your resume so that it effectively communicates your strengths to the reader. This is particularly important because the focus of one's resume is often on the first information a potential employer sees.

Try preparing two drafts of your resume, and ask your peers to choose the one that is most appealing. You may decide to design several versions of your resume, depending on the message you want to communicate based on your intended goal or overall objective.

Choosing a Resume Format

Resumes are commonly organized using either a chronological or a functional format, with most nurse recruiters preferring the chronological approach (Feery & Tierney, 2002). If you choose the traditional chronological format for your resume, arrange your information under each category in reverse chronological order, starting from the most current information to the oldest. For example, organize your professional experience section by listing your most recent job and description first, followed by the jobs you held earlier. Your oldest job should be listed last.

Although nurses commonly use the chronological format, choose this approach only if it meets your particular professional needs. Some experts suggest a chronologically formatted resume for graduate or novice nurses who are just beginning the job search process or for nurses who have been continually employed throughout their professional careers. Because information listed first within a category on your resume is likely to receive the most attention by the reader, the chronological format also may be appropriate for nurses who are seeking positions at a level higher than their previous ones.

A functional resume centers on experiences such as professional skills or competencies (i.e., management skills or special technology skills that you may have developed in previous positions) (Feery & Tierney, 2002). These strengths are stated at the beginning of the resume and accompanied with examples from your various experiences. This focal section is followed by usual information such as job positions, dates, employers, and locations.

Because functional resumes focus more on achievements and less on dates, this approach may benefit nurses with particular work experiences. These resumes may be an approach to consider if you have gaps in your professional work history, are seeking a position unrelated to your previous job, have experienced many jobs with similar responsibilities, or have held several brief jobs (Welton & Morton, 1995).

Relying on Resources

If you choose to prepare your own resume, be sure that you have access to computer word-processing software and a quality laser printer. If your budget permits, rely on the graphic expertise of a professional resume service. If you choose to use a professional firm, be sure to choose one with a good reputation. Ask others who have used this company about the quality of the resume produced and the service provided. Finally, investigate some word-processing software packages that provide resume templates in which you simply enter the content. Although various organizations on the Internet also offer assistance in preparing your resume, investigate their confidentiality policy related to the data you supply.

Regardless of the approach you choose, you as the author of your resume need to provide accurate, complete, and current content. Once you have developed your resume, keep it updated on a regular basis. Consider updating your resume each year, maybe prior to your performance evaluation at work.

Preparing the Layout: Aesthetic Considerations

Now that you have planned and organized the content of your resume, focus on its overall appearance. The first impression that your resume makes to others is important, as in the case with professional posters discussed previously in Chapter 10. Try to think from the perspective of the viewer, and develop a resume that requires the least amount of effort to read. Target developing a resume that can be read in fewer than two minutes (Straka, 1996) or can be scanned in about 20 seconds (Markey & Campbell, 1996). Because you are competing against other nurses with similar credentials, every element of your resume is vital. Although you do not want to exaggerate your experiences, you also do not want to underestimate them, either.

Characteristics of the Resume Paper

Carefully choose the quality, color, and weight of the paper for your resume. Although a variety of attractive colors and textures are available for a reasonable cost at most paper supply stores, be sure that the one you select captures a professional image. Neutral shades, such as white, off-white, beige, and ivory are appropriate selections for resume paper (DeMello & Pagragan, 1998; Feery & Tierney, 2002). Avoid the use of pastel colored papers. Although these may be attractive, they may be the deciding factor in eliminating your resume. Consider using good-quality bond paper, at least a 20-pound weight, letter size paper (Feery & Tierney). Office supply stores sell paper especially designed for resumes.

Use of Print and Special Effects

Similar to preparing a poster presentation, pay special attention to the size and type of print used in your resume. By using computer software–generated print, you can choose a font size and style that are both readable and professional, such as a 12-point font (Feery & Tierney, 2002). A resume is not the place to experiment with extreme graphics. Use a laser-quality printer to produce a crisp and attractive output. Use features such as boldface fonts, capitals, underlining, and larger type sizes selectively. Try outlining essential points, such as job responsibilities, with bullets. Avoid adding handwritten comments or corrections on your typed resume (Feery & Tierney).

Length

Most sources advise limiting your resume to two pages or fewer (Feery & Tierney, 2002). Let the essential information guide the length of your resume, not the page restrictions. If you have just one or two lines on page two, reorganize your content to make your resume fit on one sheet of paper. For example, you can choose to make earlier job experiences more concise, or combine two entries into one. Whatever your approach, review your resume and exclude unnecessary information.

Grammar, Spelling, and Punctuation

Pay close attention to grammar, spelling, and punctuation when developing your resume. These need to be perfect. Similar to the techniques described when refining a manuscript for publication discussed in Chapter 9, read your resume aloud or ask your colleagues to proofread it. Be consistent and concise when listing points, such as your major work responsibilities or accomplishments. For example, start each responsibility with an action verb and limit it to one or two lines. Figure 12-2 provides a list of action-oriented words that may be helpful for this part of your resume.

Margins and Spacing

Pay close attention to the margins and spacing on your resume. Allow at least a one-inch margin or more around the borders. Be sure to single space within an entry and double space between entries. You may need to be creative with this option if you are limited to space. Center your name and demographic information, or creatively align it to the left side of the page.

Evaluate the Results

Once you have prepared the polished draft of your resume, ask several colleagues and family members to critique it again for both appearance and content. Ask them about their first impression of your resume. Was the layout attractive and professional? Did the print direct their attention to the essential points? Was the content relevant and action-oriented? Did it reflect a valuable potential employee? Enter their suggestions into the final editing of your resume.

Pay attention to details. Record the date at the end of your resume to help you maintain its currency. Include your name on each page and record page numbers. Print original copies of your resume, rather than making photocopies (Feery & Tierney, 2002). Keep a master version and copies of your resume along with the computer disk (plus an extra disk copy) in a safe place, such as with your files or with your portfolio materials.

Creating a Cover Letter

Prepare a cover letter to accompany your resume, unless directed otherwise (Cardillo, 2002). Because the content of this letter will vary depending upon your purpose or intention, be sure to tailor this letter carefully to the receiver. The basic guidelines are similar to the instructions given in preparing a query letter as described in Chapter 9 on publishing. Figure 12-4 provides an example of a cover letter used for employment purposes.

Organization of Content

A cover letter consists of three primary parts: the opening, the body, and the closing (Cardillo, 2002). Because this letter is commonly limited to one page, you need to carefully plan the content so it captures the message you intend.

Figure 12-4.
Sample Cover Letter for a Job Application

EMILLIE M. BROOKS, BSN, RN, OCN®
126 Oaktree Drive
Pittsburgh, PA 35871
(617) 333-8979 (Work) (617) 987-4957 (Home)
E-mail: brooksem@cmm.org

September 15, 2004

Ms. Joan Kenneth, Personnel Director
Oncology Home Care, Gateway Center
Pittsburgh, PA 35871

Dear Ms. Kenneth:

This letter is in application for the position of Oncology Home Care Nurse that was advertised in the September 14th issue of the *Pittsburgh Post-Gazette*. You are seeking a BSN prepared registered nurse certified in oncology nursing to provide direct nursing care to medical oncology patients within the community in which I currently reside.

I am presently employed as a Clinical Nurse II on a medical oncology unit at University Medical Center. My career goal is to obtain a homecare position that utilizes both my professional experience and leadership abilities. As a nursing student, I had the pleasure of having my community practicum at your agency and admired the professionalism of your nursing staff.

Enclosed is my resume, which details my professional background. Should you need any additional information, please feel free to contact me by e-mail or telephone. I can be reached at work during the day or at home during the evening. My contact information is listed in the letterhead. Thank you for your time. I look forward to hearing from you.

Sincerely,

Emillie M. Brooks

Emillie M. Brooks, BSN, RN, OCN®

The opening of your letter should contain the date and your mailing address, along with the exact name, title, and address of the receiver. Be sure to spell the name correctly and include appropriate credentials. Some nurses develop their own letterhead paper by centering their name, address, and contact information at the top of the page (Cardillo, 2002).

The body of the letter consists of several essential elements. Start with a brief statement regarding the purpose of the letter. For example, if you are applying for a nursing position, include the title of the position, how you became aware of it, and briefly describe your interest. Next, introduce yourself and highlight your essential experiences. Focus on how they match the requirements for the position. Include why you want to work for this organization. Perhaps you had the opportunity to visit this organization during one of your clinical experiences as a student. When addressing your professional qualities, try using self-descriptive words such as those listed in Figure 12-5. Finally, explain how and when they can contact you for an interview. For example, you may ask them to call you at work or at home during hours when you may be at the phone; you may instruct them to leave a message; or suggest your e-mail address, if appropriate. Close the letter with your name, credentials, and title (if appropriate). Be sure to sign your name in blue or black ink above the typed version.

Figure 12-5.
Action Words to Describe Yourself

These words can be used throughout the resume or cover letter to describe yourself.

active	efficient	pleasant
adaptable	energetic	positive
ambitious	enterprising	practical
analytical	enthusiastic	productive
assertive	extroverted	proficient
attentive	fair	realistic
broad-minded	forceful	reliable
conscientious	imaginative	resourceful
consistent	independent	self-reliant
constructive	logical	sense of humor
creative	loyal	sincere
dependable	mature	sophisticated
determined	methodical	systematic
diplomatic	objective	talented
disciplined	optimistic	will relocate
discrete	perceptive	will travel
economical	personable	

Note. From *The Career Services Center 1997 Career Guide, Duquesne University* (p. 7), by Duquesne University, Career Services Center, 1997, Atlanta, GA: Career Publishing Network. Copyright 1997 by the Career Publishing Network. Reprinted with permission.

Layout and Aesthetics

Follow the guidelines described earlier for preparing your resume. Pay close attention to spacing, paper quality, and font size and style. Have your colleagues critique your cover letter along with your resume, and have them examine it for its layout and attractiveness. Be sure that the content is carefully distributed over the entire paper. Often, nurses make the mistake of crowding the text at the top third of the paper. Pay close attention to the quality of the envelope and text. Mail your resume or hand-deliver it. Then, sit back and wait for the results.

Summary

This chapter described the essential components of a resume and cover letter. Specific suggestions for organizing and developing a resume also were included.

References

American Nurses Association. (1994). *Standards for nursing professional development: Continuing education and staff development.* Washington, DC: Author.

American Psychological Association. (2001). *Publication manual of the American Psychological Association* (5th ed.). Washington, DC: Author.

Brooks, B., Barrett, S., & Zimmermann, P.G. (1998). Beyond your resume: A nurse's professional "portfolio." *Journal of Emergency Nursing, 24,* 555–557.

Cardillo, D. (2002). How to write an effective cover letter. In C.L. Saver (Ed.), *Nursing Spectrum Student Career Fitness Tool Kit 2002–2003* (pp. 14–15). Hoffman Estates, IL: Nursing Spectrum.

Clarke, L.K. (2000). Of specialty interest: Writing a resume. *ORL-Head and Neck Nursing, 18*(1), 24.

DeMello, A.B., & Pagragan, C.S. (1998). Development of professional excellence puts best foot forward. *AORN Journal, 67,* 214–216, 219–221.

Feery, B., & Tierney, C.M. (2002). Resumes: The recruiter's perspective. In C.L. Saver (Ed.), *Nursing Spectrum Student Career Fitness Tool Kit 2002–2003* (pp. 18–21). Hoffman Estates, IL: Nursing Spectrum.

Freed, P.E., & Kettler, D. (1999). Nightingale's resume: A student career-teaching strategy. *Nurse Educator, 24*(5), 14–15.

Markey, B.T., & Campbell, R.L. (1996). A resume or curriculum vitae for success. *AORN Journal, 63,* 192, 195, 197–200.

O'Connor, S.A. (1999). Your curriculum vitae is a snapshot of you. *AORN Journal, 69,* 398, 400–401.

Straka, D.A. (1996). And what about you? Are you your resume? *Advanced Practice Nursing Quarterly, 2*(1), 75–77.

Webster's third new international dictionary (unabridged). (1976). Springfield, MA: Merriam-Webster.

Welton, R.H., & Morton, P.G. (1995). Management strategies for writing an effective resume. *Critical Care Nurse, 15*(3), 118, 120–126.

CHAPTER 13

Getting Involved in Nursing Research in the Clinical Setting

Understanding the Role of Clinical Staff in Nursing Research

Clinical staff nurses vary in their understanding of the research process and their ability to actively participate in research projects on their clinical unit. Research skills often are influenced by nurses' exposure to the research process during their basic educational preparation. For example, student nurses are introduced to the research process through required courses in a bachelor's nursing (BSN) program, and nurses prepared in associate degree and hospital-based diploma programs also may receive some exposure to nursing research. Formal research courses in BSN programs usually consist of classroom lectures, discussions, and projects aimed to assist nursing students in understanding the basic steps of the research process, recognizing and retrieving published research articles in nursing journals, and understanding the value of research findings in clinical nursing practice. Sometimes, undergraduate nursing students receive practical experience in research projects during their education by working with school of nursing faculty who are actively engaged in a specific research project. Regardless of a nurse's initial educational preparation, most new graduates possess very novice skills related to research when they accept their first nursing job.

Following completion of their BSN degree, nurses who continue their formal studies in a master of science degree in nursing (MSN) program continue developing their skills related to the research process through more required courses and hands-on research practicum with experienced nurse researchers. While in school, graduate students have an opportunity to work as research assistants with school of nursing faculty on a specific project. In graduate school, nurses learn how to critique published research studies and often focus their attention on published research related to a particular clinical problem. Some schools of nursing require graduate students to plan and implement a small research project, called a thesis, under the direction of faculty with expertise on the topic and in research. Students are required to present their project as a formal presentation and often are encouraged to write and submit an article with their results to a nursing journal.

In addition to these types of formal instruction in the research process, clinical staff nurses employed in healthcare settings also can engage in a variety of informal strategies after graduation to increase their understanding of research. Most often, clinical nurses are involved in clinical research, which involves patients as subjects/participants and is "designed to generate knowledge to guide nursing practice" (Polit & Hungler, 1999, p. 697). Some nurses may be employed in institutions in which clinical trials are conducted with large numbers of subjects (patients) to "test the effectiveness of a clinical treatment" (Polit & Hungler, p. 697). Research that is planned and implemented on a clinical unit often is referred to as unit-based clinical research. Other nurses may participate in research investigating educational problems in teaching and learning or in studies that focus on problems related to the role of administration. Many of these opportunities will be discussed in this chapter.

Regardless of how staff nurses develop their skills in nursing research or in what type of research they become involved, it is important for them to understand the benefits of participating in research, ways to overcome barriers, and how to develop a personal plan to strengthen their research skills. These strategies will help you not only on an individual basis but also if your responsibility is to organize and promote research activities on your clinical unit(s).

Reasons for Participating in Nursing Research

Nurses who work in clinical settings possess strengths that make them excellent candidates to participate in clinical nursing research projects. Because nurses provide direct care to patients on a daily basis and develop close relationships with them, they are in unique positions to identify issues or problems that exist in the clinical setting. Nurses, because of their clinical expertise, can realistically evaluate the clinical significance of research reports and determine if the findings are appropriate to their practice. They also can design creative ways to incorporate research findings into their nursing practice. Through such involvement in research, clinical nurses can make a positive impact on the patients and families for whom they provide nursing care, the nursing profession, their workplace, and themselves as essential healthcare providers.

Nurses work in clinical environments that differ based on a variety of factors, including the patient acuity level (e.g., ambulatory care departments, intensive care units), clinical specialty (e.g., operating room, oncology, obstetric, psychiatric unit), patient's developmental stage (e.g., newborn, adolescent, adult, geriatric), and type of health care provided (e.g., hospitals, long-term care, industry, home care, nurse-managed wellness center). These diverse work settings provide rich environments in which nurses, as primary caregivers, can design and implement a variety of research studies. The results of these studies have the potential to strengthen the way nurses care for patients and families and to improve the work environment.

Positive Impact on Patient and Family Health Outcomes

Nursing care provided to patients and families needs to reflect current "best practices," be based on sound research results, and result in positive patient outcomes. This process of applying published research findings to your clinical unit is an example of research utilization (Polit & Hungler, 1999). Research-based modifications in practice can positively impact the quality of care that patients receive, improve their health status, and subsequently influence their recovery and healthcare outcomes. However, some nursing interventions may be based on customs or rituals and lack scientific support. Some nurses may feel comfortable doing things the way they always have done them, so some practices may lack the rationale or documentation of their effectiveness on patient outcomes.

Nurses need to strengthen their research skills to accomplish the goal of research utilization. They need to read and understand a research report in order to critically evaluate if the results can be incorporated in their daily nursing practice. Policies, procedures, standards of care, and clinical protocols used on clinical units should be grounded in research findings. Nursing practice that is based on proof documented in research reports is referred to as "evidence-based practice" (Polit & Hungler, 1999, p. 645).

For example, findings that result from a unit-based clinical research study conducted on a head and neck surgical unit can help nurses who care for total laryngectomy patients develop the most effective way to prevent airway obstruction caused by mucous plugs. A practice protocol that describes the optimal way to prevent mucous plugs in patients after a total laryngectomy can be developed based on research findings. This research-based protocol can be used by nurses caring for patients during their hospitalization. This practice has the potential to reduce a patient's risk of partial or complete airway obstruction caused by a mucous plug, minimize the anxiety and stress experienced by the patient during an airway obstruction, and minimize the expense of unnecessary interventions, supplies, and time (e.g., saline, suction catheters, nursing care).

Expected Professional Performance and Influence on Nursing Profession

Participating in research endeavors is a professional responsibility of nurses (Boswell & Sevcik, 2002) and included among the Standards of Professional Performance developed for clinical nurses by the American Nurses Association (ANA, 1998). In its *Standards of Clinical Nursing Practice,* ANA states that "the nurse uses research findings in practice" (p. 15). One way nurses can implement this standard is by using the "best available evidence, preferably research data, to develop the plan of care and interventions" for patients and their families (ANA, p. 15). Another way a nurse can meet this standard is by participating "in research activities as appropriate to the nurse's education and position" (ANA, p. 15). Incorporating nursing research into nursing practice also may enable nurses to advance to a higher level of nursing practice (Boswell & Sevcik). Examples of such activities will be discussed throughout this chapter.

In addition to these standards described by ANA, specialty nursing organizations such as the Oncology Nursing Society and the Association of Operating Room Nurses also emphasize the role of the nurse related to research. Review your professional nursing organization's documents to determine its expectations, such as its scope and standards of care, certification examination test blueprints, and position papers.

Finally, because professional nurses play an essential role in providing quality healthcare services to the public, they need to assume a leadership position in shaping health care and nursing practice. Nurses need to realize their responsibility to participate in clinical research and the potential influence they have on clinical practice (Grady, 2001). Findings generated from clinical research contribute to the knowledge base that is used to develop and change nursing practice (Polit & Hungler, 1999). Research studies designed to clarify or answer problems that exist with patients and families in clinical practice attempt to minimize the "gaps" that exist in nursing practice. Publications of research reports contribute to the body of knowledge we have in nursing and support or challenge the way that we care for patients. This body of published work also influences what we teach nursing students and practicing nurses. Without sound nursing research, few advances based on evidence can be made in nursing practice.

Benefits to Employers and the Workplace

Healthcare organizations across the nation struggle to survive in today's market characterized by financial constraints, managed care, and restructuring activities. Employers seek various ways to market themselves in a positive light in order to attract potential patients and to be at an advantage over other settings. One strategy that your employer may emphasize is its support of research-based patient care that focuses on positive outcomes. Organizations that encourage their nurses to actively participate in research can market themselves as having the "best practices" and providing nursing care that is cost-effective, cutting-edge, and evidence-based. These outcomes may include patient data such as decreased length of hospital stay, effective management of treatment side effects following chemotherapy, fewer rates of complications following surgery, or low rates of drug administration errors. Nurses need to assume a proactive role in confronting these challenges in health care. All of these outcomes can be the product of nursing research in which you may have an opportunity to be involved.

Our cost-conscious healthcare environment suggests that nurses need to evaluate the impact of their nursing care on patient outcomes. This task can be accomplished through research. For example, studies can be designed to focus on alternative ways to perform nursing procedures, such as administering tube feedings that can result in quality patient outcomes with reduced expenditures on supplies and equipment. Money saved by innovative nursing practices supported through research can be redirected to other patient-centered needs.

Nursing departments that are applying for the Magnet Nursing Services Recognition Program for Excellence in Nursing Services (Magnet Designation) must demonstrate that their clinical practice is based on academic and experiential knowledge (Hudson-Barr, Weeks, & Watters, 2002). If your employer is seeking this designation, you will be expected to sharpen your research skills so that you can not only critically evaluate published research findings but also apply them to your daily nursing care practice on your clinical unit.

Personal and Professional Rewards

Nurses can gain both personal and professional rewards by participating in research in their work settings. For example, some nurses receive a great deal of personal satisfaction in knowing they played a key role in helping solve a clinical problem, making things on the clinical unit function smoother, or improving the quality of nursing care they provide to patients and families on their unit. Some nurses obtain personal rewards by strengthening their beginning skills in nursing research and playing a key role in research projects.

In addition to personal rewards, nurses can obtain professional rewards through their participation in the research process. These gains may relate directly to job expectations in a current position, plans for promotion at your organization, and career goals. Check your current position description to determine your employer's expectations of you regarding participation in nursing research. Review the descriptions of positions above your current role and its requirements for promotion.

Nurses who develop their research skills, plan and implement unit-based clinical research projects, and use research-based findings in their nursing practice are a great asset to their employers. These nurses have the potential to assume a leadership role in changing nursing practice and validating the significant role of the professional nurse within their organizations.

If your career goal is to continue your formal education or to assume a faculty position in a school of nursing, strengthening your skills in nursing research will help you move in the right direction. Developing your research expertise also may help you acquire a position as a research nurse in institutions (universities) that manage funded research studies, such as clinical trials.

Overcoming Barriers to Participating in Research

This chapter has provided several reasons why clinical staff nurses should be involved in the research process following graduation from nursing school; take some time to list personal and professional reasons that may prevent you from attaining this goal. Next, develop realistic strategies that will help you minimize these barriers. The following section of this chapter will help you develop and implement such strategies.

Lack of Time: When Can I Add Research to My Busy Day?

Lack of time may be a reason why some clinical nurses claim they do not participate in nursing research. In the work setting, nurses spend the majority of their day focusing on providing nursing care for patients and families. Your immediate learning need might be organizing your day so that you can complete your assignments in a timely manner. Perhaps you are focusing on administering medications safely. You feel that little time remains for getting involved in research.

One way to overcome a goal that is perceived as large and overwhelming is to break it down into small pieces that are more realistic to accomplish. Try approaching your goal of learning more about nursing research in a similar manner. For example, start by talking with your agency's librarian or a nursing faculty member who has students on your clinical unit. Ask them to help you retrieve nursing research articles on a clinical topic of interest, such as studies investigating how new nurses perceive their first clinical job, how nursing students feel about their clinical experiences, or medication errors that occur on the clinical unit.

Next, plan to read at least one article per week when you have a few free minutes. Keep a small collection of articles on the nightstand or the end table by your favorite chair. You may want to read during a quiet lunch or while waiting for your appointment at the physician's office or hairdresser. This activity will not only help pass the time but also will help you in the areas in which you have job concerns. Think about how the findings in these research articles can be applied to your work setting. Discuss the findings with your coworkers, supervisor, or faculty member to see if they can be applied on your clinical unit. Over time, you will develop a better understanding of the latest research in a specific area and can become your unit's "resident expert" on a clinical issue.

Lack of Knowledge: How and Where Do I Begin?

Lack of knowledge and experience with the research process may be a barrier cited by new nurses. As mentioned at the beginning of this chapter, this reason is a common and expected one and often is related to your limited exposure to nursing research in your educational program. Most beginning research courses offered by schools of nursing focus on research methodology, with little or no emphasis on helping students learn how they can conduct research in their daily routine as a staff nurse (Dykeman & Despotes, 1999).

It is important to remember that your employer does not expect you to be a "pro" at nursing research following graduation; however, you should understand your responsibilities in your role at your workplace and investigate what specific behaviors related to nursing research are expected of you. Meet with your supervisor to clarify these expectations. Be sure to review your employer's guidelines for promotion to determine what skills related to nursing research exist. Then, together with your supervisor, develop a personal plan to attain these expectations.

Lack of Interest: It's Not My Job

Some nurses may claim that participating in the research process is not part of their role as a professional nurse or do not favor research. If these statements reflect your attitude, it is important to understand why you feel this way. Try to gain some insight into your feelings. Perhaps your negative outlook regarding research may be a result of your lack of understanding of professional nursing standards, such as those of ANA mentioned previously. They could relate to being unclear about your employer's expectations of you as they relate to nursing research. Finally, your feelings may reflect your lack of beginning research skills.

Regardless of the reasons, try to make the most of the situation. Start by reviewing the professional standards and those of your specialty organizations that apply to you. Next, clarify your role with your supervisor to determine what expectations exist in nursing research. Perhaps you envisioned an unrealistic goal of independently conducting a unit-based clinical study. Rather, you may be expected to understand select studies and incorporate helpful findings in your organization's standards of care or nursing procedures.

Remember that it takes time to build your research skills, and your employer understands this. Your situation is not a unique one, and many of your colleagues probably possess the same level of skills in research as you do. You have time to develop these skills with help, just as you are strengthening your current clinical skills. What is important is that you begin to develop your skills now and take advantage of learning opportunities as they arise. Doing this has the potential to also strengthen your nursing practice and make a significant contribution to patients.

How to Begin: Assessing Your Learning Needs

Although many clinical nurses are somewhat familiar with the research process, few nurses have had experience in designing and implementing research projects. Rather than letting this challenge be an overwhelming one, it is important for you to develop an optimistic approach and view this experience as an opportunity. This can be accomplished through several ways, whether you are doing this as a staff nurse for your own professional development or if you are a unit-based educator responsible for the development of research skills of your staff on your clinical unit. Specific unit-based strategies will be addressed later in this chapter.

Compare Your Learning Curve About Research With Clinical Practice

Place this challenge of learning more about nursing research in its proper perspective by comparing it with your past experience learning about nursing practice as a student nurse or new graduate. Try to recall how difficult it was for you to master your clinical nursing skills or to understand nursing concepts in school. After repeated practice, hours of studying, and guidance from your nursing instructors and mentors, you were able to master these nursing skills and knowledge. This process is very similar to that of becoming a competent nurse researcher. Mastering the steps of the research process can be accomplished using similar strategies, such as hands-on experience in research, study, and guidance from an experienced researcher. Over time, you can strengthen your research skills in small increments until you develop a strong list of research competencies. Attempt to learn a little more each day.

Compare Research to Things With Which You Are Familiar

Remember that the research process is not something totally unfamiliar to you. Boost your confidence by comparing elements of unit-based clinical research with knowledge and skills in other areas with which you are already familiar. You will be surprised in discovering the amount of knowledge and skills related to research that you already know.

For example, examine the similarities of the research process with those of the nursing process outlined in ANA's standards of care (ANA, 1998) (see Table 13-1). Although you may not fully understand these research activities right now, you can see how the research steps coincide with the nursing process you use daily in clinical practice. The research process is also similar to activities in which nurses are engaged when participating in quality improvement activities with patients on the clinical unit. The results of the nursing process and quality care activities, such as research, lead to changes in nursing practice and healthcare systems (ANA).

Think about your active involvement in research projects that you already have encountered, such as recruiting eligible patients on your clinical unit for studies conducted by physicians or collecting patient data, such as blood samples, based on a research protocol. Perhaps you volunteered as a subject in a research study and experienced informed consent and the data collection process. All of these experiences will help you strengthen your research skills.

Table 13-1. Comparison of Nursing and Research Processes	
Nursing Process (ANA, 1998)	**Research Process**
Assessment	Defining a research problem/clinical issue
Diagnosis	Clarifying the problem and its significance through the review of literature
Outcome identification	Developing purpose, aims, and research questions/hypotheses
Planning	Developing a research proposal or plan (design)
Implementation	Conducting the research study
Evaluation	Analyzing data and discussion of findings

Conduct a Self-Assessment of Research Activities

Now that you realize that playing an active role in research on your clinical unit is a realistic goal and one with which you may be already somewhat familiar, conduct a systematic self-assessment of your research talents. A self-assessment will help you determine what research skills you have already mastered, skills that you have encountered but need further strengthening, and skills that you have never performed and need to learn.

The self-assessment tool depicted in Figure 13-1 can help you determine your baseline competencies related to research participation. The first column lists key research activities that may be expected of clinical nurses. You are asked to indicate, using the next three columns, which activities you feel you (a) have mastered and need no review, (b) are familiar with, but need review, and (c) have never experienced and need to learn. This exercise will help you identify which research activities you need to include in your professional career plan.

Remember that your educational background and experience in nursing will influence the results of your baseline assessment. It is not uncommon for you to discover that you will need to learn more about all of the listed activities. Modify the list of research activities according to your employer's expectations of you as they relate to research at your workplace. Adapt this list to fit your professional and personal goals. Details about these steps will be explained later in this chapter.

Developing a Realistic Plan to Strengthen Skills in Nursing Research

After completing the self-assessment activities in Figure 13-1, reflect upon your employer's expectations and your personal and professional goals as they relate to research. Keep these goals in mind as you develop a realistic plan to learn these skills over time. Start by prioritizing some of the activities listed in the *Self-Assessment of Research Activities*. Organize the list from the skills you would like to attain first to those (e.g., serving as a principal investigator) you may develop within the next five years as you advance your formal education. For example, suppose you do not feel comfortable with reading and understanding a research article. If this is so, rank this activity among your top priorities to learn this year.

After ranking these activities, place them within a realistic career plan that can help you improve your research skills. For example, you may list two activities to learn this year and three the following year, until you have reached your long-term goals. Chapter 15 will help you learn how to incorporate research goals into your career plan.

Next, develop strategies to attain these goals by examining possible resources or opportunities to which you have access. Be sure to inventory your personal and professional environment for resources, such as individuals who have expertise in nursing research, research-based literature, and educational offerings that can help you be successful in your research endeavors. Be sure to include both specific content dealing with research as well as hands-on experience with actual projects. Many of these strategies will be discussed in this chapter.

Be flexible and take advantage of research opportunities that may arise, and reorganize your priorities if they were not part of your plan. For example, you may have a chance to learn how to collect data for a research project being conducted on your clinical unit. Although this research activity may not have been on your

Directions: Place an (x) in one of the last three columns to indicate your degree of comfort related to the described research activity. Use the results to develop your personal plan for strengthening your research skills. Use the following rating scale to indicate your skill level: Column 1 = You have mastered this activity and need no review; Column 2 = You are familiar with this activity, but need review; and Column 3 = You have never experienced this activity and need to learn it.

Research Activities	1	2	3
Conduct a literature review to locate nursing research articles.			
Recognize nursing journals that publish research articles in your clinical specialty.			
Distinguish between a research and theory/practice article.			
Read and understand a research study (abstract) published in a nursing journal.			
Evaluate (critique) the quality of a research report.			
Apply (utilize) research findings, as appropriate, in your clinical practice.			
Participate in key aspects of a research project:			
Identify a clinical problem to study.			
Conduct and organize a literature review.			
Clarify the purpose and specific aims (research questions/hypotheses).			
Develop a research design.			
Recruit subjects/participants.			
Schedule subjects/participants for appointments.			
Obtain informed consent from subjects.			
Collect data through instruments, samples, interviews, chart review, and measurements.			
Administer a research intervention (e.g., educational program, counseling session, treatment, drug) according to a protocol.			
Assist with data analysis or calculation of results.			
Clarify study findings and discuss relevance to clinical practice.			
Actively participate in a research project as a			
Subject			
Team member			
Principal investigator (leader)			
Student			
Serve as member of a research review committee:			
Review research proposals.			
Review research abstracts.			
Participate as a member of a work/professional committee related to research.			
Present research findings at a conference:			
Paper presentation			
Poster			
Prepare a research abstract.			
Publish a research report in a nursing journal.			

list for this year, take advantage of the learning opportunity and rethink your plan. Suppose a graduate student is presenting a unit-based in-service program describing his or her research project on a clinical unit at your organization. Try to attend that presentation to learn more about research as it relates to your clinical area. Finally, regardless of your plan, allow yourself sufficient time to practice these research skills before you evaluate your progress.

Nurses can assume a variety of roles in research based on their skills and past experiences in research activities. As a clinical nurse, you may choose to assume the role of a research subject, as mentioned earlier, or collect data as a member of the research team. Your role in the research process will be defined by your education, experience, and current position.

Seek Formal and Informal Instruction

Expand your research skills through formal and informal learning opportunities. For example, enroll in a college-level undergraduate or graduate course that focuses on nursing research methods. Courses that offer more flexibility, such as a research practicum or a self-designed directed/independent study, can provide you with excellent hands-on experience in learning about the research process under the direction of a faculty mentor who is involved in a specific project.

Opportunities for learning more about research also exist through informal educational offerings such as in-service or continuing education programs sponsored by healthcare agencies, such as hospitals and professional nursing organizations. Some colleges and universities offer workshops or certificate programs on research-related topics that are open to the nursing community. Many specialty professional nursing organizations sponsor instructional sessions on research, as well as research roundtables, research forums, and reports on specific projects at their national and local meetings. Some organizations offer membership in special groups or committees whose focus is on nursing research. Usually these subgroups sponsor educational sessions prior to or during their national conferences. Check if these sessions are audiotaped, in the event you cannot attend.

If research presentations are not available from your organization, suggest this topic to the education committee as a future program. For example, if you belong to the local chapter of a professional nursing organization, ask the education committee to sponsor a program on a research topic. When listening to these presentations, determine how they apply to your clinical setting. Think about the steps of the research process and how they were addressed in the presentation. Finally, experience the research process first hand from a subject's perspective by volunteering as a subject in a research study.

Use Print and Media Resources

Printed information, such as books and journals, along with other instructional media, such as audiotapes, videotapes, and CD-ROMs, are excellent resources from which you can learn more about research. Basic nursing research texts can be purchased through your local health professions bookstore or through advertisements in nursing journals and nursing conference proceedings. Many books provide a "how to" approach to nursing research and vary in their level of difficulty. Ask faculty who have students on your clinical unit for advice in selecting the appropriate text for your learning needs.

Many professional nursing organizations sell audiotapes of research sessions presented by speakers at their national conferences, along with research-related materials. Research resources also may be available on loan from libraries at your agency or in a nearby school of nursing.

Include various resources that exist on the Internet to help you develop your skills in nursing research. This media can be a way for you to not only focus on particular research topics but also to learn them in a cost-effective, flexible way. For example, the National Institutes of Health has an online tutorial for nurses interested in clinical research (http://cme.nci.nih.gov) (Grady, 2001). Other organizations, such as ANA and Public Responsibility in Medicine and Research (www.primr.org), also list information on their Web sites about available educational programs on research. Resources that focus on the ethical considerations in nursing research, such as ANA's *Ethical Guidelines in the Conduct, Dissemination, and Implementation of Nursing Research*, can be accessed through the American Nurses Publishing Web site (www.nursesbooks.org).

Locating Research Articles

Make a special effort to read research-based articles in professional nursing journals. This strategy can help you become more familiar with the language and steps used. Avoid getting overwhelmed at first by starting with research reports in clinical nursing journals such as the *American Journal of Nursing (AJN), Nursing,* or journals in your specialty, such as the *American Journal of Operating Room Nurses* or the *Oncology Nursing Forum.* The practical approach to research used in these journals often helps clinical nurses relate research studies to nursing practice issues.

Begin by reading research briefs like "Their Presence is Requested," recently published in the "News" department of *AJN* (Ferri & Sofer, 2003). This brief describes the key points of a recent study published in the *American Journal of Critical Care.* It indicated that despite the Emergency Nurses Association's resolution to allow families to be present during cardiopulmonary resuscitation (CPR) and other invasive procedures, many hospitals lack written policies supporting this practice. After reading this brief, reflect on how the findings affect your workplace. Investigate if your organization has a policy supporting family presence during CPR. If it does not, then share your concerns with your supervisor and volunteer to investigate it.

Although some nursing journals focus primarily on publishing research-based articles, others include only a few or none at all. The titles of some journals such as *Nursing Research* can give you a hint as to whether a journal contains research-based articles. Author guidelines discussed earlier in Chapter 9 will help you determine if research articles are among the manuscripts considered for publication in a specific journal. The list of nursing journals provided in Chapter 9 also can help you with this.

Once you find an article, determine whether it is a research-based report rather than a description about something else, such as nursing theory, concepts, or clinical practice. Some nursing journals, such as the *Oncology Nursing Forum,* use symbols (such as "R") next to each article in their table of contents to help their readers recognize a research article from other articles that focus on administration, clinical practice, or education. When in doubt as to whether or not an article is a report of a research study, try locating several key terms of the research process that will serve as cues. A list of these research terms is presented in Table 13-2.

Start by searching for the primary headings, such as Introduction, Methods, Results/Findings, or Discussion. Next, focus on the subheadings located within

Table 13-2. Key Terms to Search in a Research Article	
Section of Article	**Key Terms**
Introduction	Purpose and specific aims (research questions/hypotheses) Background Significance Theoretical/conceptual framework Literature review
Methods	Design Sample/participants and setting Instruments Data collection procedures Protection of human participants Data analysis
Results/Findings	Values of statistical tests/content analysis Interpretation of significance
Discussion	Interpretation of results Limitations Implications for nursing practice Implications for future research

the Methods section if you are in doubt. Often the title, abstract, or text of an article communicates to readers that the article is about a research study. With experience reading research articles, you will become familiar with the appearance of titles that indicate the article may be about a study. Nonresearch or theoretical-based articles are not structured in this manner.

As your understanding of the research process increases, try reviewing research-based articles published within your clinical specialty. The knowledge you possess in your clinical area may help you better understand these studies and place them within the proper context of nursing practice. You can review recent issues of these journals manually, or conduct a computerized literature search by using key words on a topic that interests you. If you have little experience in doing this, ask your local librarian for assistance in using electronic databases, such as the Cumulative Index for Nursing and Allied Health Literature (CINAHL®) for obtaining nursing and allied health literature or MEDLINE for accessing articles that focus on medicine, nursing, dentistry, and other healthcare professions. Search databases in other disciplines such as psychology, sociology, and education, as needed. The Internet also can be a source for information about nursing research, but evaluate the accuracy of the information you retrieve by reviewing its source.

Learn How to Read and Understand a Research Article

Increase your comfort with reading and understanding published nursing research reports before evaluating (research critique) a study or making a decision to apply (research utilization) research findings to your practice. Reading published articles will help you discover opportunities in which you can actively participate in the research process.

Start this process by finding a recent research article published in a nursing journal that focuses on your clinical practice area or an area of interest. For example, if your clinical specialty is adult health, try locating research articles in journals such as *MEDSURG Nursing.* Use the suggestions that were provided earlier in this section for retrieving a research article.

Next, match your reading style with your general purpose for reading the article. Experts suggest using three different reading styles when reading a research article. Each reading style increases in its complexity and time required to accomplish it. For example, start by skimming a research article if your goal is to determine if an article is research-based or to obtain a general sense about the project. This is an approach you may have used in school if you needed to read many pages and had little time to accomplish this task.

Second, read with comprehension in mind if your purpose is to understand the research study. Table 13-3 lists the key sections of a research article and its primary purpose. These descriptions will not only provide you with important infor-

Table 13-3. Key Parts of a Research Article Matched With Its Purpose	
Key Part	**Purpose**
Title	Presents key *variables/concepts* examined in the study; also may indicate *population* and *setting* under study and *research design* used.
Abstract	Provides a *general overview of the entire study*; includes problem studied, significance of study, purpose and aims, information about sample and setting, design, instruments, data collection and analysis used, results/findings, discussion, and implications for nursing.
Introduction	Sets the stage for the research study; includes *background* information about the problem under study, *significance* (why it was important to conduct the study), *purpose and specific objectives* of the study (posed as *research questions/hypotheses*), *review of related literature*, and (if appropriate) *theoretical/conceptual framework/model* used to guide the study.
Methods	Describes the details of the *plan/blueprint* for the actual study; includes an explanation of the *design* chosen to organize the study, description of the *sample* (subjects/participants), such as why they were included in the study and size, description of the *setting* in which the study was conducted, main *variables/concepts* under study and means to measure the concepts (instruments, interview guides, observations), procedures used to *collect these data*, how *informed consent* was obtained from subjects/participants, and procedures used to *analyze the data* collected.
Results/Findings	Describes the *results/findings* according to the research questions/hypotheses posed in the Introduction section of the article; includes which findings are *significant* and which are not meaningful. This section may include the results of statistical tests or content analysis procedures.
Discussion	Provides possible *explanations/interpretations* for the results/findings of the study within the context of past published research on that topic or experience; includes *limitations* of the study that were beyond the control of the researcher, how the findings/results can be used by nurses in *clinical practice, education, or administration* roles, and possible ideas for *future research* studies on this topic.
References	Listing of *resources* used by the researcher in developing the research article; provides readers with other sources of past research that relate to this topic.
Tables/Figures	Visuals that provide a ready reference for the primary data included in the study; readers can refer to tables/figures to quickly summarize details of study results/findings.

mation about the study but also can help you realize potential roles that you can assume in research projects. Refer to Figure 13-1 to match these key sections (Table 13-3) with opportunities to participate in research studies.

Finally, if your purpose in reading an article is to critique the study in order to determine its quality or evaluate whether its findings are applicable to your clinical situation, then read it with analysis in mind. Figures 13-2 and 13-3 are examples of checklists that can guide you in the critique of a research study. Figure 13-2 is a tool that was designed especially for staff nurses to help them evaluate nursing research based on quantitative methods and to serve as a teaching tool (Carlson, Kruse, & Rouse, 1999). Figure 13-3 is an example of a traditional critique guide that is helpful in evaluating studies that use qualitative research methods (e.g., phenomenology, grounded theory, ethnography, historical research, participatory action research). Critiquing a study is a more advanced research skill that you will need to develop over time. Be sure to include this skill as part of your career plan.

Link With Experts in Nursing Research

If possible, seek the advice and expertise of mentors who have experience in nursing research, especially nurses who have earned MSN or doctoral degrees (PhD). Start by identifying possible experts employed within your work setting, such as advanced practice nurses, clinical nurse specialists, staff development educators, or nurse researchers. If your agency is affiliated with a college or university, try approaching nursing faculty who bring nursing students for their clinical experience to your unit. Students enrolled in MSN and PhD programs in nursing are also good sources with whom to collaborate. Expand your search for experts through professional nursing organizations, such as specialty and nursing alumni organizations, or through research teams led by nursing faculty in schools of nursing.

Be sure to communicate your interest in becoming involved in a research project to the appropriate persons, such as your supervisor, school advisor, or colleagues. If these learning opportunities do not currently exist, suggest the development of a mentor program in research through the local chapter of your nursing organization.

Use Resources in Professional Nursing Organizations

As mentioned earlier in this chapter, professional nursing organizations can offer excellent resources to help you learn about nursing research, such as educational offerings, printed and media resources, and opportunities to network with experts in research. If research is your focus, be sure to select organizations that identify research activities in their mission. Take advantage of their support by joining the research committee on the local, regional, or national level. Chapter 8 provides a list of professional nursing organizations from which you can choose.

Obtain Hands-On Experience in Research

Having hands-on experience with the research process is helpful to gain a better understanding of research. Let your supervisor know about your interest in assuming a leadership position on your unit regarding clinical research. Ask for

	YES	NO
1. Title		
Could you tell what the article was about by reading the title?		
2. Abstract		
The abstract is a summary of all points of the study. It usually is presented at the very beginning of the article. The abstract generally includes a brief description of the problem, how the study was done (methodology), what the authors found (results), and what conclusions were drawn from the results. After reading the abstract, respond to the following statements/questions.		
• The topic is interesting.		
• The topic is pertinent to your work.		
• Is the article worth your time to read carefully?		
If you answer NO to ANY or ALL, then stop and look for another article.		
COMMENTS:		
3. Problem		
Is it clear what problem the authors are trying to solve? (If the problem is not in the introduction, look in the review of literature.)		
The research question is stated in the article.		
The significance of this problem to nursing practice is stated.		
Pertinent terms are defined.		
COMMENTS:		
4. Review of the literature		
Do the articles in the review of literature pertain to the problem?		
Is the review of literature presented in an organized fashion, from broad to specific?		
Does it tell a story?		
The reference list is comprehensive.		
The reference list is current. (At least three to five sources dated within the past five years should be included.)		
COMMENTS:		
5. Design		
Two basic types of study designs exist.		
a. In experimental, comparative, or randomized studies, the sample is divided into two groups. One group (called the experimental group) receives the experimental therapy, drug, or treatment, whereas the other group (called the control group) does not receive it. Random assignment is needed for experimental studies. Studies that use randomly assigned groups and treatments for comparison yield more credible results in terms of being able to generalize the findings to others like those studied.		
b. In observational or descriptive studies, characteristics about the sample are studied through methods such as interviews, questionnaires, surveys, and direct observation. Conclusions are made about the sample from the observations. The sample may or may not be divided into groups. If the sample is divided, it is not necessarily done in a random manner.		
The design of the study is stated.		
Did the authors explain the reason(s) for the choice of the research design?		
COMMENTS:		

Figure 13-2.
Guide to Critiquing a Research Article (Quantitative)

(Continued on next page)

Figure 13-2.
Guide to Critiquing
a Research Article
(Quantitative)
(Continued)

6. Sample	YES	NO
Is the population (i.e., the large group from which the sample was obtained) described?		
How the sample (small group) that was chosen was described.		
The sample size is important if any sound conclusions are to be drawn from the results. Larger samples generally yield stronger results than smaller samples.		
The sample size used for final analysis is appropriate.		
Standards for protection of human subjects were discussed (e.g., anonymity, confidentiality, informed consent, patient rights).		
COMMENTS:		

7. Tool		
The tool is the instrument that the authors used to gather data. Examples of tools include a questionnaire, survey, or the script to an interview. The authors should discuss the reliability and validity of the tool(s) used. These areas determine to what extent the tool measures what it is supposed to measure (validity) and how consistently the tool measures what it is supposed to measure when used over and over again (reliability). Reliability and validity are established through statistical calculations. Tools with established reliability and validity hold more scientific value than those created for one-time use by the researchers.		

	AUTHOR	BORROWED
Was the tool created by the author of this research study or borrowed from another source?		
Is a copy of the tool included in the article?		
Reliability of the tool is discussed.		
Validity of the tool is described.		
COMMENTS:		

8. Methodology		
Methods of data collection are sufficiently described. (Could you repeat this study based on the information stated in the article?)		
The time frame during which the study occurred is described.		
COMMENTS:		

9. Data analysis		
The most commonly used statistical tests for the data analysis are descriptive tests such as frequencies, percentages, means, ranges, and standard deviations; correlational statistics, which use tests of relationships or associations; and statistics that show the differences between the mean of two or more groups using *t* tests and analysis of variance (ANOVA). Statistical tests report a level of significance. The two most common levels of significance (*p* value) in nursing and medical research are 0.05 and 0.01. A *p* value of 0.05 means that there was a 5% possibility that the results obtained in the study were only due to chance. Similarly, a *p* value of 0.01 means that there was a 1% possibility that the results obtained in the study were only due to chance.		
Information presented is sufficient to answer the research questions.		
Statistical tests are used to analyze the data.		
Values obtained from the data analysis are included.		
The results are explained.		
Tables and figures are presented in an easy-to-understand and informative way.		
COMMENTS:		

*(Continued on
next page)*

	YES	NO
10. Discussion		
Is a discussion section presented?		
If YES, are the results compared with the literature review?		
COMMENTS:		
11. Conclusions		
Conclusions are clearly stated.		
Conclusions are directly related to the results presented.		
Do the findings of the study add to present nursing knowledge?		
Limitations of the study are identified.		
Recommendations are made for further research.		
COMMENTS:		

Figure 13-2.
Guide to Critiquing a Research Article (Quantitative) *(Continued)*

Note. From "Critiquing Nursing Research: A User-Friendly Guide for the Staff Nurse," by D.S. Carlson, L.K. Kruse, and C.L. Rouse, 1999, *Journal of Emergency Nursing, 25,* pp. 331–332. Copyright 1999 by the Emergency Nurses Association. Reprinted with permission.

guidance in developing a plan that can help you develop your role on the unit. Gain experience in research by spending time with staff in your organization's nursing education and research center.

If you decide to make a career change to gain research experience or to totally submerge yourself in a research role, seek a nursing position within an organization that has a research-focused environment. Start by inquiring through your human resources department. They can direct you to opportunities in research-related positions or to clinical positions that emphasize research activities. These opportunities may include working as a protocol nurse on government-funded research projects, as a clinical nurse working with patients enrolled in clinical trials, or working with an expert researcher as a research assistant.

Search the literature for creative ways to help nurses on your unit learn more about the research process and play an active role in research. For example, Warren and Heermann (1998) described a research nurse intern program they designed at their medical center. This program was intended to support research-based nursing practice at their organization and to help their staff nurses develop professionally. This two-year program combined efforts to help nurses learn how to use nursing research in their clinical practice (research utilization) and ways to communicate research findings to others (research dissemination).

Hudson-Barr et al. (2002) described an innovative project aimed at introducing hospital-based staff nurses to the research process. This project was a replication of a previous study that was documented in the nursing literature (Long & Reider, 1995; Thiel, 1987). The hospital's nursing research committee assumed the lead in this project by planning the project, recruiting nurses as subjects, and implementing the project. Subjects were asked to judge the quality and preference for two chocolate chip cookies, each prepared using different ingredients. Results were shared through the hospital's newsletter and nursing journals. The project was successful in helping nurses understand nursing research in light of their active involvement.

Fostering a Research Environment on the Clinical Unit

While you focus on your personal and professional learning needs as they relate to research, your role also may include helping other nurses on your unit enhance their research skills. If this is the case, use Figure 13-1 in developing the learning needs of staff on your unit. Follow the strategies described in Chapters 6 and 7 in order to include research activities in your unit's educational plan.

Figure 13-3.
Guide to Critiquing
a Qualitative
Research Article
(Using Phenom-
enology)

Focus/Topic
1. What is the focus or the topic of the study? What is the researcher studying? Is the topic researchable? Is it focused enough to be meaningful but not too limited so as to be trivial?
2. Why is the researcher using a qualitative design? Would the study be more appropriately conducted in the quantitative paradigm?
3. What is the philosophical tradition or qualitative paradigm upon which the study is based?

Purpose
1. What is the purpose of the study? Is it clear?

Significance
1. What is the relevance of the study to what is already known about the topic?
2. How will the results be useful to nursing and/or health care?

Method
1. Given the topic of the study and the researcher's stated purpose, how does the selected research method help to achieve the stated purpose?
2. What research method(s) has the researcher identified to conduct the study?
3. Based on the material presented, how does the researcher demonstrate that he or she has followed the method?
4. If the researcher used any form of triangulation, explain how he or she maintained the integrity of the study.

Sampling
1. How were participants selected?
2. Explain how the selection process supports a qualitative sampling paradigm.
3. Are the participants in the study the appropriate people to inform the research? Explain.

Data Collection
1. How does the data collection method reported support discovery, description, or understanding?
2. What data collection strategies does the researcher use?
3. Does the researcher clearly state how human subjects were protected?
4. How was data saturation achieved?
5. Are the data collection strategies appropriate to achieve the purpose of the study? Explain.

Data Analysis
1. How were data analyzed?
2. Based on the analysis reported, can the reader follow the researcher's stated processes?

Findings/Trustworthiness
1. How do the reported findings demonstrate the participants' realities?
2. How does the researcher relate the findings of the study to what is already known?
3. How does the researcher demonstrate that the findings are meaningful to the participants?

Conclusions/Implications/Recommendations
1. How does the researcher provide a context for use of the findings?
2. Are the conclusions drawn from the study appropriate? Explain.
3. What are the recommendations for future research?
4. Are the recommendations, conclusions, and implications clearly related to the findings? Explain.

Once you have determined your learning needs related to the research process and have identified supports to help you become successful at research, apply these concepts to your clinical unit or department. One way to begin this process is by organizing a brainstorming session with coworkers who also want to be involved in unit-based clinical research. If your clinical unit does not have a nursing research committee, create one. Join forces with other nurses who work on other units within your agency and who share similar clinical research interests. It is important to let everyone have an opportunity to participate to make it work. The following section will provide you with a variety of strategies to enhance your research skills both as an individual and as a coordinator of unit-based research initiatives.

Develop a Strategic Plan

Create an environment on your unit that is conducive to nursing research. Start by developing a strategic plan for the nursing staff on the unit that is based on ideas generated from the brainstorming session and feedback from the Self-Assessment of Research Activities tool (Figure 13-1). Include specific goals or outcomes that deal with research for your unit. Be sure that these goals are in harmony with the goals of your unit and those of the organization. Depending on the staff's abilities and available resources, goals may range from initiatives such as helping the nursing staff learn how to read research articles to implementation of an actual unit-based research project.

Set a realistic timeline for these unit-based efforts. Anticipate the staff's possible barriers to participation in nursing research that may result in their initial hesitation to play an active role. Be prepared to help staff realize the potential impact that research can play in their professional and personal lives. Keep the activities open to staff who may choose to become involved at a later time. Schedule research forums on your unit in which nurses can discuss their concerns about being involved in research (Carlson et al., 1999).

Mobilize Supports and Resources

Once you developed a plan for your unit, seek support systems to assist your research endeavors, such as the ones described earlier in this chapter. Obtain support from your supervisor to maximize your success in this endeavor, especially in allotting resources such as time and financial support for programs and projects.

Partnerships that your healthcare organization holds with other agencies may be a valuable resource and source of support for fostering nursing research on your clinical unit. Thompson, McNeill, Sherwood, and Starck (2001) described the benefits of a research collaboration that was developed between a school of nursing and a healthcare organization. This partnership was an effective strategy in producing quality, cost-effective clinical research. Benefits were described for undergraduate nursing students involved on the research teams and for both organizations.

Implement Projects Gradually

As with introducing any new change, start with the implementation of small projects and ones that pose little threat. Once the nursing staff develop their skills and confidence, gradually proceed to more advanced unit-based projects. Implement these initiatives slowly, and try to integrate them into the daily work schedule and activities as much as possible.

Start a Journal Club

Start a journal club on your clinical unit. A journal club is a group of nurses that meets on a regular basis to review and critique nursing research articles on a particular clinical topic of interest (Polit, Beck, & Hungler, 2001). Members of the journal club also examine whether the findings can be applied to their clinical setting.

Select a research article that is of interest to the staff on your unit. Ask everyone to read the article, then meet to discuss it. Provide a set of questions for the staff to reflect upon before they attend the meeting. Focus the group's efforts on reviewing the steps of the study first, then discussing its quality and applicability to your clinical setting. Figures 13-2 and 13-3 can assist you with this process.

Brainstorm about possible ways the study could be replicated on your unit, or discuss what the next study should investigate. Take turns among staff finding articles, developing questions, and leading the group discussion. Gradually advance to reviewing a set of articles that study similar topics, and compare and contrast their approaches and findings.

Share Personal Research Experiences

Ask staff to share their research experiences with each other during unit-based programs. Topics can include their experience as a subject or reports on research-based conferences.

Seek Available Research Roles

As mentioned earlier in this chapter, seek opportunities that exist at your workplace and at nearby schools of nursing that can help staff develop their research skills through hands-on experiences. These include being a team member of a research project whose tasks are to recruit subjects, conduct a literature review, collect data, and assist as needed. Work with your human resources department, which can help you organize these opportunities and provide you with a mechanism to communicate them to staff. Share your endeavors with faculty from schools of nursing who bring students to your unit. Faculty often seek individuals who can help them develop or implement research projects on a part-time or full-time basis. Explore the possibility that your clinical unit can serve as the setting for their future projects.

Include Research Topics in Your Unit's Education Plan

Include research topics in your unit's in-service plan (see Chapters 6 and 7). Invite nurse researchers to talk about their research projects with staff. In addition to focusing on the project itself, ask speakers to describe how the idea originated and how the findings impact nursing practice. Start a special "research series" of unit-based in-service programs that focus on the research process. For example, a topic may include identifying a clinical problem to study, types of research designs, sampling techniques, and protecting human participants. Consider reviewing the basics of a research critique using a research article with which the staff is familiar. Refer to Table 13-3 for more ideas, or ask nursing staff to take turns developing a 30-minute presentation or poster on each topic. Chapters 6 and 7 will help staff develop an in-service program, and Chapter 9 will assist them in developing posters.

Try to incorporate research in all of your unit-based programs. For example, when conducting clinically oriented in-service programs, such as managing nausea and vomiting experienced by patients following chemotherapy, include one or two recent research articles on this topic. Discuss research findings as they apply to standards of care for managing these symptoms in patients on your unit.

Develop a Unit-Based Research Project

As mentioned earlier in this chapter, one way for clinical nurses to understand the process and value of nursing research is by playing an active role in the research process. Once their confidence and understanding of the research process increases, challenge their skills by involving interested nurses in a unit-based research project. Unit-based nursing research, mentioned at the beginning of this chapter, is a successful clinical research activity described nearly two decades ago in the nursing literature (Hoare & Earenfight, 1986).

In unit-based clinical research, staff nurses design and implement a nursing research project under the guidance of an experienced nurse researcher who serves as a mentor (Burns, 2002). The research project addresses a problem, such as a patient care issue, that exists on the clinical unit. Findings have the potential to be incorporated into patient care on your unit. Results of the study are shared with other nurses through unit-based in-service programs, formal presentations or posters sponsored by professional nursing organization, and publications in nursing journals.

Mentors usually are prepared in nursing at the master's or doctoral level. These nurse researchers may be employed at your healthcare organization or at a local agency. They may hold positions such as a staff development educator, clinical nurse specialist, or nurse researcher. Faculty employed at affiliating university or college-based schools of nursing can serve as excellent research mentors for clinical nurses planning a unit-based research project. Regardless of the source, the research mentor needs to understand the knowledge, skills, and time constraints faced by clinical nurses involved in a research project and provide support (Burns, 2002).

Under the direction and guidance of this research mentor, determine how interested staff can participate in the study. Consider inviting other members of the healthcare team, such as social workers, nutritionists, and physical therapists, to join the project, if appropriate. Success of the project can be maximized by allowing staff to have ownership of the project. Implementing a research study on a clinical unit can be a challenge, so suggest ways that nursing staff interested in the project can participate. Use the Self-Assessment of Research Activities to carefully match the research skills of each participant with the tasks to be accomplished. Plan a schedule of research team meetings in advance. Identify an effective means that can be used to foster ongoing communication among team members, especially in light of conflicting work schedules. Consider using e-mail as a communication method, if available.

Before you begin planning your project, work with the research mentor in identifying resources you will need to successfully complete the project (Dykeman & Despotes, 1999). Resources may include services of a reference librarian to help with the literature review, access to a library to retrieve references, fees assessed to duplicate references, fees charged to use instruments, and assistance with data analysis. Some of these services are available to employers of healthcare organizations at no charge, so check with your supervisor.

Gaining support for this project from your employer can help the project succeed (Dykeman & Despotes, 1999). Organizational support for research, with research seen as part of the work culture, was suggested as having a positive influence on hospital-based staff nurses' participation in a clinical nursing research project (Tranmer, Lochhaus-Gerlach, & Lam, 2002). Start by discussing the project with your supervisor before your begin the planning phase. Your employer may be able to help you obtain the financial resources previously mentioned and provide you with other resources. For example, your supervisor may permit you to dedicate a portion of your daily work schedule to focus on the project. Regular discussions and open communication with your supervisor about the project can serve as a source of encouragement for you and the research team.

Think about choosing a problem of interest to staff that may be fairly easy to complete. Consider designing a pilot study or replicating a previously published study before you decide to implement an original research project. Once you have a list of possible research ideas, ask the staff to prioritize them. Consider selecting a topic that is on the top of the list for most staff, critical to patient care, causes the most distress for staff, or is least costly to implement. Because of their close involvement in patient care, clinical nurses can be extremely helpful in identifying a clinical problem to study and clarifying the purpose and specific aims of a research project. Continue to develop the remaining steps of your research proposal, your plan for conducting the study.

After developing your proposal, submit the proposal to your employer's institutional review board (IRB). The IRB is a group of individuals that will review the ethical implications of the study. Your supervisor or research mentor can help you determine if other committees at your agency are required to review your proposal and provide approval. Following approval from these groups, implement the project. Continue to meet regularly as a research team to monitor the progress of the study and to discuss concerns or issues that may arise.

Following completion of your study, meet as a team to evaluate this new experience and to prepare final reports. Carefully examine the results of your study and compare them to similar past studies. Determine whether the results of your study should be used to change patient care on your unit or be incorporated into clinical documents such as policies, procedures, and standards of care. The research team should develop plans for the next unit-based research project, considering comments obtained from the evaluation meeting.

Develop plans to share the study results with others through publications and presentations. Details about these professional activities are discussed in Chapters 9 and 10. Be sure to use a variety of approaches in disseminating your research findings in a timely manner so that they reach the audience of nurses who can understand and best utilize the findings in their nursing practice. In addition to refereed publications, consider sharing information about your project in your organization's newsletter or through a poster on your unit. Think about the target audience when submitting your abstract for presentation at professional nursing conferences. Be sure to include unit-based in-service programs in your dissemination plans.

Finally, recognize and celebrate the efforts of your research team. Talk with your supervisor about awarding certificates of recognition or providing other means of recognition. Consider planning these awards during National Nurses Week or at an annual nursing research event.

Summary

This chapter describes clinical research and the process involved in developing and implementing unit-based clinical nursing research projects. Practical suggestions are offered to help staff nurses overcome potential barriers to participating in research. Methods to develop research skills such as critiquing studies, using research in practice, and disseminating findings are included. Suggestions for unit-based educators who may be responsible for strengthening the research skills of clinical nurses are provided.

References

American Nurses Association. (1998). *Standards of clinical nursing practice* (2nd ed.). Washington, DC: Author.

Boswell, C., & Sevcik, L. (2002). Invest in yourself. Start a clinical research project. *Nursing Forum, 37,* 30–32.

Burns, S.M. (2002). Clinical research is part of what we do: The experience of one medical intensive care unit. *Critical Care Nurse, 22*(2), 100–113.

Carlson, D.S., Kruse, L.K., & Rouse, C.L. (1999). Critiquing nursing research: A user-friendly guide for the staff nurse. *Journal of Emergency Nursing, 25,* 330–332.

Dykeman, M., & Despotes, J. (1999). The unexpected challenges of clinical research or what they do not tell you in school. *Journal of the Association of Nurses in AIDS Care, 10*(5), 98–101.

Ferri, R.S., & Sofer, D. (2003). Their presence is requested. *American Journal of Nursing, 103*(6), 17.

Grady, C. (2001). Clinical research: The power of the nurse. *American Journal of Nursing, 101*(9), 26–31.

Hoare, K., & Earenfight, J. (1986). Unit-based research in a service setting. *Journal of Nursing Administration, 16,* 35–39.

Hudson-Barr, D., Weeks, S.K., & Watters, C. (2002). Introducing the staff nurse to nursing research through the Great American Cookie Experiment. *Journal of Nursing Administration, 32,* 440–443.

Long, C.M., & Reider, J.A. (1995). The cookie experiment revisited. *Nurse Educator, 20*(3), 13.

Polit, D.F., Beck, C.T, & Hungler, B.P. (2001). *Essentials of nursing research: Methods, appraisal, and utilization* (5th ed.). Philadelphia: Lippincott.

Polit, D.F., & Hungler, B.P. (1999). *Nursing research: Principles and methods* (6th ed.). Philadelphia: Lippincott.

Thiel, C.A. (1987). The cookie experiment: A creative teaching strategy. *Nurse Educator, 20*(3), 8–10.

Thompson, C.J., McNeill, J.A., Sherwood, G.D., & Starck, P.L. (2001). Using collaborative research to facilitate student learning. *Western Journal of Nursing Research, 23,* 504–516.

Tranmer, J.E., Lochhaus-Gerlach, J., & Lam, M. (2002). The effect of staff nurse participation in a clinical nursing research project on attitude towards, access to, support of and use of research in the acute care setting. *Canadian Journal of Nursing Leadership, 15*(1), 18–26.

Warren, J.J., & Heermann, J.A. (1998). The research nurse intern program: A model for research dissemination and utilization. *Journal of Nursing Administration, 28*(11), 39–45.

CHAPTER 14

Marketing the Talents of Clinical Nurses Through Continuing Education Programs

As mentioned in Chapter 2, continuing education (CE) is one of the three main professional development activities included in the American Nurses Association's (ANA's) Framework for Nursing Professional Development, along with staff development and academic education (ANA, 2000). Although CE exists as a separate entity, portions of it overlap with staff development and academic education. The overlap of CE with staff development indicates that CE offerings can be a part of staff development activities.

ANA defines CE as the "systematic professional learning experiences designed to augment the knowledge, skills, and attitudes of nurses" (ANA, 2000, p. 5). CE activities not only help nurses provide quality care to patients but also assist nurses in attaining the goals identified in their professional career plan. Therefore, CE activities that exist within the domain of staff development often focus on nurses' continuing competence in their specific role within the work setting.

As mentioned in Chapter 2, professional nurses are expected to actively participate as learners in CE activities. This expectation is true for all nurses, regardless if they are staff development educators, clinical nurses, or unit-based educators. In addition to assuming the role of the learner in CE activities, your responsibilities may include designing or coordinating CE offerings for clinical nurses within your organization. You may be a speaker for a CE program. As a unit-based educator, you also may guide clinical nurses in seeking CE activities both within and outside your healthcare organization. In addition to implementing CE activities at your workplace, you may be involved in CE programs for your professional nursing organization as part of your own professional development.

Regardless of your responsibilities related to CE, it is important for you to understand the process involved in sponsoring CE activities and to be aware of the various CE opportunities that exist for clinical nurses. You also need to learn how to develop a CE program, depending on the expectations of your employer. This chapter will discuss these features of CE programs that you may develop for nurses within your organization.

Professional Standards for Continuing Education Programs

The American Nurses Credentialing Center (ANCC), a subsidiary of ANA, is responsible for implementing credentialing programs, such as the accreditation of CE activities developed and sponsored for nurses (ANA, 2000). Serving in this capacity, ANCC, through its Commission on Accreditation, establishes standards and guidelines for organizations to follow as they design and implement CE activities.

Expectations of Continuing Education Providers

Nursing organizations, such as schools of nursing and professional nursing organizations, can apply to ANCC to become recognized as a provider of CE for nurses (ANCC, 2002). These organizations can submit an application fee to obtain one of following CE provider categories: (a) apply to ANCC to become an accredited provider, (b) apply to be an approved provider through a constituent member association, such as a state nurses association, or (c) apply to one of ANCC's approvers for a specific educational offering. Organizations that are granted provider status by ANCC have the authority to conduct CE programs and award CEs with oversight by their accredited approver of CE for nurses by ANCC.

Provider organizations are expected to follow specific guidelines outlined in provider accreditation manuals. These manuals provide an overview of the accreditation program and include relevant policies and procedures and the criteria to follow when developing CE programs and submitting application forms (ANCC, 2002).

For example, CE providers must submit a biosketch and lesson plan for each speaker included in the program (Pennsylvania Nurses Association [PNA], 1998). Providers also must develop a method to verify the attendance of participants and a way for participants to evaluate the offering. The evaluation form should include feedback from each learner regarding his or her ability to attain stated objectives, as well as the effectiveness of the speakers, appropriateness of their audiovisuals and handouts, and quality of the learning environment. Adult learning principles need to be reflected in the educational design. Include a copy of the marketing brochure and evidence of any pilot testing, if appropriate.

As a unit-based educator, you need to understand the accreditation process and your specific responsibilities associated with CE program planning. It is important for you to investigate how CE programs are processed at your healthcare organization or professional nursing organization. Review these requirements with a nurse who is experienced in developing CE programs prior to developing your own CE offering.

Contact Hours Awarded

ANA specifies that CE activities, including both formal and independent approaches to CE, must meet specific criteria to be eligible for serving as a source of contact hours (ANA, 1994). A contact hour is a way that the credentialing agencies measure the amount of credit awarded to nurses for successfully completing an "approved, organized learning experience" (ANA, 1994, p. 12). One contact hour of CE is awarded to participants for every 50 minutes of CE programming they attend.

Because the amount of time that nurses directly participate in CE activities determines the number of contact hours they are awarded, educators need to carefully consider this issue when planning a CE event, scheduling speakers, and verifying participants' attendance. Participants receive a document at the conclusion of the CE event, such as a printed certificate, that serves as an official record of their contact hours awarded. A similar process is used when using more independent-learning CE approaches, such as journal articles.

Sources of Continuing Education for Nurses

A variety of CE activities exists for professional nurses. CE activities can be designed using traditional or independent approaches. Some CE activities rely on a blend of both approaches. Regardless of the approach, CE activities need to incorporate adult learning principles in their design and teaching-learning strategies (ANA, 2000). Strategies for providing these CE programs will be discussed next in this chapter.

Traditional Continuing Education Designs

Traditional CE activities are those educational offerings that require nurses to be physically present (ANA, 2000). Traditional CE programs are planned and coordinated by nurses, such as staff development educators, who determine the pace of the CE activity.

Nurses can participate in traditional CE offerings by attending workshops, programs, or conferences sponsored by their workplace, professional nursing organizations, colleges and universities, or other community agencies and groups. Although some of these offerings involve nurses being part of an audience in a classroom, other learning options exist that involve distance learning. For example, some offerings currently are available to nurses using satellite video conferencing, the Internet, and audio conferencing techniques. Some Web-based CE activities designed for advanced practice nurses include an interactive component (Hayes, Huckstadt, & Gibson, 2000).

Although many employers sponsor CE programs for their nursing staff, some organizations allow their nurses to attend CE programs that are sponsored by outside sources, such as professional nursing groups, schools of nursing, or independent firms. The employer also may assume travel costs and time.

If your employer provides this benefit to staff, it is important for you, as a unit-based educator, to develop ways that all nurses can benefit from the CE program, even if they could not attend. For example, ask nurses who attend outside CE programs to present key points of the program at a unit-based in-service, post a one-page report, or send a brief e-mail to colleagues. Be sure to include such external CE programs in developing your unit's educational plan, such as the learning needs identified in the example provided in Chapters 6 and 7.

Independent Continuing Education Activities

Independent CE activities are those offerings designed for completion by the learner, independently, and at the learner's own pace. Independent CE offerings allow learners to complete their learning at a time of their choice.

Nurses can participate in independent CE activities through a variety of options. One example of independent CE offerings is CE feature articles printed in nursing journals or provided through the Internet. To receive contact hours, nurses read the offering, answer a series of questions that pertain to the topic, complete an evaluation form, and mail it to the provider. A certificate for a specified number of contact hours is provided if the nurse attains a passing score. Many CE opportunities require a minimal processing fee. Many journals, such as the *Oncology Nursing Forum*, the *American Journal of Nursing, Nursing*, the *Association of Operating Room Nurses Journal*, and the *Journal of Continuing Education in Nursing*, sponsor independent home study or online options for nurses.

Reasons for Continuing Education for Nurses

In addition to providing opportunities for nurses to pursue their expectations for lifelong learning and continuing competence, evidence of successful completion of CE activities is a requirement for some RNs in particular situations. For example, states with mandatory CE features in their Nurse Practice Act require nurses licensed in their state to obtain a defined number of contact hours for relicensure (Huber, 2000). The overall goal of those states that support this legislation is to assure the public that RNs remain current in their nursing practice. According to ANA (2003), approximately 25 states require mandatory CE for an RN to maintain a license, and 40 states require CE for nurses who want to return to practice following a prolonged period.

Contact hours in CE are also an option provided by some national professional nursing organizations for recertification. Certification is a "process by which a professional nursing organization validates, based on predetermined standards, an individual RN's qualifications, knowledge, and practice in a defined functional or clinical area of nursing" (ANA, 2000, p. 23). Being certified means a professional nursing organization or agency has recognized you for your knowledge in a general or specialty practice area. After meeting certain eligibility criteria and clinical practice requirements, you passed an examination that validated your abilities and received initial certification.

To maintain this credential, these certification organizations offer nurses various options in addition to retesting, such as evidence of participation in specific CE programs with contact hours awarded. For example, the Oncology Nursing Certification Corporation (ONCC) developed an option called the Oncology Nursing Certification Points Renewal Option (ONC-PRO) for nurses certified in oncology nursing who are seeking renewal (ONCC, 2003). This opportunity allows nurses to earn points by submitting various sources as evidence of their professional development, including CE programs.

Developing a Continuing Education Program

As a unit-based educator, you may have the opportunity to participate as a member of a planning committee for a CE program. You may be asked to assume a leadership role and chair the planning committee. Regardless of the role you play in CE activities, it is important for you to understand the steps involved in assessing, planning, implementing, and evaluating CE programs. These steps should be familiar ones, as they reflect those involved in presenting an in-service education program discussed in Chapters 6 and 7. Each step will be discussed in detail in the section that follows.

What to Do Before the Continuing Education Program

Careful assessment and planning are essential skills for you to use when developing a CE program. Both of these aspects in organizing a CE event include a variety of steps.

Assess Learners and Learning Needs

Begin the assessment phase of developing a CE program by determining who the potential participants will be for the program and the theme (topic) for the CE program. The theme should be derived from the results of a needs assessment obtained through input from the learners (PNA, 1998). For example, if you are developing a CE program for staff nurses who work on clinical units within your organization, the need for the CE program might be reflected in the results of the staff's needs assessment you recently conducted on your unit. Chapter 6 described this process of designing an effective, comprehensive needs assessment for nurses working on various clinical units within one organization. For example, according to the needs assessment you recently conducted for your clinical units, it was evident that staff nurses needed to develop their skills in serving as preceptors for new staff nurses. The nurses on the units also expressed this need and asked for your assistance. You also realized that a local school of nursing plans to recruit staff nurses from your units to precept junior nursing students in a summer internship program. You see the need for existing staff to develop their skills and decide to plan a one-day CE program on preceptor development. Although a few nurses on your units are experienced preceptors, you realize that the majority of clinical nurses who were recently hired possess novice preceptor skills. You realize that all of these nurses cannot leave the clinical unit at the same time, so you will consider this factor in your planning phase. You are considering repeating this program so that more nurses can attend.

Determine Available Resources

Before you begin planning your CE program, identify the specific resources, or budget, that are available to you for this project. In addition to money, potential resources can include services such as typing and duplication, human resources such as expert speakers and audiovisual technicians, or physical resources such as conference rooms and audiovisual equipment. List the resources you do not have and will need for the project, including time and staff support. Keep track of the cost of each task as you move through the planning process. As a general rule, it is beneficial to overestimate the cost of each item when preparing the budget associated with a CE program (Zimmermann, 1999). Discuss your need for resources that are not available to you with your supervisor.

Develop a Detailed Plan

After you have assessed the learning needs and identified the learners who will attend the CE program, develop a detailed plan. This plan will help you organize the tasks you need to accomplish, keep you on track, and communicate the needs to others who will be involved in the project.

Organize and Orient a Planning Committee

Start the planning process by organizing a planning committee to work with you in developing the CE program. Some approvers of CE programs require at least two nurses to serve on the planning committee and expect the leader to possess specific qualifications, such as a bachelor's degree in nursing (PNA, 1998). Recruit individuals who have expressed an interest in participating in this activity and who possess the talents that you need to make the project a success. The number of additional committee members should be appropriate to accomplish the tasks.

For example, you decided to have three nurses comprise your planning committee, in addition to yourself. You include two experienced preceptors as members of your CE planning committee and one nurse with experience in leading similar CE projects.

Once you have gathered the members of the CE planning committee together, explain the committee's charge to them. Review any expectations you have of them, such as attending planning committee meetings and meeting deadlines. Next, designate specific roles and responsibilities for each member. Establish an effective communication method, such as e-mail, so that information can be shared among members in a timely manner. Establish the dates, times, and locations of future planning meetings, starting with the target date for the CE program and working backward. Spend some time helping committee members get acquainted with each other.

Determine Key Tasks of the Project

After orienting the members of your planning committee, make a list of key tasks that need to be accomplished before the date of the CE program and assign due dates when these tasks need to be completed. Figure 14-1 lists examples of activities that need to be included among your tasks, the name of the committee member responsible to accomplish the task, and the due date.

Verify the Date, Time, Location, and Facilities

Start by establishing the date, time, and location for the program and verifying the availability of the conference room. Allow yourself sufficient time to plan this event. Some experts suggest planning an event at least six to nine months in advance (Zimmermann, 1999). Choose a location that will provide a good learning environment. The room should be appropriate for the type of CE program you are planning, accessible to participants, and able to accommodate the teaching strategies you anticipate will be used (PNA, 1998). It also should be a comfortable size for the number of participants you anticipate will be attending the CE program. If you are unfamiliar with the room, make an onsite visit to examine it. Make arrangements for the physical layout of the room, such as the seating pattern and speaker facilities. Consider a room for vendors if you choose this option.

Investigate if special services, such as access to food services and audiovisual equipment, are readily available for this room. Speak with the appropriate representatives from food and technical services to plan for your needs in advance. Determine if assistance with audiovisual equipment is available or if you need to assign this task to a member of the planning committee.

Finally, consider the approximate length of the CE program. Following discussions with nurse managers about staffing issues and budget constraints, you may decide to limit the program to one day.

Estimate Audience Size and Special Needs

Determine the number of participants you will invite to the CE program. Consider a variety of factors when making this decision, such as budget constraints and the need for providing adequate staffing to remain on the clinical units to care for patients. Anticipate if participants will need special accommodations because of physical limitations, such as accessing the room using a wheelchair.

Task	Due Date	Person Responsible
Before the CE Program		
Assess learners and learning needs.		
Determine available resources.		
Develop a detailed plan.		
Organize and orient a planning committee.		
Determine key tasks of the project.		
Verify the date, time, location, and facilities.		
Estimate audience size and special needs.		
Determine the purpose and goals.		
Determine key topics.		
Recruit and confirm speakers and materials.		
Develop a brochure for the program.		
Establish a method for verifying participation and successful completion.		
Determine a method of evaluation.		
Submit CE application.		
Duplicate and organize handouts.		
Day of the CE Program		
Check accommodations.		
Set up the registration table.		
Greet participants and speakers.		
Introduce speakers.		
Maintain the time schedule.		
Orient participants and review evaluation.		
Award certificates.		
After the CE Program		
Analyze and review evaluations.		
Make revisions for future programs.		
Complete the budget process.		
Write thank-you letters and provide feedback.		
File documents in a secure location.		

Figure 14-1.
Checklist for Organizing a Continuing Education Program

Determine the Purpose and Goals of the Continuing Education Program

Although you already have decided that the theme for your CE program will be preceptor programs, you will need to develop the general purpose and goals for the program. For example, the planning committee decides that the purpose of the CE program is to assist staff nurses in learning how to effectively assume the role of a clinical preceptor for nursing staff or nursing students on the clinical unit. Next, outline objectives for the program—outcomes (knowledge, skills, and attitudes) you expect participants to attain following completion of this program. Details on developing objectives were provided in Chapter 7.

Determine Key Topics for the Continuing Education Program

After you have determined the purpose and objectives for the CE program, identify key topics that should be included in the program. Content on these topics should match the objectives and enable participants to attain the objectives. Ask experienced preceptors to help you in identifying these topics, and review the nursing literature on preceptors for additional ideas. Refer to your needs assessment to ensure that these topics are ones that the learners have not yet mastered. After listing these topics, assign an approximate time limit for them.

For example, after reviewing the literature on preceptor programs, you decided that a review of adult learning principles should be one of the topics included in the CE program. Given the time limit for the entire program, objectives, key concepts included in this topic, and contact hour specifications, you assign a 50-minute time limit to this topic. You continue to assign time limits to each topic on your list until you have developed a tentative schedule for the entire day. You will use this information later when designing a marketing brochure for the CE event.

Recruit and Confirm Speakers and Materials

After designing the format of your CE program, recruit appropriate speakers for the topics. Speakers who participate in CE offerings should possess expertise on the topic for which they are presenting (PNA, 1998). If presenting nursing content, these speakers should be nurses themselves (PNA).

Consider inviting nurses within your organization to be speakers, if appropriate. This strategy is an effective way to market the talents of yourself and your colleagues, helping everyone to develop professionally.

In communicating with speakers, provide a description of the program, its purpose, and objectives. Provide them with a brochure of the program, if available. Include the date, time, location, and information about the audience. Remind them of the audiovisuals available to them, and ask them to confirm their needs. Keep in contact with the speakers up until the time of the event. Consider purchasing small gifts for each speaker.

Ask each participant to supply you with a recent biosketch and a lesson plan for his or her topic. The lesson plan should include specific objectives, a content outline, time allotted to each portion of the topic, and teaching-learning strategies. Chapter 7 provides an example of developing a lesson plan. Provide speakers with the appropriate forms to complete these tasks, using forms designed by the representatives at your organization who will submit the CE application for approval. Encourage speakers to use active learning strategies in their presentations and to include realistic examples, such as case studies, that will pique the interest of the participants.

Ask speakers to provide you with information you can use to introduce them and with a copy of handouts they need to have duplicated for participants. Request these materials well in advance of the CE program so that you will have sufficient time to prepare and organize them into packets for participants.

Develop a Brochure for the Continuing Education Program

If appropriate, develop a brochure to market the program. Work with representatives from your public relations department to accomplish this task. If developing an official brochure is not needed for your program, you can provide this information in another manner, such as in a handout. Use samples of past brochures in developing one for your program. Be sure to include key information about the program, objectives, content, and speakers, as well as logistical information regarding registration, contact hours, sponsors, breaks, and lunch.

Establish a Method for Verifying Participation and Successful Completion

The planning phase of developing a CE program includes designing a method for verifying participants' attendance at the sessions and for determining their successful completion of the program (PNA, 1998). A variety of methods can be used to determine this, so check with representatives at your organization who are responsible for preparing the CE application. For example, some places conduct a roll call of participants, whereas others rely on sign-in sheets or self-reports of attendance (PNA). Regardless of the method, be sure it complies with requirements for gaining approval for CE programs.

Check with CE representatives regarding verification forms or certificates that can be awarded to participants after successful completion of the program. Certificates usually contain information such as the participant's name; number of contact hours awarded; name and address of the sponsor; the title, date, and location of the program; and the signature of the person administratively responsible for the event (PNA, 1998). The certificate also includes an official statement provided by the CE approval organization.

Determine a Method of Evaluation

During the planning phase for the CE program, you will need to determine the method(s) you will use to evaluate if participants met each objective. Learners also have an opportunity to evaluate the expertise of each speaker, his or her teaching strategies, and the learning environment (PNA, 1998). Participants usually are asked to supply suggestions for future programs, which will assist you in validating future learning needs. You will need to develop appropriate forms for this evaluation if they are not available to you. Sample forms may be available through your CE representative and can be adapted to reflect your specific program.

Submit the Continuing Education Application

After you have obtained the aforementioned information during the planning phase, work with your CE representative to prepare the application for contact hours. Be sure to do this well in advance of the actual event so certificates can be available to participants following the program.

Duplicate and Organize Handouts

After compiling the handouts and the brochure for the program, organize them in a packet that can be distributed to participants when they arrive on the day of the CE program. Include other essential documents, such as evaluation forms. Consider including a list of participants and speakers in the packets, along with contact information participants can use to network with each other. Include name tags that participants can wear during the conference. If lunch is not available onsite, include suggested restaurants that participants can visit.

What to Do the Day of the Continuing Education Program

Your careful planning for this event should pay off when the day of the CE program arrives. Members of the planning committee can help you oversee the day's events, coordinating the day so that it runs smoothly. Members assigned to the registration desk can greet speakers and participants, provide them with packets, and guide them accordingly. They also can acquaint speakers to the audiovisual equipment they requested and introduce them to the technician, if available. Make a last-minute check on details, such as food services and the room setup.

Start the program by introducing the planning committee and sponsors and thanking them for their assistance. Orient the participants to information provided in their packets, and provide them with logistic information, such as evaluation forms, the schedule for the day, and facilities.

As the program progresses, anticipate potential problems and be ready to manage them. Keep the program on schedule by providing speakers with cues. Consider using small red and green cards to signal speakers regarding their status within the allotted time.

Provide participants with certificates as they return completed evaluation forms to the registration desk. Thank participants, speakers, and vendors for attending the CE program. Be sure to extend your personal appreciation to members of the CE planning committee.

What to Do After the Continuing Education Program

The CE program is complete and was a success, but your responsibilities are not completed yet. Convene a meeting of the planning committee to analyze and review the evaluation comments provided by the participants. Review the planning process that was used in developing the CE events. Develop suggestions for future programs based on this feedback. Start planning the next program, incorporating these suggestions.

Be sure to send thank-you notes to individuals, such as speakers, sponsors, vendors, and planning members, who were involved in developing and presenting the program. Provide speakers with feedback about their presentations.

Organize and file essential documents that resulted from this event. Check with your CE representative to determine the type of documents that need to be filed and where they should be maintained. Be sure that these documents are kept confidential and in a place where they can easily be retrieved (PNA, 1998).

Review the final budget that was allocated for your CE program. Make sure that all receipts have been accounted for and have been submitted to the appropriate person.

Finally, consider ways to evaluate the impact that this program has had on the participants' performance. For example, consider tracking the performance of nurses who attended the program as they precept new nurses and nursing students on your unit. Share your successful project with peers through your organization's newsletter or at a conference sponsored by a professional nursing organization. Consider submitting a manuscript about the planning of your CE program for a nursing journal.

Summary

This chapter reviewed the process of developing a CE program and reviewed essential features that need to be accomplished before, during, and following the CE event. Specific responsibilities of unit-based educators are discussed.

References

American Nurses Association. (1994). *Standards for nursing professional development: Continuing education and staff development*. Washington, DC: Author.

American Nurses Association. (2000). *Scope and standards of practice for nursing professional development*. Washington DC: Author.

American Nurses Association. (2003, April 28). *States which require continuing education for RN licensure*. Retrieved January 21, 2004, from http://www.nursingworld.org/gova/state/2003/cernchrt.pdf

American Nurses Credentialing Center. (2002). *Accreditation*. Retrieved June 21, 2003, from http://www.nursingworld.org/ancc/certify/Certs.htm

Hayes, K., Huckstadt, A., & Gibson, R. (2000). Developing an interactive continuing education on the Web. *Journal of Continuing Education in Nursing, 31*(5), 199–203.

Huber, D. (2000). *Leadership and nursing care management*. Philadelphia: Saunders.

Oncology Nursing Certification Corporation. (2003). *2003 oncology nursing certification bulletin for OCN®, AOCN®, and CPON® certification*. Pittsburgh, PA: Author.

Pennsylvania Nurses Association. (1998). *Continuing education approval program*. Harrisburg, PA: Author.

Zimmermann, P.G. (1999). Planning a successful continuing education program: Pearls of wisdom. *Journal of Emergency Nursing, 25,* 324–326.

CHAPTER 15

Developing a Career Plan: Taking a Proactive Approach for the Future

You have accomplished your goal of becoming an RN and accepted a clinical nurse position at a healthcare organization. Although your current energies are focused on developing your knowledge and skills related to your current position, such as providing patient care, you need to take some time and reflect on your professional goals. You can start this process by developing a career plan for yourself.

Perhaps you are a unit-based educator on your clinical unit responsible for helping the nursing staff develop themselves as professionals. This aspect of the staff development role was explained previously in Chapters 2 and 3. You can help the nursing staff accomplish this task by developing a career plan for yourself first. This approach will help you strengthen your skills in developing career plans and prepare you to help other nurses develop their plans. For example, start by reviewing the process of developing a career plan to staff during a unit-based in-service program. Then, during individual sessions, help them create a career plan for themselves.

Understanding a Career Plan

A career plan is what the words imply. It is a personal "plan" or blueprint that is designed to help you shape the direction of your professional career. Although a written version of your career plan can be thought of as a tool or worksheet, your document is the result of an organized and systematic decision-making process that you perform, called career planning. The process involved in developing a career plan can be conceptualized as containing six key related components: assessment, diagnosis, outcomes (goals), planning, implementation, and evaluation.

This process is familiar to most nurses. Its components are similar to those of the nursing process (standards of care) outlined by the American Nurses Association (ANA) in its *Standards of Clinical Practice* (ANA, 1998). However, in this case, you are both the planner and the focus of the plan. This process also resembles the steps used in developing an educational plan for unit-based in-service programs described in Chapters 6 and 7. Table 15-1 compares the components of the nursing process with key steps used in developing a career plan. These components will be discussed in greater detail throughout this chapter.

Table 15-1. Comparing the Components of the Nursing Process and Career Plan	
Nursing Process (ANA, 1998)	**Career Plan**
Assessment	Gather data about yourself, positions, and market.
Diagnosis	Analyze assessment data and make judgments.
Outcome identification	Define long- and short-term goals.
Planning	Develop interventions and due dates for each goal.
Implementation	Accomplish interventions listed in plan.
Evaluation	Evaluate progress on plan and revise as needed.

Reasons for Developing a Career Plan

Career-long learning is an essential component of professional nursing that "must be planned, nurtured, and managed by individual nurses" (Craven & DuHamel, 2003, p. 14). Professional nurses can develop a career plan to facilitate this learning process. A career plan can help nurses focus their learning efforts within the context of their career goals and manage these efforts in a timely and organized fashion (Broscio & Scherer, 2003). This is true whether your goals relate directly to your current nursing position or to future opportunities that may arise. The following section will describe the benefits of a career plan and offers practical examples.

Focus on Career Goals in a Timely Manner

As mentioned previously, a career plan can help you not only identify your career goals but also direct them in a timely, systematic fashion. A career plan can help you focus your everyday professional decisions toward reaching your professional goals. A career plan also helps you determine the knowledge, skills, and experiences you need to master in order to attain your career goals. Because a career plan contains target dates matched with goals and interventions (strategies), it minimizes the chance that you will be distracted along the path.

For example, suppose you are a staff nurse on an adult medical-surgical unit. You feel that despite your enthusiasm in caring for these patients, your professional life does not have a focus. You lack a sense of identity compared with other nurses who work on specialty clinical units such as cardiology, oncology, or obstetrics. You regularly volunteer for various projects at your workplace and within the community, but you are not sure you are making the best professional decision in selecting these projects. You feel like you are functioning aimlessly without a professional focus. You enjoy medical-surgical nursing and would like to strengthen your knowledge and skills in this clinical area. Developing a career plan can help you clarify your professional goals and guide your daily decisions so that you can reach your goals in a timely manner.

Meet and Exceed Job Expectations

In addition to helping you focus on your career goals, a career plan can help you attain or even exceed the expectations of your employer in your current position. A career plan also can help you develop more complex behaviors required for promotion at your workplace.

For example, suppose you recently graduated from an associate's degree in nursing program and passed the licensure (NCLEX) examination before assuming a staff nurse I position at your local community hospital. You want to be the best nurse possible but feel a bit overwhelmed in your first nursing position. Each day poses a challenge for you as you focus on providing safe, quality patient care in a timely, organized way. You still are perfecting your skills in organizing your day and prioritizing your patient care activities. Regardless, you want to be sure that you will be able to meet your employer's expectations during your performance appraisal and possibly exceed in some areas. Developing a career plan that contains goals reflecting components of your position description can help you minimize your concerns and keep you on target.

Increase Your Marketability

A career plan can help you increase your marketability as a professional nurse. Given the current and future shortage of RNs (Health Resources and Services Administration, 2001), opportunities exist that will enable you not only to refocus your professional interests toward another specialty but also to develop a new, unique nursing role that fills a gap in patient services. Opportunities for professional growth may exist at your current workplace or through other healthcare or community agencies. Be creative in developing your career goals, and match them with healthcare and nursing marketing projections, if possible.

For example, your clinical unit has experienced an extremely low census rate over the past year and is scheduled to merge with another clinical unit within your organization. You will be expected to provide competent nursing care not only for patients who traditionally were admitted to your unit but also for patients with urologic conditions. You are unfamiliar with caring for patients with these needs. Although you realize that you will be learning about the nursing care for these patients in the near future, you want to get a "head start" on this, especially because a few of the new patients already have started to be admitted to your unit before the formal unit merger. Develop a career plan that will help you gain the in-depth knowledge and skills you will need to provide safe, quality care to urology patients. You may decide to develop a career plan that will allow you to refocus your career if you choose to transfer to a clinical unit with a different specialty.

Communicate Your Career Goals

Finally, a career plan can serve as an effective tool to communicate your career goals and learning needs to those who can support your plan. This may include your immediate supervisor, a faculty member in your school of nursing, the clinical specialist or educator assigned to your unit, a close friend, or a family member. Sharing your plan with these individuals can help them better understand your goals and learning needs. They may be able to provide you with emotional support or resources such as time, finances, or learning opportunities that will help you attain your goals. Because your career plan provides the impression of you being a self-directed, focused, and organized individual, consider placing a copy of your career plan in your professional portfolio. Guidelines for developing a portfolio were discussed in Chapter 11.

When You Should Develop a Career Plan

Now is the best time for you to develop your career plan, regardless of your nursing experience or educational background. Remember, a career plan can change over time, so be sure it is flexible. A career plan should be dynamic and evolving and not "written in stone."

For example, suppose an unexpected opportunity arises on your clinical unit, that of serving as a preceptor for an undergraduate junior nursing student. Although this role was not part of your original career plan, you decide to volunteer as a preceptor. You realize your employer will require you to be a preceptor for promotion to the next staff nurse level, so you decide to volunteer now and learn in advance. You also would like to determine if teaching other nurses is a role you may want to pursue in the future. You make these changes and modify your career plan accordingly.

The Process of Developing a Career Plan

As mentioned previously, the process of developing a career plan is similar to the steps involved in the nursing process. The actual "plan" can be merely a draft created with pencil and paper or a document developed with computer software or recorded in a personal digital assistant. Regardless of what method you choose to record your career plan, it needs to be easily accessible and able to be revised. The information that follows will help you proceed step-by-step through the process of developing a career plan. A case example will be used to clarify the steps.

Conduct a Self-Assessment

The first step in developing a career plan is to conduct a self-assessment. Gathering data from a variety of sources, start your assessment by conducting an inventory of yourself. Include items such as your educational background, community involvement, awards, certifications, experiences, and knowledge and skills. Use your professional portfolio (Chapter 11) and resume (Chapter 12) to help you with this step. Make a list of your personal and professional strengths, along with areas that need further improvement.

Include feedback from others who know you well, such as your supervisor, peers, and faculty, to gain their perspective of your strengths and weaknesses. Recall patient and family comments that speak to your knowledge and skills as a professional nurse.

In addition to collecting data about your current qualities, gather information about the qualifications you will need to attain your future dreams. Start by asking yourself, "What would I like to be doing in the future?" Think about your future as being in two different time spans: long-term, which can be three to five years from now, and short-term, which can be conceived as up to three years from the present. Talk with nurses who hold positions to which you aspire, and ask for their personal suggestions about qualifications you should acquire to obtain a similar position. Obtain a copy of the position description that lists the functions, qualifications, and responsibilities for those roles.

If your healthcare facility has a career center, meet with counselors to explore self-assessment tools and resources that can help you. Remember to contact your alma mater and investigate what career services are available to you as an alumnus.

Work with your local librarian to retrieve current reports that describe trends in the nursing profession and healthcare market. Be sure to investigate the strategic plan of your current healthcare organization and include key points in your assessment.

Analyze Your Assessment Data

After you have conducted a thorough assessment, organize the data and look for patterns or trends. Attempt to form some judgments (or diagnoses) about your strengths, areas for improvement, professional and personal interests, qualifications needed to gain, and nursing and healthcare trends. Your judgments will help you progress toward the next two steps of career planning: determining your goals (outcomes) and developing interventions (strategies) to help you attain these goals.

Case example: You are an RN who graduated from a bachelor's nursing program and have been working for the past two years as a staff nurse I on a medical oncology unit. You want to make oncology nursing part of your career goals. Your self-assessment reveals that you demonstrate excellent communication skills with patients and families, especially those patients experiencing end-of-life situations. Peer evaluations from a unit-based in-service program you presented on bereavement were extremely good. You enjoy caring for these patients and helping staff learn new skills.

Your discussions with role models reveal that you will need at least a master's degree in nursing (MSN) to attain the job of your dreams. You need to develop your knowledge and skills in oncology nursing, participate in professional nursing organizations, and volunteer in the community. Other skills you need to develop include formal presentations, publishing, and research. You need to regularly read key oncology nursing journals.

The review of your organization's strategic plan reveals its goal of expanding its services in cancer care by opening an outpatient chemotherapy unit within the next two years. Your employer values certification of nurses and considers this credential in promotions to advanced clinical nursing positions. A literature review describes not only a nursing shortage but also a current and impending shortage of nursing faculty (National League for Nursing [NLN], 2002). You remember your days as a student nurse and the excellent clinical instructors who mentored you. The dream of teaching in a school of nursing comes back to you now.

Develop and Prioritize Your Goals (Outcomes)

Use your analysis of assessment data to develop goals or outcomes that will provide you with direction in your professional career. These goals should be measurable and challenging, yet realistic. Your goals should be tailored to your specific situation based on your assessment data and the resources available to you, such as time and money. Identify both long-term goals (LTGs) and short-term goals (STGs). Develop a rationale, or reason, for why you selected each goal. You can accomplish this by asking yourself, "Why is this goal important to me?" or "Why should I do this?"

Although goals need to reflect what and where you want to be in your professional life, consider matching them with the goals of your clinical unit and healthcare organization. If you plan on changing jobs in the future, review the goals of the organization in which you choose to work. Reflecting on organizational goals when preparing your career plan will help you become a valued employee and help you create a unique niche for yourself.

Remember to keep your personal goals in mind when developing professional goals. Your professional life does not function in isolation from your personal life. Planned or unplanned personal life events can alter the best-laid career plans. Anticipate personal changes such as marriage, birth of a child, relocation to another state, or a family illness. Rather than view these life events as barriers to your career goals, be proactive by integrating them with your career goals. In fact, personal goals may shape your career plan into an entirely different but equally exciting one.

After you have identified your professional goals, set a target date for attainment of each goal. Whereas a target date for an LTG can be expressed by the year, STG targets should include the month and year. If you can be more specific, then include the date. Prioritize your goals in order of time and importance. Start this process with STGs, then proceed to LTGs.

Case example: Based on your assessment data and analysis, you identify and prioritize two STGs and one LTG. You assign a target date and rationale for each goal. Figure 15-1 illustrates an example of your goals, target dates, and rationale for each entry.

Develop a Plan

After you have established your goals, focus on the first goal. Develop a list of interventions, a "to-do list," that you will need to complete to help you reach that goal. Keep each goal's target date in mind as your assign a due date for each intervention. Next, reorganize your interventions according to their due date, starting with the most current. Repeat this procedure for each goal.

Interventions may vary in their complexity and in the time it may take for you to complete them. Some interventions may take little time, such as joining a professional nursing organization, or longer, such as completing a formal nursing degree. Interventions may overlap across more than one goal.

Case example: You examine your first STG and develop a list of interventions you need to accomplish in order to reach that goal. You assign realistic due dates for each intervention. Next, you reorganize your interventions by dates. You re-

Figure 15-1.
Example of Long- and Short-Term Goals, Target Dates, and Rationale in a Career Plan

Short-term goal #1: Obtain certification in oncology (OCN®) (July 2005).
Rationale: You, your employer, and the nursing profession value certification. It involves an increase in pay and professional recognition. Certification is preferred for advancement within your organization and would make you competitive in acquiring a position on the chemotherapy unit in the future.

Short-term goal #2: Obtain promotion to a staff nurse II position on an oncology unit, preferably on the outpatient chemotherapy unit (July 2006).
Rationale: Seeking promotion to next level is an obvious step in career and results in more prestige and an increase in pay. Minimal requirement for nurses in chemotherapy unit.

Long-term goal #1: Obtain a full-time faculty position in a school of nursing (2009).
Rationale: Teaching in a school of nursing has always been a dream of yours. Your self-assessment and analysis revealed that you possess many strengths as a teacher, such as oral communication skills, working with students, and teaching skills. Trend literature has identified a shortage of nursing faculty in the future, so market seems good. See ads.

peat this process with your next two goals. Figure 15-2 provides a detailed example of interventions based on your first STG.

- Obtain certification in oncology (OCN®) (July 2005).
- Obtain information for OCN testing from ONCC Web site or via mail (June 2004).
- Review OCN eligibility criteria* (June 2004):
  - Active RN license (done)
  - One year nursing experience within three years of application (done)
  - 1,000 hours of oncology nursing practice within 30 months of application (done)
  - 10 contact hours of continuing education in oncology nursing or academic elective in oncology nursing (need five more hours before application due date of April 2005).
- Seek support for testing fee from employer or Oncology Nursing Society (July 2005).
- Obtain study materials (e.g., references, study guides, sample examinations) (August 2004).
- Develop an OCN study group on your unit (September 2004).
- Take an OCN review course (Fall 2004 or Spring 2005).
- Develop a study plan (July 2005).
- Submit application form with payment (before April 20, 2005).
- Take OCN exam (July 20, 2005).

Figure 15-2.
Example of Interventions Matched With Short-Term Goal #1 in a Career Plan

*Source: Oncology Nursing Certification Corporation. (2003). *2003 Oncology Nursing Certification Bulletin for OCN®, AOCN®, and CPON® Certification.* Pittsburgh, PA: Author.

Seeking a Nursing Degree

Some nurses perceive pursuing a nursing degree as a difficult process. By breaking this process down into logical steps, you can make this endeavor a manageable one. You will need to make two key decisions: the type of degree to pursue and where to pursue it.

Start by exploring available degrees you wish to pursue. Rely on feedback from your assessment data, discussed earlier in this chapter, to help you make this decision. Be sure to include information from your mentors, literature review, and career counselors. Determine the educational preparation (degree) that is required for you to reach your career goal and best prepares you to accomplish the responsibilities in your aspired position.

Second, identify universities or colleges that offer the degree you desire. You can obtain a list of accredited schools of nursing through the Web sites of two nursing organizations that accredit schools of nursing, the National League for Nursing Accrediting Commission (NLNAC) and the Commission on Collegiate Nursing Education (CCNE). Check both sites because the two lists of nursing schools are different from each other, depending on which agency granted their accreditation status. The Web site for NLNAC is www.nlnac.org/home.htm, and CCNE's accreditation page is www.aacn.nche.edu/accreditation. You also could obtain this information from individual schools of nursing links located in a useful educational resource on the Internet called Peterson's (www.petersons.com). You can access detailed information about each school at this site and connect with each school directly through a link.

After locating accredited schools of nursing that offer the degree you wish to pursue, obtain and review information about each school. Obtain this information either through the school's Web site or by calling the school of nursing and speaking with the recruiter. Use the tool presented in Figure 15-3 to examine the features of each school, determine their match with your interests, and narrow your choice of schools.

Next, make a personal visit to these schools, if possible. Speak with faculty, current students, and alumni. Use these results in making your final decision to apply for admission to the school that is your top choice.

Figure 15-3.
Rating Scale for
Evaluating a
School of Nursing

Directions: Review the following features of a school of nursing listed in the left column. Rate your personal preference for each feature in selecting a school. Use a scale from one to three to conduct this rating, with one indicating the least amount of importance to you and three indicating the highest importance. Use the results to evaluate schools on an individual basis.

Feature	Rating
University and school of nursing	
Mission and philosophy matches my values.	
Private or public institution matches my needs.	
Accredited by university and nursing accrediting bodies (e.g., NLNAC, CCNE)	
Good reputation, locally and nationally	
Leadership of the university and school has a good reputation.	
Value on quality teaching and research	
Administration, faculty, and staff are friendly and accessible.	
Interesting community partnerships exist.	
Organization offers unique opportunities (international nursing, research, nursing centers).	
Academic program	
Offers degrees that reflect my interest	
Offers undergraduate and graduate programs	
Offers certificate programs of interest to me	
Admission requirements are clear and attainable.	
Advanced standing for previous course work and experience is valued and available.	
Prerequisites are easily attainable.	
Program of study (curriculum) is interesting, innovative, challenging, and current.	
Courses can be completed full-time or part-time.	
Required credit hours are reasonable to attain in a timely manner.	
Opportunities exist for accelerating course work.	
Courses include opportunities to pursue my interests and flexibility and interdisciplinary focus.	
Exit examinations (comprehensive exam) and final projects (thesis or dissertation) are required for graduation.	
The NCLEX pass rate of undergraduates is acceptable to me.	
Program includes international nursing opportunities.	
Student services	
Offers support with services such as advisement, registration, and orientation	
Offers various student activities	
Provides opportunities for tutors	
Effective communication flow between faculty and students	
Financial resources	
Offers opportunities for financial aid, such as loans, scholarships, awards, and graduate assistant positions	
Tuition is affordable to me.	

(Continued on next page)

Feature	Rating
Physical facilities	
Campus is conducive to foster my learning, including classrooms, computer laboratories, and skill laboratories.	
Class size is appropriate for my learning needs.	
Parking is available at reasonable cost.	
Clinical experience	
Clinical opportunities are appropriate to my needs and career interest.	
Size of clinical groups (faculty : student ratio) is acceptable.	
Opportunities to experience innovative community-based events (e.g., nurse-managed wellness centers) are available.	
Faculty	
Faculty are excellent teachers and researchers.	
Faculty have an excellent reputation regionally and nationally.	
Faculty have a record of publishing in refereed publications and conducting research in areas of my interest.	
Faculty use active learning strategies in courses.	
Faculty are accessible and friendly.	
Faculty mentor students.	
Students/alumni	
Student demographics reflect my needs, including cultural diversity.	
Students/alumni express positive comments about their learning experiences.	
Outcomes of graduates (accomplishments and competencies) are positive.	
Employers value graduates of this school and seek them for employment.	
Alumni association is active and contributes to the school.	
Student organizations are supported and valued.	
Technology	
Latest technology is used in teaching.	
Opportunity for distance learning (DL) exists.	
If course is offered through DL, campus visits are required.	
Provides access to computers and software	
Provides state-of-the-art technology to students	
Various methods of communication are available (e.g., e-mail, voice mail, office hours, newsletters).	
School's Web site is informative and inviting.	
Other resources	
Library facilities are adequate and accessible.	
Career planning services are available.	
Counseling and test-taking assistance is available.	
Recreational and social activities are available.	
Books required for courses are easily accessible.	

Figure 15-3.
Rating Scale for Evaluating a School of Nursing
(Continued)

If you already have a degree in nursing, consider enrolling in a certificate program. Certificate programs are an effective opportunity for nurses to "develop skill sets and in-depth knowledge in specialized areas of nursing practice (Craven & DuHamel, 2003, p. 14). Certificate programs exist at various degree levels and many clinical areas, such as nursing education, nursing administration, forensic nursing, and nurse practitioners. Certificate programs require a minimal number of credits for completion.

Case example: By talking with individuals mentioned earlier in this chapter, you decide to pursue an MSN in nursing at your local university. After reviewing school materials and in speaking with faculty at that school of nursing, you choose to apply to its nursing education program. Their advice supports what you recently read in the NLN Position statement regarding the preparation of nurse educators as generalists (NLN, 2002). Faculty at the school of nursing helped you develop a program of studies in which you still can focus on clinical projects in oncology nursing. The school's distance learning program will provide you with the flexibility you need in light of your busy work schedule and personal responsibilities. You access the application through the school's Web site and plan to complete the admission requirements. You are excited and looking forward to this major step in your professional career.

Implement Your Career Plan

After you have developed your goals and target dates, implement your interventions as listed, starting with the first item. Continue to implement your plan, making decisions along the way as scheduled. Even though a career plan is intended to serve as a guide, try to stay on schedule. As mentioned earlier in this chapter, you should have developed your career plan with enough flexibility to easily make changes. Remember that it is not unusual for your career plan to change because of unexpected opportunities or events. As you complete the interventions, document your accomplishments in your professional portfolio. Be sure to update your resume, as discussed in Chapter 11.

Case example: During the first year of your career plan, you have been able to accomplish the interventions in a timely manner, despite an unexpected family illness. Your workplace recently developed a clinical partnership with a local school of nursing. This change has enabled you to be a guest speaker on oncology nursing in an undergraduate nursing course. You volunteered to be a preceptor for a senior nursing student who is completing an independent study on your clinical unit in cancer nursing over the summer. You decide that these activities, although not in your original plan, can be easily added to your career plan and will significantly contribute to helping you attain your goals.

Evaluate and Revise the Career Plan

As mentioned earlier in this chapter, evaluation is an integral part of the process of developing a career plan. Monitor your career plan regularly to determine if you are on track. Conduct a more involved evaluation of your plan at least yearly. A good time to do this evaluation is when you are scheduled for your annual performance appraisal. Make any necessary modifications to your plan. For example, if your plan is not helping you meet your goals, then reevaluate it and make changes as needed. Perhaps it is taking you more time than expected to complete your interventions. Take this time to rethink your goals, target dates, and interventions.

In addition to evaluating your career plan, be sure to update the plan annually so that it always reflects a five-year span. Think about your next set of goals as you accomplish existing ones. Consider developing an alternative career plan in the event that you lose your job or need to change your job tomorrow. This plan will help you survive financially and emotionally.

Case example: Prior to you annual performance appraisal, you conduct a formal evaluation of your career plan. You feel no major changes are needed at this time. You feel pleased that you have been successful in accomplishing the interventions you identified in your career plan to help you attain your goals. You share your success with your supervisor and other nurses on your clinical unit.

Summary

This chapter presents information on how to develop a personalized career plan based on realistic long-term and short-term goals. Examples of specific interventions on implementing and evaluating a career plan are provided. Suggestions to use in selecting an advanced degree are given, including a practical tool to accomplish this task. An example of a career plan is presented based on the information provided in this chapter.

References

American Nurses Association. (1998). *Standards of clinical practice* (2nd ed.). Washington, DC: Author.

Broscio, M., & Scherer, J. (2003). Creating and implementing a reality-based career plan. *Journal of Health Care Management, 48*(2), 76–81.

Craven, R.F., & DuHamel, M.B. (2003). Certificate programs in continuing professional education. *Journal of Continuing Education in Nursing, 34*(1), 14–18.

Health Resources and Services Administration. (2001, February). *The registered nurse population: National sample survey of registered nurses, March 2000.* Washington, DC: Author.

National League for Nursing. (2002, May 18). *Position statement: The preparation of nurse educators.* New York: Author.

INDEX

The letter *f* after a page number indicates relevant content appears in a figure; the letter *t*, in a table.